Rational Psychopharmacology

A Book of Clinical Skills

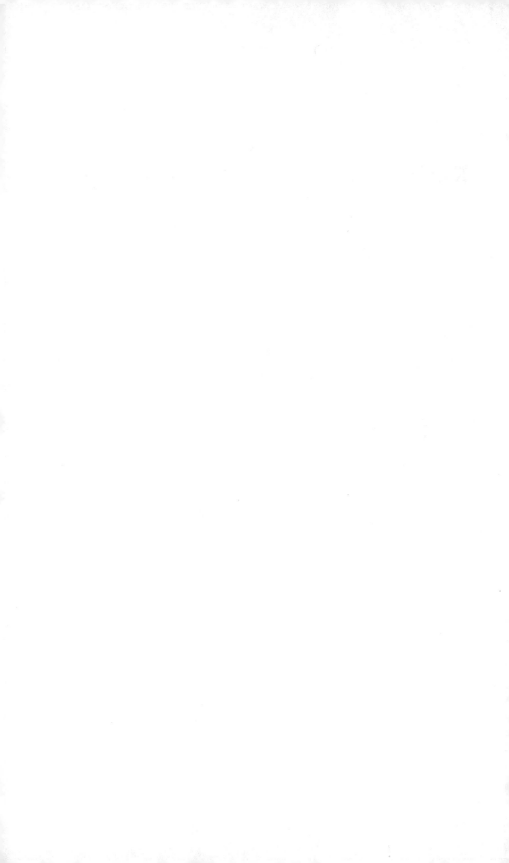

Rational Psychopharmacology

A Book of Clinical Skills

H. Paul Putman III, M.D.

Distinguished Life Fellow,
American Psychiatric Association,
Austin, Texas

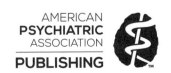

AMERICAN
PSYCHIATRIC
ASSOCIATION
PUBLISHING

If you wish to buy 50 or more copies of the same title, please go to www.appi.org/specialdiscounts for more information.

Copyright © 2020 American Psychiatric Association Publishing

ALL RIGHTS RESERVED

First Edition

Manufactured in the United States of America on acid-free paper
24   23   22   21   20   5   4   3   2   1

American Psychiatric Association Publishing
800 Maine Avenue SW
Suite 900
Washington, DC 20024-2812
www.appi.org

Library of Congress Cataloging-in-Publication Data
Names: Putman, H. Paul, III, author. | American Psychiatric Association Publishing, issuing body.
Title: Rational psychopharmacology : a book of clinical skills / H. Paul Putman III.
Description: First edition. | Washington, DC : American Psychiatric Association Publishing, [2020] | Includes bibliographical references and index.
Identifiers: LCCN 2020014016 (print) | LCCN 2020014017 (ebook) | ISBN 9781615373130 (paperback ; alk. paper) | ISBN 9781615373178 (ebook)
Subjects: MESH: Psychopharmacology—methods | Clinical Decision-Making | Problems and Exercises
Classification: LCC RM315 (print) | LCC RM315 (ebook) | NLM QV 18.2 | DDC 615.7/80835—dc23
LC record available at https://lccn.loc.gov/2020014016
LC ebook record available at https://lccn.loc.gov/2020014017

British Library Cataloguing in Publication Data
A CIP record is available from the British Library.

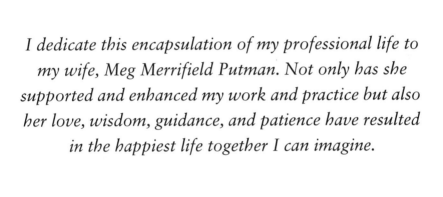

I dedicate this encapsulation of my professional life to my wife, Meg Merrifield Putman. Not only has she supported and enhanced my work and practice but also her love, wisdom, guidance, and patience have resulted in the happiest life together I can imagine.

Contents

Introduction

Many books about psychopharmacology have been published. Most focus heavily on the basic science involved and describe the currently available medications, including brief rationales for their use as well as their dosages and their side effects. Others are more for the general public, intended to help them understand how psychopharmacology might be helpful. This book is different.

What I hope to achieve is not only to teach you, the reader, what medicines are available and what their characteristics are but also to teach very valuable skills: how to think thoroughly and methodically when assessing a patient, when reviewing research data (both basic and clinical), and when thinking through, developing, and monitoring the most effective clinical recommendations for patients. Rather than a lesson in elementary patient assessment, this book is an attempt to help you identify weaknesses in your practice style and improve them where psychopharmacology is involved. Medicines will come and go, but these skills, applied alongside regular literature reviews, should keep you on the cutting edge for the length of your career, helping each patient to the greatest degree possible and enjoying high professional satisfaction for decades to come.

"Wait!" you may protest. "I understand how to identify a good research study and to analyze data. I had to demonstrate these abilities to get into medical school and then again while in medical school, residencies, and fellowships." I am certain that you did. You certainly also witnessed, however, the human tendency to not use these skills on a daily basis; to give in to hearsay, anecdotal evidence, and yes, even advertising; to not really understand the study design or statistical analysis in journals and to read non-peer-reviewed articles; and even to be lazy about asking enough questions to understand our patients.

Clinical psychopharmacology is best practiced through a routine process of ongoing thorough and complete assessments of our knowledge base and our patients. This discipline is attached to conscious application of abductive and Bayesian logic in formulating and adjusting treatment plans until they produce outcomes desired by both patient and practitioner. This text attempts to explicate the necessary techniques, in detail, in the hope of elevating clinical practice. Participation in a therapeutic alliance with a patient is a privilege practitioners honor by providing only their very best—time, patience, safety, undivided attention, and goodwill—plus the rational steps stressed in this book.

Therefore, should you embark on this process, please read the entire book, even if it seems elementary in some cases. Chapter 1 begins with a description of the various methods humans have used to structure rational thought, ultimately defining the most useful practices for the medical field. Chapter 2 explores the nature of data and outlines tools for the best analysis of basic and clinical research. Chapter 3 is a detailed discussion of what information is necessary to obtain from patients and the skills for eliciting it. Chapter 4 demonstrates how combining the lessons from the first three chapters can help physicians structure optimal treatment planning sessions with their patients.

Chapter 5 explores how errors in learning and thinking across scales can affect medication selection. Chapter 6 quickly reviews pharmacokinetics, pharmacodynamics, and pharmacogenomics, before plunging into a historical and broad review of psychotropic medications in Chapter 7 and commonly used supplements in Chapter 8. Essential patient lifestyle elements necessary for good pharmacological outcome are covered in Chapter 9. Although this is a book on pharmacology, Chapter 10 provides an update on somatic treatments that are also available to patients. Very importantly, Chapter 11 discusses adverse event awareness, assessment, and response. The final chapter, Chapter 12, focuses on effective techniques for the ongoing assessment of patients and treatment plans and how any necessary alterations may be formulated and best approached.

Self-assessment questions are included at the end of each chapter, as are topics to consider individually or to discuss in seminars or journal clubs. Suggestions for additional reading are provided. I encourage you to use the description of statistical methods covered in Chapter 2 to evaluate the references included with each chapter. Remember, this process is both thorough and methodical; skipping around is neither. That is where many would-be clinicians begin to fail. Commitment to a standardized routine is the beginning of success. If you work through each chapter completely, my hope is that you will be rewarded with not only new insights but also a commitment to return to best practices learned from others that may have been forgotten, devalued, or discarded during busy and hectic practice. With effort, we not only may "do no harm"—we also may do some good.

Acknowledgments

My career in psychiatry has been stimulated and nurtured by many generous teachers and colleagues; I thank them and those who encouraged my idea of writing this book. Mr. Joe Wood, my high school government teacher, and Professor Shelton Williams, Ph.D., at Austin College (AC) most impressed in me the process of thinking rationally. Professor Henry Gorman, Ph.D., let me into his AC January term course in psychopharmacology, although I was a sophomore, and followed it with "The Physiological Basis of Behavior." Obviously, it stuck. During my residency at the Medical University of South Carolina, Thomas Steele, M.D., stressed the importance of avoiding "chronic undifferentiated therapy," while Alberto B. Santos Jr, M.D.; James C. Ballenger, M.D.; Raymond F. Anton, M.D.; and Charles Kellner, M.D., also took me under wing and imparted their best. Thanks also to Bruce Lydiard, M.D., Ph.D., who was kind enough to treat a lowly resident as a friend and colleague. I was fortunate to benefit early in my career from association with many at the American Psychiatric Association (APA) but particularly from the wisdom, knowledge, and guidance of Carolyn B. Rabinowitz, M.D.

I want to thank my early teachers and eventual colleagues in psychiatry, Albert Singleton, M.D.; Ahmed Zein-Eldin, M.D., Ph.D.; and William Bondurant III, M.D., a fellow AC grad. My colleagues in Austin, James Kreisle, M.D.; Simone Scumpia, M.D.; and Rex Wier, M.D., supported the proposal for this book to the APA. Special thanks to John McDuffie, publisher; Laura Roberts, M.D., M.A., editor-in-chief; and Erika Parker, acquisitions editor, of APA Publishing for their belief in and acceptance of this project. Thank you to Greg Kuny, managing editor; Jennifer Gilbreath, senior editor; Susan Westrate, production manager; and Zoe Boyd, marketing associate, all at APA Publishing, for shepherding me through the publication process. Your guidance and suggestions were invaluable.

I mostly thank, however, my family: particularly my wife, Meg, whose love and support made devoting a year to this project possible. I thank my computer scientist sons, Houston and Alex, for their advice on the future of computerized scientific publishing, and my daughters, Bonnie and Charlotte, for their love and encouragement. I also thank the patients who, during my 35 years in psychiatry, allowed me to participate in their lives at vulnerable moments and satisfy my dream of becoming a practicing physician.

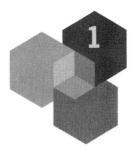

Thinking Thoroughly
and Methodically

We seek to describe the clinician as the ultimate algorithm—a tool for decision making with a solid grounding in available research regarding treatment outcomes, knowledge of pharmacology and medicine, and a complete assessment of the patient. Extending the introductory comments, this chapter hopes to expand your mind's vision of how clinicians fit into the world of information and can make the best use of it.

Algorithms and Memes

Today's culture increasingly alludes to *algorithms*—a set of rules or processes to be followed in calculations or problem solving. These underlie the computer programs and applications ("apps") that we use daily but are really nothing more than equations and step-by-step instructions humans have always used to achieve goals. The process of becoming the finest clinical psychopharmacologist you can be will involve developing and internalizing your own algorithm—the most useful set of instructions to follow, every time, step-by-step, to produce the best outcome for patients.

Associated with algorithms is the concept of *memes*: systems of behavior that are passed from one person to another—not genetically but by imitation. The word was coined more than four decades ago (Dawkins 1976). Given our current internet and social media milieu, "meme" has itself become "viral" and has evolved to refer not to ideas but rather to a group of items created with an awareness of each other (Shifman 2013). In this chapter, *meme* refers to its original usage and definition in evolutionary biology. Our goal is to describe algorithmic changes you can make to your practice and carry forward as a meme that can be imitated and shared with the profession at large, improving the practice of psychopharmacology.

Reasoning and Development of the Scientific Method

As we interact with the world of data, we seek to refine it into the world of knowledge. All data are not knowledge, just as all knowledge might not be wisdom. The clarification of knowledge from data, followed by its judicious use, is the source of wisdom. The most useful tool we have as clinicians in sorting knowledge from data is the modern scientific method.

Ancient philosophers explored the process of rational thought, seeking to develop reason so that human cognition could achieve a greater understanding of the world. Plato believed all knowledge could be obtained through *pure reasoning*. Aristotle influenced centuries of scholars by combining observation and measurement into *inductive reasoning*, realizing that rational thought had to be supported by data from the real world. Using inductive reasoning, an observation is made, and the mind attempts to draw a conclusion from the data observed. For example, every bald man you see might be geriatric. Therefore, inductive logic would lead to the theory that all bald men are of advanced age, a theory we know is not true when placed beside further observation or testing of this hypothesis. This represents a *sampling error*, which is solved with *frequentism* (discussed later).

Aristotle's work was preserved and expanded upon by Islamic scholars such as Ibn al-Haytham, who formalized the first modern scientific method based on observation, hypothesis, and experimentation; Al-Biruni, who appreciated the opportunity for bias and stressed replication of results; and Ishaq bin Ali al-Rohawi, the first to utilize peer review. Progress continued with the Europeans Roger Bacon and Francis Bacon, who further used inductive reasoning in early Western forms of the scientific method. Renée Descartes is remembered for returning Platonic deductive reasoning to the Western method, which could then involve observable testing (Shuttleworth 2009b). *Deductive reasoning* is the use of hypothesis to predict observations, valid only if the hypothesis is true. For example, a hypothesis states that all As are Bs; if this is correct, then if C=A, then C=B. Deductive predictions can be logical yet false if the hypothetical premise is false (Bradford 2017).

Using various parts or forms of deductive and inductive reasoning, the scientific method was developed and improved, and knowledge advanced. Copernicus used his actual measurements and mathematical calculations to shift thought away from our egocentric cosmology and toward a heliocentric solar system. The tale of Galileo dropping his spheres from the tower of Pisa to show how experimentation triumphed over theory is well known, but he is also important for his standardization of measurements among experiments. Francesco Redi laid to rest the centuries-old debate over spontaneous generation by performing the first known controlled experiments. Isaac Newton formalized the synthesis of inductive and deductive reasoning into our modern scientific method (Shuttleworth 2009b). Louis Pasteur's experiments led the world into a deeper understanding of microbiology, and Robert Koch's postulates advanced the understanding of infectious disease transmission.

Physiology advanced through the work of rational scientists such as William Harvey (1628/1995), the first to describe completely how blood circulates through the body, who wrote, "I do not profess to learn and teach Anatomy from the axioms of Philosophers, but from Dissections and from the fabrick of Nature" (p. XIII), and Robert Hooke (1667), known not only for his description of the cell but also for his clever experiments testing Galen's hypothesis about how the movement of air through the lungs was necessary to sustain life through its support of circulation.

Yet by the twentieth century, scientific philosophers such as Karl Popper had come to realize that science still was not infallible, that some disciplines advanced without using the scientific method and others that used it came to quite erroneous conclusions. He redefined *scientific fields* as those whose hypotheses could be tested through conjecture and refutation or "falsification." These did not include psychology and social sciences until empirical methods were developed (Shuttleworth 2009a). Thomas Kuhn (1962) usefully explained how paradigm shifts described scientific revolutions: how stubbornly scientific communities hold onto current beliefs (strong priors in Bayesian logic, see Chapter 4) and the enormity of data required to dislodge them. Paul Feyerabend observed that not all scientific disciplines are able to follow the same rules. When it is very difficult to control all the variables necessary to form a clear test of a hypothesis, inductive reasoning must be relied upon more heavily in the balance—as Copernicus, Galileo, Charles Darwin, and Albert Einstein found when they developed hypotheses that took years to fully test (Shuttleworth 2009a).

In psychopharmacology, we are called to be rational and to use the same scientific method that led to the discovery of the Higgs boson and the structure of the atom. As we wait for our field to further improve empirical methods and to build enough data to solidify or tear down our current paradigms, however, patients are waiting for relief. We are obliged to offer them only the information that we have been able to test and should not rely on highly inductive guesses that will wait decades for verification.

As I discuss later in Chapter 4, we rely on *probability theory*, which was initiated in the seventeenth century by Blaise Pascal and Pierre de Fermat, advanced by Jacob Bernoulli and Pierre-Simon Laplace (names you would probably associate with other areas of scientific advancement), benefited from significant revision by Thomas Bayes and Ronald A. Fisher, and is still developing. Fisher is most associated with defeating the null hypothesis with *P* values and with advancing the frequentist approach that any outlying finding is likely to eventually be subsumed by larger and larger data sets. Unfortunately, not all knowledge can be obtained by restricting truth to a rigid cutoff for significance in order to defeat the null hypothesis: far too many theories must be tested, and our resources, especially for many possible randomized controlled trials (RCTs), are limited (see Chapter 2). Bayes's prior probability (Chapter 4) can help rationally inform our use of the degree of significance in our abductive logical creation of treatment decisions. *Abductive reasoning*, explored further in Chapter 5, is what we often use when forming diagnoses and treatment plans: we develop theories from partial information, such as examination results and RCTs, and make temporary hypotheses that are then tested.

Threats to Reason

We must also take into account unconscious biases that may distort our interpretation of data and cause us to reject important information that we need in our knowledge base. The same may happen in our patients. Haidt (2012) wrote of how an emotional response, such as that linked to morality, will lead a person to cherry-pick data of varying quality to justify that response rather than evaluate the data objectively and seek more data to form or alter opinions. The use of reason, in this case, is in service of supporting the emotional reaction rather than the best objective knowledge. Furthermore, Schulz (2010) explored how social pressures shield individuals in groups from contrary data, exaggerating support for our own ideas and discouraging internal and external disagreement.

These influences are in addition to the cognitive confirmation bias that we attempt to eliminate in clinical research by, for example, blinding ourselves to the nature of samples during experiments. As I discuss further in Chapter 5, we strive to make treatment recommendations based on the *results* of controlled clinical trials, not on the hypotheses upon which they are based. Awareness of these emotional confounding factors in our assessment of data is the first step in minimizing their influence. Read broadly and discuss often with those who disagree with you on clinical issues, not so that you will automatically adapt your own thinking to theirs (they might be wrong as well) but so that you are exposed to the greatest amount of information, and attempt to consider it all value free (beyond the highest regard for the scientific method and good study design).

Although we might expect that clinicians' knowledge base and wisdom only improve during medical education, data show otherwise. Misconceptions about the biomedical information to be absorbed and collated develop alongside more correct conceptions (Badenhorst et al. 2015). Furthermore, research about how we learn scientific information spotlights additional potential roadblocks to useful knowledge. It appears that learning new scientific theories does not result in the simple displacement of the original naive and, presumably, inaccurate theories but rather is added to them, requiring our brains to actively suppress the older theories for many years in order to recognize the new. The extended length of time this requires is measurable (Foisy et al. 2015; Shtulman and Valcarcel 2012). Even the best intentions must overcome many unconscious and potentially conscious barriers to understanding and using only the best knowledge.

Artificial Intelligence and Human Reasoning

It is unlikely that human clinical psychopharmacologists will be completely replaced by artificial intelligence (AI) in the foreseeable future, but tools to supplement our work involving machine learning and AI are already here. "Big data" also offers the promise of unexpected knowledge and speed of response. From the simple use of the internet to look up studies and dosages, to computer-assisted scans for drug–drug interactions, to electronic medical records and even email for clinical communication, algorithms developed by others are already sharing the workload with us. We must make sure that our own contributions are as reliable.

Our current situation really is not any different than when physicians looked up pharmacological data in hardbound reference books such as *Drug Facts and Comparisons* (Facts and Comparisons 2016), kept notes and prescription logs in paper charts, and stored paper copies of favorite journal articles in physical filing cabinets. The processes are similar; only the equipment has changed. A similar change occurred in the 1950s with the introduction of the copy machine and in the 1970s with the introduction of the answering machine. What we did and aspired to did not change, the processes just improved and made it a bit easier for practitioners to make decisions.

The president of Northeastern University, Joseph E. Aoun, Ph.D., has explored how higher education may adapt to preparing students to remain relevant as AI takes over more tasks previously performed by humans. He suggests that although knowledge alone will not be sufficient to reserve a place for the effort of the human mind, the ways we think about the world may remain our contribution. He suggests emphasizing not only entrepreneurship and cultural agility but also *systems thinking* or making integrated connections (Aoun 2017). He proposes that AI may analyze complex problems well, but it cannot yet understand how to apply the results in a creative and useful way through critical thinking. Although *convergent thinking* (identifying the single best answer) may sometimes be handled by AI, *divergent thinking* (generating multiple responses in a free flow of ideas) remains a skill humans might master. We can learn to understand and apply the context in which data are gathered and answers are formed, thus using well-analyzed ideas and information most effectively.

Penitus et Methodice, Omni Tempore

While we look at the cutting edge of the future with AI, algorithms, and memes, let us also carry forward the concept of a *motto*: a phrase guiding the ideals of an individual or institution. Visualize a scroll containing the Latin phrase *penitus et methodice, omni tempore* (thoroughly, methodically, all the time). Imagine this motto when you think of yourself practicing psychopharmacology.

The words *thorough* and *methodical* recur often throughout this book, and to that is added the imperative to perform to this level habitually. The best clinical practice involves repetition—repetition of all the known best practices, completely, every time. The clinical environment of excellence we are creating has no room for shortcuts—no hunches, no cutting corners "just this once." As I cover in Chapter 2, we can never achieve certainty in science, and we can approximate it only with a rigorously applied scientific method. Probability will play a large role in the treatment recommendations we make to patients. Uncertainty and probability are inherent in our process, so we must leave no room for unnecessary expansion of uncertainty through incomplete assessments, inadequate knowledge of the literature, unrecognized bias, and the lack of a plan. The goal is to do things the right way the first time and every time to benefit our patients.

It can be useful to consider the best practices of successful practitioners in other fields. In a recent interview with Dinah Eng, the celebrated architect Frank Gehry discussed the importance of always being your professional best. He tackles each project, even small ones, the same way, as though it were the most important. He tries to avoid expectations in a project and tests relentlessly, not just following the first idea that comes to mind (Eng 2018). He is thorough and methodical.

To achieve this yourself, you must develop and refine your list of "best practices," just as hospital quality and improvement committees do, and you must promise yourself that you will adhere to them, adopting them *in toto* as your algorithm and therefore demonstrating a meme—a system of behavior you can pass on. Identify your tools: trusted sources of information (your knowledge base), adequate resources for patient evaluation and monitoring (time, space, safety), and sufficient resources for treatment planning (trust, a good therapeutic alliance, clinical judgment). Patients bring to the therapeutic alliance their trust in us, their disclosure of information, and their agreement to comply with a mutually agreed-upon treatment plan. Clinicians bring not only their attention, goodwill, and common sense but also their tools: trust in their patients and the alliance, a database, safety, time, space, and clinical judgment guided by critical thinking.

By pledging to yourself that you will apply these tools *thoroughly, methodically,* and *consistently,* you create the boundaries and structure of your algorithm and enter the flow of information in medicine as a positive influence: the rational psychopharmacologist. The chapters that follow will fill in the details.

Summary

The best algorithm for the clinical practice of psychopharmacology is a defined set of thorough steps, followed completely each and every time, that may be passed on as a cultural meme, improving overall practice. The modern scientific method is our best tool for developing wisdom from data using a combination of inductive, deductive, and abductive reasoning: observation, hypothesis generation, and experimentation resulting in new observations that restart the process. Probability theory further informs the practice of psychopharmacology.

Clinicians must be ever alert for unconscious biases, both emotional and cognitive, that restrict access to information and rational conclusion. As technology takes over many of providers' traditional tasks, divergent thinking may yet still lead to the creative and useful application of knowledge beyond the conceivable capabilities of AI. Habitually thorough and methodical, rational psychopharmacologists consciously define best practices as the elements of their algorithm: their database, space and time for safe and adequate evaluation, development of a therapeutic alliance, and application of clinical judgment guided by critical thinking.

Key Points

■ Adherence to the modern scientific method offers better clinical outcomes.

■ Consistently use thorough and methodical assessments of research data and patients.

■ Be alert to unconscious cognitive and emotional biases during each assessment.

Self-Assessment

1. The concept of God is an example of

    A. A meme
    B. An algorithm
    C. Neither
    D. Both

2. *Therapeutic alliance* refers to (choose all that apply)

    A. The provider making the final treatment decisions for a patient
    B. The patient making the final treatment decisions
    C. A contract of mutuality where both patient and provider work together to improve the health of the patient
    D. A multispecialty treatment team directing a patient's care

3. An *algorithm* is

    A. A set of rules to help artificial intelligence learn on its own
    B. A list of steps to solve a problem or accomplish a goal
    C. A small procedure that solves a current problem in computer science or mathematics
    D. All of the above

4. *Abductive reasoning* refers to

    A. Drawing conclusions from a single observation
    B. The use of hypothesis to predict observations
    C. Developing theories from partial information, forming hypotheses, then testing them
    D. The belief that all knowledge may be obtained through pure reason

5. Unconscious biases that distort our rational consideration of data may be

   A. Emotional responses linked to morality
   B. Group dynamics restricting the consideration of contrary information
   C. Cognitive confirmation bias
   D. All of the above

6. *Divergent thinking* involves

   A. Generating multiple responses in a free flow of ideas
   B. Identifying the single best answer
   C. Playing devil's advocate with the ideas of another
   D. Identifying a response no one else has thought of

Discussion Topics

1. Consider the clinical psychopharmacologist's role in upholding the highest clinical and scientific standards for patient care. How can inconsistent or uninformed care affect the quality of clinical care provided by others?

2. With increasing use of electronic databases, big data, machine learning, and artificial intelligence in clinical medicine, how will the role of the human practitioner evolve? What opportunities exist for enhancing patient care and provider satisfaction?

3. Identify examples of emotional, societal, and cognitive biases that influence our perception of knowledge. What tools can we use to minimize their influence in clinical practice?

Additional Reading

Christian B, Griffiths T: Algorithms to Live By: The Computer Science of Human Decisions. New York, Henry Holt, 2016 (This detailed work provides examples of how algorithms and human judgment must work together for effective problem solving.)

Ellenberg J: How Not to Be Wrong: The Power of Mathematical Thinking. New York, Penguin Press, 2014 (A superb review of mathematical thinking for exact results as well as the value of estimation. Also, a good review of statistical concepts discussed in Chapter 2 and Bayesian influence in Chapter 4.)

Lynas M: Seeds of Science: Why We Got It So Wrong on Gmos. London, Bloomsbury Sigma, 2018 (Chapter 9 is an excellent discussion of the moral, emotional, and cognitive biases against scientific data that even the most intelligent
human minds must overcome to obtain objective knowledge; also discusses
the work of Haidt and Schulz referenced in this chapter.)

McInerny DQ: Being Logical: A Guide to Good Thinking. New York, Random
House, 2004 (A 135-page quick read covering the basic principles of logic.
"Part Five: The Principal Forms of Illogical Thinking" and the afterword are
particularly helpful to review.)

Pagel M: Wired for Culture: The Natural History of Human Cooperation. New
York, Penguin Books, 2012 (This work is an excellent introduction to and exploration of cultural memes as used by evolutionary biologists.)

Stephens-Davidowitz S: Everybody Lies: Big Data, New Data, and What the Internet Can Tell Us About Who We Really Are. London, Bloomsbury, 2017 (An en-
tertaining yet eye-opening description of what big data may someday offer us.)

References

Aoun JE: Robot-Proof: Higher Education in the Age of Artificial Intelligence.
Cambridge, MA, MIT Press, 2017

Badenhorst E, Mamede S, Hartman N, et al: Exploring lecturers' views of first-
year health science students' misconceptions in biomedical domains. Adv
Health Sci Educ Theory Pract 20(2):403–420, 2015 25099944

Bradford A: Deductive reasoning vs. inductive reasoning. Live Science, July 24, 2017.
Available at: https://www.livescience.com/21569-deduction-vs-induction.html.
Accessed September 23, 2019.

Dawkins R: The Selfish Gene. New York, Oxford University Press, 1976

Eng D: Frank Gehry: the award-winning architect tells Fortune how he got
started. Fortune 178(5):47–48, 2018

Facts and Comparisons: Drug Facts and Comparisons 2017. Philadelphia, PA,
Lippincott Williams and Wilkins, 2016

Foisy L-MB, Potvin P, Riopel M, et al: Is inhibition involved in overcoming a common physics misconception in mechanics? Trends Neurosci Educ 4(1–2):26–
36, 2015

Haidt J: The Righteous Mind: Why Good People Are Divided by Politics and Re-
ligion. New York, Penguin Books, 2012

Harvey W: The Anatomical Exercises: De Motu Cordis and De Circulatione San-
guinis (1628). New York, Dover, 1995

Hooke R: An account of an experiment made by M. Hook, of preserving animals
alive by blowing through their lungs with bellows. Philosophical Transactions
2:539–540, 1667

Kuhn TS: The Structure of Scientific Revolutions. Chicago, IL, University of Chicago Press, 1962

Schulz K: Being Wrong: Adventures in the Margin of Error. London, Portobello
Books, 2010

Shifman L: Memes in Digital Culture (Essential Knowledge Series). Cambridge, MA, MIT Press, 2013

Shtulman A, Valcarcel J: Scientific knowledge suppresses but does not supplant earlier intuitions. Cognition 124(2):209–215, 2012 22595144

Shuttleworth M: History of the scientific method. Explorable, August 18, 2009a. Available at: https://explorable.com/history-of-the-scientific-method. Accessed September 23, 2019.

Shuttleworth M: Who invented the scientific method? Explorable, April 23, 2009b. Available at: https://explorable.com/who-invented-the-scientific-method. Accessed September 23, 2019.

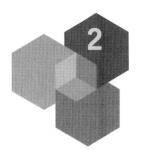

Evidence-Based Medicine in an Era of Sparse Evidence

Assessment of Data

Problems With Validity

Recently, health care has become particularly focused on the evidence-based practice of medicine. This might lead one to wonder just what we thought we were using previously—tea leaves? Clearly, we have always been using what we thought was evidence in making treatment decisions. This leads us to consider the nature of data and information. We are taught early in our careers to eschew "anecdotal" evidence and to seek data obtained only from randomized, double-blind, controlled trials. Although we may have had an elementary discussion of statistics at some point in our education, it has recently been demonstrated that the majority of statistical analyses published in peer-reviewed journals are inadequate (Ercan et al. 2015).

In the past two decades, journals in science and medicine have frequently reported failure of study design and statistical analysis (Hebert et al. 2002; Nieuwenhuis et al. 2011; Strasak et al. 2007a). Overreliance on the simplified methods of statistical analysis we all learned in school has led to many erroneous conclusions; study designs have become more complicated, rendering the simple methods inadequate. Consider also that peer reviewers may lack the necessary statistical sophistication to adequately assess the analyses of submissions (Strasak et al. 2007b).

The problem has become particularly grievous in behavioral science, where a high rate of irreproducibility has been demonstrated (Open Science Collaboration 2015). Many medical and scientific journals have answered by reviewing their own published articles in honest self-assessment and by responding to the poor results by hiring outside statisticians to review analyses of proposed articles. Some have formalized new standards and checklists to guide potential authors and reviewers in avoiding erroneous conclusions. Attempts also have been made to improve the quality of information contained in the abstracts of articles (Hays et al. 2016). Although we as practitioners have been schooled in study design, the many pitfalls in assessing both basic and clinical scientific research behoove us to strengthen our understanding of the commonly used, and in some cases increasingly sophisticated, methods of data analysis we are likely to encounter (Horton and Switzer 2005). The data we use to help our patients are obtained solely from treatment outcome studies, so our correct assessment of these data is the very beginning of providing the best and most hopeful care for our patients.

As we observe that many studies published in peer-reviewed journals suffer from inadequate design or analysis, let us start with the idea that some of this is actually intentional. It is quite common for us to read a case report of one, two, or even three patients that alerts the field to potential problems or solutions requiring further study. This might then lead a researcher to design and carry out a limited open-label study of the problem, at moderate to low cost. The results, again, if adequately assessed, provide further information on whether it is reasonable to seek funding from third-party sources to carry out expensive randomized controlled trials (RCTs) that will, it is hoped, be the first step in answering the questions raised in the case reports. It is incumbent upon the reader, of course, to remember that case reports and open-label studies are the early part of the data-gathering process and not the final word.

A successful study must combine good design with adequate methods and assessment. This means that the design must match the type of statistical analysis being applied and that the methods must be adequate to provide the data to be examined. Common study design errors include inadequate numbers of patients included in a study to justify the chosen method of statistical analysis; an excessive number of variables that overwhelms elementary statistical analysis; and, given the cost of RCTs, the very short length of observation time commonly used. Only the fine print under "methods" will disclose ancillary treatments that were allowed for humane reasons but that certainly may have muddied the clarity of the results. For example, it is quite common to allow what some people might consider liberal use of benzodiazepines in evaluations of major tranquilizers or mood stabilizers used to treat acute mania. Their use would not be taken into account in the final analysis of efficacy. Choice of placebo, active or not, and of the relative dosages of the studied agent and the comparator may not reflect real-world use and therefore may skew the findings. Consider whether the dosages being given in clinical research are fixed or variable, what criteria allow them to vary, and whether serum levels have been measured. Do the dosages and the serum levels reflect those used in clinical practice? Are the clinical scales used both published and standardized, and do the measurements using them reflect standard use and understanding? Are patients who did not complete the study included in the analysis?

Another problem is the definition of the endpoint to be measured (Yu et al. 2015). Are we measuring a cause, a correlation, or an unrelated and possibly insignificant event as the treatment outcome, and then extrapolating inaccurately and assuming clinical benefit? The famous Clinical Antipsychotic Trials of Intervention Effectiveness study by the National Institute of Mental Health (Lieberman et al. 2005) considered discontinuation of treatment for any cause as the primary outcome measurement, and clinical scales as secondary measurements, as it attempted to compare the relative value of traditional with atypical antipsychotic medications.

Missing from much of published science, in any field, are studies that report they cannot show a statistically significant outcome (Turner et al. 2008) and studies that repeat the work of others, including those that may or may not demonstrate the same statistical significance. It has recently been reported that researchers are unlikely to even write up a study, or submit it for publication, unless it fails to support the null hypothesis, demonstrating a positive effect or outcome and supporting an alternative hypothesis (Franco et al. 2014). This bias appears to have less hold over conference and poster submissions but significantly curtails publication of important data, although journals and other databases are now seeking such studies. Additionally, because much research in our field is currently proprietary, it is difficult to discern whether studies have been performed that resulted in disappointing data or whether such studies have not actually been done. Head-to-head studies are far too rare due to proprietary fear of the loss of market share. All too often, the most interesting and important questions are not asked.

Along these lines, it is encouraging to know that efforts are under way to correct some of these problems, including the Cochrane Collaboration (Herxheimer 1993) study registries and the AllTrials petition. The Cochrane Collaboration provides ongoing reviews of RCTs, published online as the Cochrane Library (www.cochranelibrary.com), and includes the *Co-*

chrane Database of Systematic Reviews, the *Cochrane Handbook for Diagnostic Test Accuracy Reviews*, consumer summaries, and the *Cochrane Handbook for Systematic Reviews of Interventions*. Initiatives seeking to first register all new clinical trials prior to enrollment (in addition to all past trials performed) and to require publication of results within 1 year of study completion began in the United States in 1997, when Congress passed a law mandating a registry database (National Institutes of Health 2018). As a result, ClinicalTrials.gov was launched in 2000, initially requiring only National Institutes of Health–funded studies to be registered.

In 2005, the International Committee of Medical Journal Editors initiated registration of clinical trials as a prerequisite to publication and updated their recommendations for registration and publication in 2017 (International Committee of Medical Journal Editors 2018). The World Health Organization (WHO) decreed in 2006 that all trials should be registered and proposed a minimum amount of data that must be collected in a study (updated in 2017 [World Health Organization 2019]). WHO followed up in 2007 by establishing its own registry for studies, the International Clinical Trials Registry Platform, which provided a single source for locating studies in several international registry databases, including ClinicalTrials.gov. Also, that year, the FDA updated its own requirements for reporting, requiring more types of studies and specific information that must be included in ClinicalTrials.gov.

In 2008, the World Medical Association defined prospective study registration as an ethical requirement and in 2013 further clarified that registration must precede patient recruitment (World Medical Association 2018). The European Medicines Agency in 2013 updated the European Clinical Trials Database, making summary clinical results from registered studies available in the European Union Clinical Trials Register, which is aligned with ClinicalTrials.gov (National Institutes of Health 2018). The registration number of a trial should be found on both abstracts and full-text articles when published.

Beyond registration, however, is the goal of actually getting the data from registered studies published and made available to all for review. Both the United States (Zarin et al. 2016) and the International Clinical Trials Registry Platform (World Health Organization 2015) have since clarified rules requiring publication of data from registered studies within 12–36 months of study completion. Explicitly stated is the intention that all trials ever conducted publish their data, even if registration followed the actual study. Efforts are proceeding to include smaller databases so that all of the available data can be considered as we draw scientific conclusions, reducing the number of type I errors (discussed later).

Data have shown that 64.1% of studies registered on ClinicalTrials.gov from academic medical centers had still not published data within 24 months of study completion (Chen et al. 2016). The AllTrials campaign, begun in 2013, is attempting to improve these numbers through a petition calling for "all past and present clinical trials to be registered and their full methods and summary results reported" (AllTrials 2019). To date, more than 93,000 individuals, companies, and organizations have signed the petition. The latest rules from the United States, Europe, WHO, and publishers and international efforts such as AllTrials show promise in increasing the rate of registration and publication in the coming decades.

Clinical Gossip

Lest we place all the blame on researchers, however, we must also look at how even those who primarily see patients, rather than do research, might compound the problem of valid evidence without proper self-vigilance. We have all known peers who are inclined to exaggerate, to remember incorrectly, or even, sadly, to lie about studies during rounds or other clinical discussions. Even the best-intentioned individuals might propagate misinformation unless circumspect about their contributions. For example, a clinician might share a case report or open-label study with peers without clarifying that well-designed and analyzed controlled studies have yet to be done. Treatments effective for one problem are commonly tried for many other problems. It might be said that a certain pharmacological agent is "being used" to treat a particular clinical problem, when the more correct and important phrasing would be "being studied." This commonly leads to other clinicians assuming the best and using the treatment without assessing the data for themselves. Hardly textbook behavior, but we all know that this is too common. Clinical "gossip" not only is disappointing but also can be harmful for our patients.

Study Design and Data Analysis

We are left with a paucity of seemingly accurate information in order to make treatment recommendations to patients. To ascertain the best data available, clinicians must be knowledgeable in study design and data analysis. Both must be chosen by a researcher in tandem because the methods of data analysis must match the structure of the study. Emphasis on registration of studies prior to recruitment also encourages commitment to the data analysis method chosen prior to seeing the results, so that outcomes cannot be massaged statistically to fit some eventual significance (Lancee et al. 2017). Familiarity with the contemporary methods of study design and data analysis that may be encountered is essential so that a reader can adequately evaluate the validity of the data, including phase I–IV studies, prospective and retrospective analyses, meta-analysis, intention to treat (ITT), risk ratio or relative risk, odds ratio, confidence interval, *P* value, absolute risk reduction (ARR), number needed to treat (NNT), and number needed to harm (NNH).

Studies that attempt to seek FDA approval for marketing are ranked by Phases I–IV. Following studies with animal models for efficacy and safety, Phase I studies give an investigational medication, usually identified only by a research number, to "healthy volunteers" who do not have any diagnosis; they agree to take the medication for a few days to weeks so that investigators can determine the "maximum tolerated dosage." If extensive physical and laboratory examinations fail to demonstrate toxicity, then Phase II trials are begun. In these RCTs, the test medication is given specifically to volunteers who have the illness the medication is hypothesized to treat, while further tests on safety are conducted. If enough success and safety are found, Phase III trials are carried out, which also test for efficacy and safety, but this time against standard treatment. Phase III trials are large, multicenter studies also using a randomized, double-blind, placebo-controlled design. To obtain FDA approval for marketing, the proposed treatment must usually show efficacy and safety in at least two Phase III studies. Phase IV studies are performed after FDA approval and can focus on long-term trials for safety and efficacy or use of the study medication in expanded populations, such as in pregnant women (Suvarna 2010).

Much criticism has been leveled in the past several decades about the tradition of testing primarily males in pharmacological studies (originally due to worries about teratogenicity) and assuming that the results can be extrapolated accurately to females. As a result, the National Institutes of Health in 1993 issued guidelines requiring that females and minority groups be included in all Phase III studies. The latest revision was published in 2017 (National Institutes of Health 2017). Awareness that gender identity may also have an impact on outcome, particularly in psychiatry, has led the European Association of Science Editors to develop the Sex and Gender Equity in Research Guidelines (Heidari et al. 2016; Lancet Psychiatry 2016).

Researchers must make choices about how to gather and analyze data prior to enrolling and testing participants, so study design is crucial. Several models have become commonplace, including ITT, which determines, in advance, which patients enrolled in a study will be subjected to final statistical analysis. In an ITT study, every patient who reaches randomization will be analyzed, regardless of compliance or any other factor that might prevent the patient from completing the study. If a patient passes the initial screening and starts the study, his or her results will be analyzed, even if many data points are missing. Advantages of ITT include preserving the original power of the study, because the number of patients in each cell remains static during analysis. ITT also accepts the real-world issues of less-than-perfect compliance, protocol errors, and deviations. Shortcomings of ITT include the possibility that head-to-head comparisons are not actually being made, because an immediate dropout subject may be compared with a study completer (Gupta 2011).

The most commonly used technique for evaluating ITT studies is last observation carried forward (LOCF). The *final* data point for a participant, which may occur just after randomization or at any point through the end of the study, is evaluated as though the participant completed the study. LOCF may, however, lead to biased estimates of treatment effect and biased tests of the null hypothesis when no treatment effect is assumed (Liu and Gould 2002). A similar technique, baseline observation carried forward (BOCF), analyzes the final outcome using the *starting* data for a participant, collected prior to treatment, although this is more likely to lead to a type II error. Another approach, modified BOCF, attempts to minimize the distortion of a participant dropping out for a nonclinical reason: LOCF is used for participants who either complete the study or who drop out for nonclinical reasons, and BOCF is used for those who fail to complete for treatment-related reasons. Adverse events BOCF was also developed to be even more specific about discontinuation of the study related to adverse events (Liu-Seifert et al. 2010).

If the data missing in ITT analyses from treatment and nontreatment groups are about the same, then the bias is against finding an effect; bias could also exist, in either direction, from more uneven distributions of missing data (Lane 2008). Lachin (2016) demonstrated that if gaps in data are truly random and the data analyzed have the same distribution as the missing data, then bias may be avoided. Because this can never be known by someone evaluating the data, however, it is well to assume that bias is always introduced when LOCF is used. Although alternative solutions to using LOCF in ITT studies have been proposed since 2010 (Little et al. 2012; National Research Council 2010), most papers published in peer-reviewed journals continue to employ this method (Lachin 2016). Many other arguments have been brought forward in attempts to minimize skewed evaluation, including proposals of how some randomized patients might be removed from analysis (Fergusson et al. 2002; Hollis and Campbell 1999; White et al. 2012). Still, LOCF is so likely to add a bias that many authors eschew its use, and the FDA now discourages it as well. Ultimately, bias in ITT studies is best guarded against by following all study participants thoroughly and as long as possible so as to include the maximal amount of data, especially whenever LOCF or BOCF is to be used.

Another study design is *retrospective analysis*, in which patients are enrolled after a clinical event, such as being recruited for inclusion or chosen at random in a chart review. This type of design is common when big databases are available to mine but may also be chosen when the data are skimpier. Scandinavian countries publish many of these reports in light of their deep national databases and, until recently, relatively homogeneous populations. The shortcoming of this approach, however, is sampling error. In selecting, say, 100 out of 5,000 charts, seemingly at random, it is still possible one might choose all 20 cases of good or poor outcome found in the 5,000 charts, leading to an observed incidence of 20% rather than the actual 0.4%. You have no way to determine that the event you are studying is evenly distributed. The same error may be made by recruiting patients who have experienced bad outcomes from treatments, termed *retrospective registries*. Those who come forward may certainly be counted, but how can we count those who are problem free and did not tell us? Patients who had a bad outcome are more motivated to consider enrollment than are those who have recovered and moved on.

In a clinical aside, we used to make this mistake when we assumed that manic episodes could be provoked by stress in a patient's life, because our patients with manic outbreaks would come to our attention and often would report a stressful preceding event. After several years of more careful observation, we realized that far more patients with bipolar affective disorder were actually at home, well stabilized, handling stress just fine, who did not feel the need to rush to the office to tell us. We learned, then, that response to stress is a measurement of mood stability, not a single or clear cause of a manic episode. Our literature is rife with retrospective studies, which are also often reported in the media, so consider them carefully and explain them to your patients.

Alternatively, a *prospective* study is considered more valid because we enroll patients prior to an observable event, be it trying a new medication or having a baby while receiving medication. We then have the opportunity to learn what actually happened to everyone. In addition to well-designed studies that use this method, prospective patient registries are another form of data collection often used to gather accurate information on effects in pregnancy, including fetal response to illness and treatment.

When evaluating a single variable through a prospective registry, such as the safety of the fetuses of pregnant mothers who received fluoxetine during pregnancy, we usually need around 750 prospective cases to ensure valid statistical analysis. If more than one variable exists, then the number goes higher. Patient registries are wonderful sources of data, but the data arrive slowly and are not regularly reported at fixed intervals. Also, not every problem is studied with a registry. Some researcher must have an interest in a project, set it up, and maintain it. Regular reporting is not required, and obtaining the data when you want them can be difficult. Nevertheless, the data are often very useful.

A discussion of how the perception of lithium-induced teratogenicity was influenced by the use of these two methodologies illustrates how they can be used more or less effectively. The first assessments of the effect of lithium on fetuses used the Register of Lithium Babies, data that started in Scandinavia and then was supplemented by other countries, including the United States. It must be pointed out that although this was a registry, it was a retrospective one. Clinicians were asked to submit cases of in utero lithium exposure post delivery. The frequencies of any abnormalities reported in the infants were then compared with expected incidences in the general population. By the late 1970s, this resulted in the assessment that a fetus exposed to at least one prescription of lithium in utero during the first trimester carried a 3% chance of developing Ebstein's anomaly, a right ventricular outflow abnormality. This represented an increased relative risk by a factor of 400 over the general population (Schou et al. 1973; Weinstein and Goldfield 1975). It was not until almost two decades later that data from controlled studies and prospective registries demonstrated a much lower relative risk of this abnormality, ranging from 1.2 to 7.7, significantly lower than 400 and illustrating the bias that retrospective reports may carry (Cohen et al. 1994). This estimate has been replicated at a 2.6 adjusted risk ratio in a recent study using retrospective case review, but this time it was through a review of *all* pregnancies resulting in a live birth that were paid for by Medicaid during a 10-year period (Patorno et al. 2017). It did not rely upon random report gathering, which tends to increase the estimate of the variable being measured. The change in relative risk from 400 to an adjusted risk ratio less than 3 based on the methodology of the research is one important example of how critical evaluation of journal articles by the practitioner is essential in providing the best medical care for patients.

These studies used the measurement of risk ratio, or relative risk: the ratio of the proportion of patients who experience a bad outcome when exposed to that risk divided by the proportion of patients who had the same bad outcome without exposure to the risk. Absolute risk, relative risk, odds, and odds ratio may all be used in the literature to judge the outcome of exposures and treatments, so it is important to understand the differences (Table 2–1).

TABLE 2–1.   Risk and odds

Absolute risk	Number of events in group divided by number of people in group
Relative risk or risk ratio	Number of bad outcomes with exposure divided by number of bad outcomes without exposure
Odds	Number of subjects with event divided by number of subjects without event
Odds ratio	Odds of x in presence of y divided by odds of x in absence of y

Risk is the number of patients experiencing an event divided by the total number of patients. *Odds* is the number of patients experiencing an event divided by the number of patients who did not experience the event. The *odds ratio*, then, is the odds of one group compared to the odds of another, in ratio form. Odds ratios are often cited with a confidence interval, which attempts to justify a small sample with the general population, and *P* values, which estimate the degree of statistical significance. The three taken together often give a better chance of evaluating the validity of a research finding when they are not contradictory.

Although odds ratio is frequently used to estimate the risk of exposure to a threat, such as smoking or use of alcohol, it is also used as a relative comparison of the results of treatment versus nontreatment: the odds of obtaining a particular outcome with a treatment compared with the odds of that same outcome without the treatment. Treatment result odds is placed as the numerator and the comparison placebo, or control, result odds as the denominator (see Table 2–1). If the outcome result is identical for the experimental (or intervention) group and the placebo (or control) group, OR = 1. If the treatment group is superior to control, OR > 1; it follows that an OR < 1 shows the control group to be superior.

The interpretation of odds ratio is clearest when only two factors are being compared, such as whether a patient is better with or without a single treatment or potentially dangerous exposure. If additional factors or variables are introduced, such as gender or age, then a logistic regression analysis may have been performed in order to clarify an accurate odds ratio. In small sample sizes, the relative risk and odds ratio might appear similar, but as sample sizes increase, the odds ratio might be of more value, especially because the logistic regression may be applied (Frick et al. 2011).

The confidence interval is used to estimate the accuracy and the size of the effect of the odds rato. A broader confidence interval is less accurate, and a smaller confidence interval is more accurate. Basically, the confidence interval estimates the probability that the odds ratio will fall within a certain range in the general population, even though it may have been determined from a small sample size. A confidence interval of 95% is commonly accepted, although you may find 90% or 99%. In the 2017 study of lithium-induced fetal risk mentioned earlier (Patorno et al. 2017), the authors reported a relative risk of 2.6 with a 95% CI of 1.00–7.06, meaning a 95% chance that the relative risk determined from the entire population would fall within 1.00–7.06. Confidence interval does not estimate statistical significance, just accuracy and scale.

Statistical significance is described by the *P* value, and explaining this requires a review of the null hypothesis (signified as H_0 in equations) and type I and type II errors in statistics. The null hypothesis (from nullify) asserts that no true statistical difference exists between two experimental groups. This null hypothesis is either disproven (rejected) or *fails* to be disproven. If disproven, then an alternative hypothesis (H_a) may explain the statistically significant difference between the experimental groups. A null hypothesis fails to be disproven when the confidence interval includes a value of *no difference*, or CI=1. Failing to reject the null hypotheses means that researchers have not gathered enough data to do so, which can occur for many reasons, including sample size, design flaws, and errors in data collection in addition to the possibility that the two groups really demonstrate no difference. In a type I error, the null hypothesis is incorrectly rejected—a difference is detected that is not true. In a type II error, a difference that is true is not detected.

The *P* value gives us a guide as to how strongly our data support the null hypothesis. A low *P* value is very supportive of rejecting the null and therefore points to a significant difference in the results. A high value is less supportive of rejection and therefore indicates a higher likelihood that no difference between the groups exists. What is very important to realize is that no absolute value for the *P* conclusively rejects or fails to reject the null. It has become common among many to accept a $P<0.05$ as proof of statistical significance, yet this is a misunderstanding of the value. The *P* value represents a scale along which statistical significance increases or decreases but is never definitive (Sterne and Davey Smith 2001). For this reason, many authors now encourage reporting the actual value of *P*, or reporting to at least three decimal places, rather than a cutoff at 95% (or <0.05) (Habibzadeh 2013). The error, or false discovery, rate is actually still quite high at $P<0.05$ and can become significantly lower as the *P* value drops further, such as to $P<0.001$ (Colquhoun 2014). Therefore, the most helpful articles include the *P* value to as many decimal places as needed. To illustrate, $P<0.01$ does not indicate the actual error rate but tells us that in similar studies we would see a type I error of the same degree or greater 1% of the time due to sampling error.

Determining statistical significance, however, does not fully describe the magnitude or clinical effect we are seeking to determine for our patients—in other words, how likely we are to see results in our patients. The NNT can provide a measure of this expectation, as long as the time interval of treatment and the appropriate confidence interval accompany this number (Flechner and Tseng 2011). NNT is the number of patients you would need to treat with the new treatment to see one more patient improve than you would from the older treatment. It is determined by taking the inverse of the ARR, which is the difference in event rate between a control and a treatment group (Table 2–2) (Laupacis et al. 1988). A lower NNT indicates a more robust effect, but the value of NNT must be taken into context. Comparison groups must be similar in baseline risk, stage of illness, time allowed for treatment, and comparison of the multiple outcomes that may arise from a treatment (McAlister 2008). If properly standardized, however, NNT can give the reader a quick estimate of how much better an outcome the new treatment can offer our patients, taken as a group.

Related to NNT is NNH, which estimates the number of exposures to a risk it takes to produce one additional bad outcome. This can be useful when evaluating the safety of a pharmacological treatment, but again, only when properly applied. NNH represents the inverse of attributable risk (incidence in exposed minus incidence in nonexposed). A higher NNH indicates greater safety than a lower number. A recent review of the literature has suggested that improper use of this statistic may be rife, thus misleading readers; NNH in current usage appears inferior to postmarketing surveillance and case management (Safer and Zito 2013).

Meta-Analysis

Now we move to the slippery slope of meta-analysis. A traditional study compares one group of individual patient outcomes with another group's individual outcomes, searching for statistical significance. Meta-analysis, however, applies statistical techniques to a collection of completed studies. The smallest data point in a typical study is one patient. The smallest unit in a meta-analysis may be the summary data from one study. The hope is to observe a possible treatment effect that is consistent through the studies examined or to show that the effect is not present. Whereas at one time a clinician had to read literature review summaries that were published in peer-reviewed journals to be brought up to date quickly on the latest thinking, meta-analyses offer quick assessments in statistical form. Their

TABLE 2–2. Magnitude measurements

Absolute risk reduction	Absolute risk of control group minus absolute risk of treatment group
Number needed to treat	1 divided by absolute risk reduction
Number needed to harm	1 divided by attributable risk

use has expanded exponentially in the past five decades (Haidich 2010), eventually becoming cited by authors more often than traditional randomized studies (Patsopoulos et al. 2005).

As with any method of analysis, however, many possible flaws can introduce bias and distort the outcome in meta-analysis (Naylor 1997). Any conclusions drawn are, of course, dependent upon the quality of the underlying studies. The quality of meta-analysis can be further weakened by a myriad of factors, including some studies not being included in the analysis; the size of the studies varying greatly (often giving weight to the larger studies); summary data, rather than individual patient data, being analyzed; differences in outcome measurements occurring among the studies; attempts to measure a small effect size and rare or random effects; not balancing the number of patients and control subjects well; and studying different target populations. Analysis of the complete, actual patient data is referred to as *integrated data analysis*, or pooled data, and is preferable to the analysis of summary data in meta-analysis (Curran and Hussong 2009).

Sample bias (selection error) is an important confounding factor. Ideally, a meta-analysis would analyze all the data that were ever present on an issue; this is, of course, unlikely. Prior to any analysis, a systematic review should be undertaken to make sure the research team is aware of all available data; it is strongly encouraged that unpublished studies be included, given the publication bias for positive results among authors, reviewers, and publishers. Standards for attempting to ensure the fullest unbiased review and selection possible have been published (Higgins and Green 2011). Great care must be taken in choosing the studies to compare. The funnel plot (Egger et al. 1997; Figure 2–1) has been used to try to determine the bias introduced by publication and other sampling biases. As with any technique, its limitations have also been characterized, and caution has been urged against its own assumption of accuracy (Lau et al. 2006).

Once an adequate systematic review is complete, meta-analyses are usually performed according to either a fixed effects or random effects model. Fixed effects analyses assume a common treatment effect in each study, whereas random effects analyses do not. Any difference in treatment

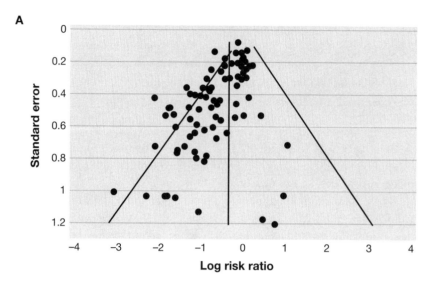

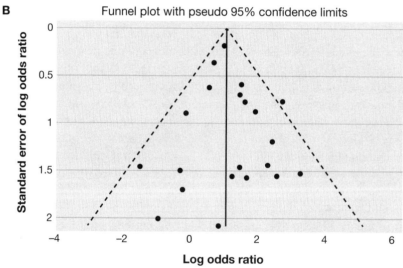

FIGURE 2–1.   Funnel plot.

Asymmetric and symmetric funnel plots. **A,** Asymmetric funnel plot indicating possible publication bias. **B,** Symmetric funnel plot consistent with lower likelihood of publication bias.

Source.   **A,** Reprinted from Ritchie ML, Romanuk TN: "A Meta-Analysis of Probiotic Efficacy for Gastrointestinal Diseases." *PLoS One* 7(4):e34938, 2012. Used with permission. **B,** Reprinted from Liyanage SS, Rahman B, Ridda I, et al: "The Aetiological Role of Human Papillomavirus in Oesophageal Squamous Cell Carcinoma: A Meta-Analysis." *PLoS One* 8(7):e69238, 2013. Used with permission.

effect among the studies in a fixed effects analysis is assumed to be attributable only to chance. No allowance is made, therefore, for the possible distortion of data from larger studies. To help determine, then, if this will be a valid technique, the degree of similarity or homogeneity among the studies should be measured. The Cochran Q test has been employed to determine the degree of heterogeneity among the studies chosen for analysis. This refers to how dissimilar the studies are by measuring the difference in each study's treatment effect compared with the average effect calculated by the meta-analysis (Cochran 1954).

More recently, however, the Q test has been found inadequate, especially when only a few studies are analyzed; the improved I^2 measurement has largely replaced it (Higgins and Thompson 2002; Higgins et al. 2003). I^2 attempts to quantify the *degree* of study variation due to nonrandom heterogeneity and to intuitively aid judgment. Roughly, $I^2 < 50$ indicates low heterogeneity or, rather, homogeneity (better similarity and speaking well for the results); $I^2 > 50$ is consistent with high heterogeneity (or more questionable results from the meta-analysis). Again, it is important not only to determine heterogeneity, but also to estimate the degree (Higgins et al. 2009). At one time it was thought that testing for homogeneity could be used as a simple guide to choosing between use of the fixed effects or random effects analysis, but that has also been called into question, especially when comparing large studies with low rates of the observed event, for which random effects analysis may give a more accurate result (Shuster et al. 2007).

Random effects analysis, assuming that the treatment effect is not consistent throughout the studies being analyzed, attempts to measure its average by weighing all the studies included equally, eliminating the size effect of a large study (Riley et al. 2011). This can help account for unexplained heterogeneity in the data by adding a predictive value rather than focusing solely on the mean effect (Higgins et al. 2009). This predictive value attempts to measure how likely the common treatment effect will be observed in future studies with new groups. One of the promises of this form of meta-analysis is that it may allow the determination of a moderate-sized effect by analysis of at least three small studies that, alone, each has insufficient power to demonstrate the effect. Again, however, many factors may distort the results.

A forest plot (Figure 2–2) is often used to visually demonstrate the nature and results of the meta-analysis, particularly illustrating heterogeneity and pooled result. It displays the studies chosen for analysis, their size power and confidence levels, their relative weight in the analysis, the reported relative risk for each study, and the meta-analysis total, depicted

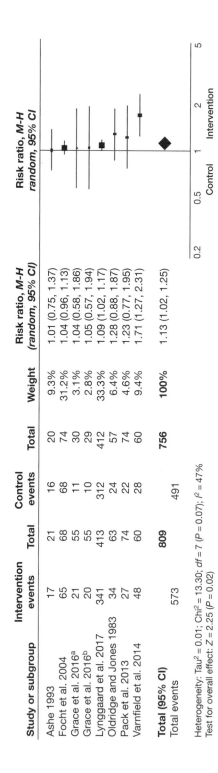

Study or subgroup	Intervention events	Total	Control events	Total	Weight	Risk ratio, M-H (random, 95% CI)	Risk ratio, M-H random, 95% CI
Ashe 1993	17	21	16	20	9.3%	1.01 (0.75, 1.37)	
Focht et al. 2004	65	68	68	74	31.2%	1.04 (0.96, 1.13)	
Grace et al. 2016[a]	21	55	11	30	3.1%	1.04 (0.58, 1.86)	
Grace et al. 2016[b]	20	55	10	29	2.8%	1.05 (0.57, 1.94)	
Lynggaard et al. 2017	341	413	312	412	33.3%	1.09 (1.02, 1.17)	
Oldridge and Jones 1983	34	63	24	57	6.4%	1.28 (0.88, 1.87)	
Pack et al. 2013	27	74	22	74	4.6%	1.23 (0.77, 1.95)	
Varnfield et al. 2014	48	60	28	60	9.4%	1.71 (1.27, 2.31)	
Total (95% CI)		**809**		**756**	**100%**	**1.13 (1.02, 1.25)**	
Total events	573		491				

Heterogeneity: Tau² = 0.01; Chi² = 13.30; df = 7 (P = 0.07); I² = 47%
Test for overall effect: Z = 2.25 (P = 0.02)

0.2   0.5   1   2   5
Control   Intervention

FIGURE 2–2. Forest plot—the effect of cardiac rehabilitation utilization interventions on program completion.

Boxes represent the risk ratio for individual trials. The boxes are proportional to the weight of each study in the analysis. The *lines* represent their 95% confidence interval. The *diamond* represents the pooled risk ratio, and its width represents its 95% confidence interval.
M-H = Mantel-Haenszel odds ratio.
[a]Women-only cardiac rehabilitation.
[b]Home-based cardiac rehabilitation.
Source. Pio CSA, Chaves G, Davies P, et al: "Interventions to Promote Patient Utilization of Cardiac Rehabilitation: Cochrane Systematic Review and Meta-Analysis." *Journal of Clinical Medicine* 8(2):E189, 2019. Copyright © 2019 by the authors. Licensee MDPI, Basel, Switzerland. Used with permission.

both numerically and graphically. If the total relative risk touches the vertical line representing RR = 1 or "no effect," then the meta-analysis shows no difference between experimental and control groups within the given parameters. A relative risk to the left of the vertical line would demonstrate that an intervention designed to avoid an undesirable outcome is helpful. A relative risk to the right of the vertical line indicates that an intervention designed to treat a problem appears successful, as long as the line is not touched. Note that I^2, predictive value, and P test values are often included.

Another significant issue with meta-analysis has been the move beyond analysis of the original questions to efforts to answer new questions not intended or not feasible for analysis in the original studies. A common method for attempting this is called *subgroup analysis.* As an example, subgroup analysis has been used to search for variations in responses to selective serotonin reuptake inhibitors (SSRIs) compared with serotonin-norepinephrine reuptake inhibitors (SNRIs) (Anderson and Tomenson 1994; Thase et al. 2001). It may indicate whether treatment outcomes will vary in subpopulations of the original study group (e.g., gender, age, or those with concomitant illnesses), including whether a treatment may be riskier for one subgroup. As with all analyses, confounding factors may easily distort the results, often in favor of a type I error. Standards have been proposed and implemented to try to preserve the value of this type of review while minimizing erroneous conclusions. The subgroups to be studied should be selected prior to the analysis, based on sound biological reasons, as well as clearly stated in the methods of analysis. Also, only a small number of subgroups should be examined with each analysis (Sun et al. 2014; Tanniou et al. 2016; Wang et al. 2007). The goal is to resist never-ending data mining that eventually creates a spurious conclusion.

The most recent statistical tool that may impact our delivery of patient care is the network meta-analysis (Figures 2–3 and 2–4). Network meta-analysis is an indirect method in which items not compared head to head in the original studies can be compared through one or more common comparators. For example, if almonds are compared with walnuts in one study and walnuts with pecans in another, this technique allows us to compare almonds with pecans without having to perform a third study. Hopefully, more than one comparator (walnuts) can be used, thus a "network." When the network is thick, both direct and indirect evidence can be combined for mixed evidence that should be more statistically robust (Leucht et al. 2016). This technique faces all the limitations of other meta-analyses and can be performed with fixed effects and random effects techniques, although the overall complexity, as you might imagine, is greater. As a

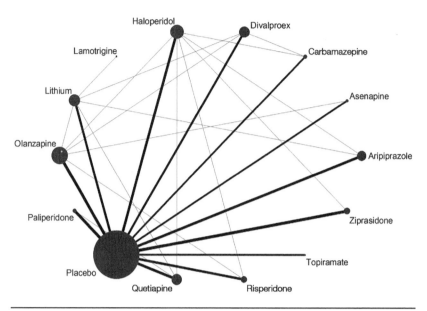

FIGURE 2–3.   Network meta-analysis plot of efficacy.

Network plot of the acute mania network (efficacy outcome). *Nodes* are weighted according to the number of studies, including the respective interventions. *Edges* are weighted according to the mean control group risk for comparisons between placebo and active treatment. Edges connecting two active treatments have been given minimal weight.

Source.   Reprinted from Chaimani A, Higgins JPT, Mavridis D, et al: "Graphical Tools for Network Meta-Analysis in STATA." *PLoS One* 8(10):e76654, 2013. Copyright © 2013, Public Library of Science. Used with permission.

newer technique, guidance for standardized reporting of network meta-analysis has not been fully accomplished (Bafeta et al. 2014).

Ultimately, the results of well-designed and analyzed controlled trials are preferable to meta-analysis results, unless we are seeking a rare or small treatment effect that is logistically difficult to demonstrate in one large study or we need to identify an important variation in a subgroup. Notable reports have been made of large trials refuting previous conclusions of meta-analyses, highlighting the statistical error that resulted in the apparently erroneous conclusion and illustrating how all of our data must be always be considered *in toto* (LeLorier et al. 1997; Sivakumar and Peyton 2016).

As a summary of this discussion of study design and data analysis, consider this review of the investigation of the use of olanzapine to potentiate the effectiveness of fluoxetine in treatment-resistant major depression,

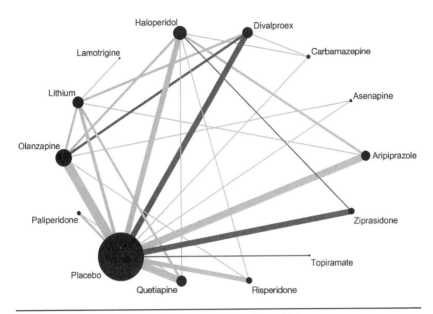

FIGURE 2–4.   Network meta-analysis plot of bias.

Plot of the acute mania network (efficacy outcome) using edges shaded according to adequacy of allocation concealment estimated as the level of bias in the majority of the trials and weighted according to the number of studies in each comparison. *Source.* Reprinted from Chaimani A, Higgins JPT, Mavridis D, et al: "Graphical Tools for Network Meta-Analysis in STATA." *PLoS One* 8(10):e76654, 2013. Copyright © 2013, Public Library of Science. Used with permission.

which occurred mostly in the late 1990s and early 2000s. The first mention in the literature of such a treatment were case reports—two, part of a series in a peer-reviewed journal (Weisler et al. 1997). This was followed by a very small and short study combining open-label and double-blind randomized phases with flexible dosing that appeared to show efficacy for this combination over each medication alone with placebo, using an ITT analysis and LOCF (Shelton et al. 2001). An open-label study by another team assessed long-term safety and efficacy over 76 weeks (Corya et al. 2003). An 8-week randomized, double-blind, placebo-controlled, multi-center study was performed that included a subgroup analysis, but the authors admitted that several methodological questions were raised (Shelton et al. 2005). Replication attempts proceeded with additional randomized, double-blind, controlled studies (Brunner et al. 2014; Corya et al. 2006; Thase et al. 2007).

By this time, researchers had branched out to explore similar effects from other antidepressants and atypical antipsychotics in both open-label and randomized, controlled, double-blind studies (Gharabawi et al. 2006; Hellerstein et al. 2008; Ostroff and Nelson 1999; Papakostas et al. 2004; Pitchot and Ansseau 2001). Eventually, integrated data analysis (Trivedi et al. 2009) and meta-analysis of many of these studies were performed, with random effects (Papakostas et al. 2007) and fixed effects analyses (Nelson and Papakostas 2009). Some made use of funnel plots and I^2 to determine the use of relative risk as the effective measure, rather than odds ratio, when heterogeneity was detected (Wen et al. 2014). Review articles began to describe the state of the art with this procedure (Bobo and Shelton 2009; Shelton et al. 2010). Theories were proposed to explain what appeared to be a treatment effect by the preponderance of clinical data (Koch et al. 2004; Marx et al. 2006; Seager et al. 2004; Zhang et al. 2000). Science does not flow smoothly, or directly, to a clear conclusion, but many branches and curves appear. Appreciating the organic process of how our knowledge is determined helps assess the value of each step in the process.

I hope that this very basic discussion of the statistical analysis of clinical research data has provided you with tools to better evaluate the peer-reviewed articles upon which clinical practice must be based. Using them allows a better idea of what "evidence" is; remember, though, that no single statistical tool or study design is perfect or can give the reader the absolute answer to the validity of a result. We hope to see studies repeated, at least several times, and to see all of the results obtained made available for us to compare. Replication of results is one of best clues to help determine evidence that we can use. Set the bar high for assigning new data the exalted rank of "evidence," just as you would posit a hypothesis before proposing a theorem, before advancing it to a law. Treat all new findings as Trojan horses that lie in wait to destroy your patient care. That is what good statistics, flawed though they may be, attempt to do. Only the best data should survive; seldom do we find easy answers. The best practitioners will perform regular literature reviews. When evaluating the literature, use all of your intellectual tools in your assessment: knowledge of the underlying science; the broader review of the literature, including comparative and replicated studies; the purpose and meaning of statistical measurements; and an understanding of study design.

Summary

Evidence-based medicine requires good evidence. Journals, however, are rife with erroneous conclusions and irreproducible data based on poor study design, improper statistical analysis, and publication bias. Because treatment planning is based on RCTs and meta-analyses, a strong knowledge of study design and analysis is essential. Research follows a progression: from case report to open-label studies to RCTs and then, usually, to meta-analysis. Evaluation of the evidence must heed its context and what can be expected from each step in the process. Clinical gossip, or passing on partial or invalid information without clarifying its limitations, harms patient care. Researchers must make choices about how to gather and analyze data and register studies prior to enrolling and testing participants and analyzing the data; publication of results must be timely. The profession must have access to all studies performed, even those that fail to show support for the working hypothesis or to replicate previous findings.

In an ITT study, every patient who reaches randomization will be analyzed; modified BOCF may be superior to exclusive use of either LOCF or BOCF in the analysis of an ITT study. LOCF is so prone to bias that the FDA currently discourages its use. Retrospective analysis, although popular, is prone to sampling error. Prospective analysis of studies and registries is considered more valid. Absolute risk, relative risk, odds, and odds ratio are often used to measure effects of exposure to risks and treatments. Odds ratios, confidence intervals, and P values, taken together, help clarify the validity of a research finding when they are not contradictory. No absolute value for the P conclusively rejects or fails to reject the null hypothesis. The null hypothesis asserts no true statistical difference between two experimental groups. In a type I error, a difference is detected that is not true; in a type II error, a difference that is true is not detected. NNT and NNH can help estimate the magnitude of a treatment effect in practice. NNT is the number of patients you would need to treat with a new treatment to see one more patient improve than with previous treatments. NNH is the number of exposures to a risk it takes to produce one additional bad outcome, although it is inferior to postmarketing surveillance.

Meta-analysis attempts to determine clinical outcome by grouping studies and analyzing the data. High heterogeneity, or dissimilarity, among the studies will distort the outcome; methods such as funnel plots and I^2 describe this. Integrated data analysis is preferable to the analysis of summary data; forest plots visually describe the data and conclusions that may be drawn from this pooled data. Subgroup analysis may help answer questions that single studies cannot, if the questions are defined prior to analysis and are limited in scope. Network meta-analysis compares items not compared head to head in the original studies through one or more common comparators. Well-designed and -performed RCTs are preferable to meta-analyses, unless a rare or small treatment effect is sought. New data should always be interpreted in the context of previous knowledge, and replication of results is an invaluable step. Regular critical literature review is essential for rational psychopharmacologists.

Key Points

- Many studies published in peer-reviewed journals suffer from inadequate design or analysis.
- Practitioners need an understanding of the statistical methods used in randomized controlled trials and meta-analyses.
- Broad current knowledge of the literature is essential.
- It is the practitioner's responsibility to critically evaluate the validity of conclusions.
- Be cautious of, and do not spread, clinical gossip.

Self-Assessment

1. The following methods of data analysis are prone to bias (choose all that apply):

   A. Last observation carried forward
   B. Baseline observation carried forward
   C. Intention to treat
   D. Meta-analysis

2. Usually, clinicians might favor a new treatment that has (choose two)

   A. A low number needed to treat
   B. A high number needed to treat
   C. A high number needed to harm
   D. A low number needed to harm

3. A P value

   A. <0.05 is always proof of statistical significance
   B. Is never proof of statistical significance
   C. <0.005 is always proof of statistical significance
   D. Need only be reported to two decimal places

4. Which two statements are true for the null hypothesis?

   A. Fails to be disproven when the confidence interval includes a value of *no difference* or CI=1
   B. Can be proven

    C. Asserts that true statistical difference exists between two experimental groups

    D. Asserts that no true statistical difference exists between two experimental groups

5. Which two types of data collection are the most valid?

    A. Retrospective studies

    B. Prospective studies

    C. Retrospective registries

    D. Prospective registries

Discussion Topics

1. A patient is concerned because the media has reported a Scandinavian study that appears to indicate one antidepressant has a greater risk of teratogenicity than another. When you locate and review the original peer-reviewed article, what will you look for in the study design and data analysis? How will you discuss your assessment with your patient?

2. In a discussion among your peers, one colleague reports that a new atypical antipsychotic is being used for the treatment of OCD. What questions should you ask the colleague, and what investigation should you undertake on your own? How would you share the information you find with others?

Additional Reading

Ioannidis JPA: Why most published research findings are false. PLoS Med 2(8):e124, 2005

Jüni P, Altman DG, Egger M: Systematic reviews in health care: assessing the quality of controlled clinical trials. BMJ 323(7303):42–46, 2001

Szumilas M: Explaining odds ratios. J Can Acad Child Adolesc Psychiatry 19(3):227–229, 2010

Ten Have TR, Normand S-LT, Marcus SM, et al: Intent-to-treat vs. non-intent-to-treat analyses under treatment non-adherence in mental health randomized trials. Psychiatr Ann 38(12):772–783, 2008

Tonin FS, Rotta I, Mendes AM, et al: Network meta-analysis: a technique to gather evidence from direct and indirect comparisons. Pharm Pract (Granada) 15(1):943, 2017

Walker E, Hernandez AV, Kattan MW: Meta-analysis: its strengths and limitations. Cleve Clin J Med 75(6):431–439, 2008

References

AllTrials: All Trials Registered, All Results Reported (petition). London, AllTrials, 2019. Available at: http://www.alltrials.net/petition. Accessed September 24, 2019.

Anderson IM, Tomenson BM: The efficacy of selective serotonin re-uptake inhibitors in depression: a meta-analysis of studies against tricyclic antidepressants. J Psychopharmacol 8(4):238–249, 1994 22298630

Ashe ED: The effects of a relapse prevention program on adherence to a Phase II cardiac exercise program. Ph.D. thesis, Florida State University, Tallahassee, FL, 1993

Bafeta A, Trinquart L, Seror R, et al: Reporting of results from network meta-analyses: methodological systematic review. BMJ 348:g1741, 2014 24618053

Bobo WV, Shelton RC: Olanzapine and fluoxetine combination therapy for treatment-resistant depression: review of efficacy, safety, and study design issues. Neuropsychiatr Dis Treat 5:369–383, 2009 19590732

Brunner E, Tohen M, Osuntokun O, et al: Efficacy and safety of olanzapine/fluoxetine combination vs fluoxetine monotherapy following successful combination therapy of treatment-resistant major depressive disorder. Neuropsychopharmacology 39(11):2549–2559, 2014 24801768

Chaimani A, Higgins JPT, Mavridis D, et al: Graphical tools for network meta-analysis in STATA. PLoS One 8(10):e76654, 2013 24098547

Chen R, Desai NR, Ross JS, et al: Publication and reporting of clinical trial results: cross sectional analysis across academic medical centers. BMJ 352:i637, 2016 26888209

Cochran WG: The combination of estimates from different experiments. Biometrics 10:101–129, 1954

Cohen LS, Friedman JM, Jefferson JW, et al: A reevaluation of risk of in utero exposure to lithium. JAMA 271(2):146–150, 1994 8031346

Colquhoun D: An investigation of the false discovery rate and the misinterpretation of P-values. R Soc Open Sci 1(3):140216, 2014 26064558

Corya SA, Andersen SW, Detke HC, et al: Long-term antidepressant efficacy and safety of olanzapine/fluoxetine combination: a 76-week open-label study. J Clin Psychiatry 64(11):1349–1356, 2003 14658950

Corya SA, Williamson D, Sanger TM, et al: A randomized, double-blind comparison of olanzapine/fluoxetine combination, olanzapine, fluoxetine, and venlafaxine in treatment-resistant depression. Depress Anxiety 23(6):364–372, 2006 16710853

Curran PJ, Hussong AM: Integrative data analysis: the simultaneous analysis of multiple data sets. Psychol Methods 14(2):81–100, 2009 19485623

Egger M, Davey Smith G, Schneider M, et al: Bias in meta-analysis detected by a simple, graphical test. BMJ 315(7109):629–634, 1997 9310563

Ercan I, Karadeniz PG, Cangur S, et al: Examining of published articles with respect to statistical errors in medical sciences. UHOD Uluslar Hematol Onkol Derg 25(2):130–138, 2015

Fergusson D, Aaron SD, Guyatt G, et al: Post-randomisation exclusions: the intention to treat principle and excluding patients from analysis. BMJ 325(7365):652–654, 2002 12242181

Flechner L, Tseng TY: Understanding results: P-values, confidence intervals, and number need to treat. Indian J Urol 27(4):532–535, 2011 22279324

Focht BC, Brawley LR, Rejeski WJ, et al: Group-mediated activity counseling and traditional exercise therapy programs: effects on health-related quality of life among older adults in cardiac rehabilitation. Ann Behav Med 28:52–61, 2004 15249259

Franco A, Malhotra N, Simonovits G: Social science. Publication bias in the social sciences: unlocking the file drawer. Science 345(6203):1502–1505, 2014 25170047

Frick K, Milligan R, Pugh L: Calculating and interpreting the odds ratio. American Nurse Today, March 11, 2011. Available at: https://www.americannursetoday.com/calculating-and-interpreting-the-odds-ratio. Accessed September 24, 2019.

Gharabawi GM, Canuso CM, Pandina GJ, et al: A double-blind placebo-controlled study of adjunctive risperidone for treatment-resistant major depressive disorder. Eur Neuropsychopharmacol 16:S562, 2006

Grace SL, Midence L, Oh P, et al: Cardiac rehabilitation program adherence and functional capacity among women: a randomized controlled trial. Mayo Clin Proc 91:140–148, 2016 26682921

Gupta SK: Intention-to-treat concept: a review. Perspect Clin Res 2(3):109–112, 2011 21897887

Habibzadeh F: Common statistical mistakes in manuscripts submitted to biomedical journals. Eur Sci Ed 39(4):92–94, 2013

Haidich AB: Meta-analysis in medical research. Hippokratia 14(suppl 1):29–37, 2010 21487488

Hays M, Andrews M, Wilson R, et al: Reporting quality of randomised controlled trial abstracts among high-impact general medical journals: a review and analysis. BMJ Open 6(7):e011082, 2016 27470506

Hebert RS, Wright SM, Dittus RS, et al: Prominent medical journals often provide insufficient information to assess the validity of studies with negative results. J Negat Results Biomed 1:1, 2002 12437785

Heidari S, Babor TF, De Castro P, et al: Sex and gender equity in research: rationale for the SAGER guidelines and recommended use. Res Integr Peer Rev 1:2, 2016 29451543

Hellerstein DJ, Batchelder S, Hyler S, et al: Aripiprazole as an adjunctive treatment for refractory unipolar depression. Prog Neuropsychopharmacol Biol Psychiatry 32(3):744–750, 2008 18164528

Herxheimer A: The Cochrane Collaboration: making the results of controlled trials properly accessible. Postgrad Med J 69(817):867–868, 1993 8290433

Higgins JPT, Green S (eds): Cochrane Handbook for Systematic Reviews of Interventions, Version 5.1.0. The Cochrane Collaboration, New York, Wiley, 2011. Available at: http://handbook.cochrane.org. Accessed September 24, 2019.

Higgins JP, Thompson SG: Quantifying heterogeneity in a meta-analysis. Stat Med 21(11):1539–1558, 2002 12111919

Higgins JPT, Thompson SG, Deeks JJ, et al: Measuring inconsistency in meta-analyses. BMJ 327(7414):557–560, 2003 12958120

Higgins JPT, Thompson SG, Spiegelhalter DJ: A re-evaluation of random-effects meta-analysis. J R Stat Soc Ser A Stat Soc 172(1):137–159, 2009 19381330

Hollis S, Campbell F: What is meant by intention to treat analysis? Survey of published randomised controlled trials. BMJ 319(7211):670–674, 1999 10480822

Horton NJ, Switzer SS: Statistical methods in the journal. N Engl J Med 353(18):1977–1979, 2005 16267336

International Committee of Medical Journal Editors: Recommendations for the Conduct, Reporting, Editing, and Publication of Scholarly Work in Medical Journals. International Committee of Medical Journal Editors, December 2018. Available at: http://icmje.org/icmje-recommendations.pdf. Accessed September 24, 2019.

Koch S, Perry KW, Bymaster FP: Brain region and dose effects of an olanzapine/fluoxetine combination on extracellular monoamine concentrations in the rat. Neuropharmacology 46(2):232–242, 2004 14680761

Lachin JM: Fallacies of last observation carried forward analyses. Clin Trials 13(2):161–168, 2016 26400875

Lancee M, Lemmens CMC, Kahn RS, et al: Outcome reporting bias in randomized-controlled trials investigating antipsychotic drugs. Transl Psychiatry 7(9):e1232, 2017 28895941

Lancet Psychiatry: Sex and gender in psychiatry. Lancet Psychiatry 3(11):999, 2016 27794374

Lane P: Handling drop-out in longitudinal clinical trials: a comparison of the LOCF and MMRM approaches. Pharm Stat 7(2):93–106, 2008 17351897

Lau J, Ioannidis JPA, Terrin N, et al: The case of the misleading funnel plot. BMJ 333(7568):597–600, 2006 16974018

Laupacis A, Sackett DL, Roberts RS: An assessment of clinically useful measures of the consequences of treatment. N Engl J Med 318(26):1728–1733, 1988 3374545

LeLorier J, Grégoire G, Benhaddad A, et al: Discrepancies between meta-analyses and subsequent large randomized, controlled trials. N Engl J Med 337(8):536–542, 1997 9262498

Leucht S, Chaimani A, Cipriani AS, et al: Network meta-analyses should be the highest level of evidence in treatment guidelines. Eur Arch Psychiatry Clin Neurosci 266(6):477–480, 2016 27435721

Lieberman JA, Stroup TS, McEvoy JP, et al: Effectiveness of antipsychotic drugs in patients with chronic schizophrenia. N Engl J Med 353(12):1209–1223, 2005 16172203

Little RJ, D'Agostino R, Cohen ML, et al: The prevention and treatment of missing data in clinical trials. N Engl J Med 367(14):1355–1360, 2012 23034025

Liu G, Gould AL: Comparison of alternative strategies for analysis of longitudinal trials with dropouts. J Biopharm Stat 12(2):207–226, 2002 12413241

Liu-Seifert H, Zhang S, D'Souza D, et al: A closer look at the baseline-observation-carried-forward (BOCF). Patient Prefer Adherence 4:11–16, 2010 20165594

Liyanage SS, Rahman B, Ridda I, et al: The aetiological role of human papilloma-virus in oesophageal squamous cell carcinoma: a meta-analysis. PLoS One 8(7):e69238, 2013 23894436

Lynggaard V, Nielsen CV, Zwisler AD, et al: The patient education—learning and coping strategies—improves adherence in cardiac rehabilitation (LC-REHAB): a randomised controlled trial. Int J Cardiol 236:65–70, 2017 28259552

Marx CE, Shampine LJ, Khisti RT, et al: Olanzapine and fluoxetine administra-tion and coadministration increase rat hippocampal pregnenolone, allopreg-nanolone and peripheral deoxycorticosterone: implications for therapeutic actions. Pharmacol Biochem Behav 84(4):609–617, 2006 16996120

McAlister FA: The "number needed to treat" turns 20—and continues to be used and misused. CMAJ 179(6):549–553, 2008 18779528

National Institutes of Health: NIH Policy and Guidelines on the Inclusion of Women and Minorities as Subjects in Clinical Research. Bethesda, MD, National Insti-tutes of Health, December 6, 2017. Available at: https://grants.nih.gov/grants/funding/women_min/guidelines.htm. Accessed September 25, 2019.

National Institutes of Health: 2013: European Medicines Agency expands clinical trial database to include summary results. ClinicalTrials.gov: History, Policies, and Laws, 2018. Available at: https://clinicaltrials.gov/ct2/about-site/history#EmaExpands. Accessed September 25, 2019.

National Research Council: The Prevention and Treatment of Missing Data in Clinical Trials. Washington, DC, National Academies Press, 2010

Naylor CD: Meta-analysis and the meta-epidemiology of clinical research. BMJ 315(7109):617–619, 1997 9310553

Nelson JC, Papakostas GI: Atypical antipsychotic augmentation in major depres-sive disorder: a meta-analysis of placebo-controlled randomized trials. Am J Psychiatry 166(9):980–991, 2009 19687129

Nieuwenhuis S, Forstmann BU, Wagenmakers E-J: Erroneous analyses of interac-tions in neuroscience: a problem of significance. Nat Neurosci 14(9):1105–1107, 2011 21878926

Oldridge NB, Jones N: Improving patient compliance in cardiac exercise rehabil-itation: effects of written agreement and self monitoring. J Card Rehabil 3:257–262, 1983

Open Science Collaboration: Estimating the reproducibility of psychological sci-ence. Science 349(6251):aac4716, 2015 26315443

Ostroff RB, Nelson JC: Risperidone augmentation of selective serotonin reuptake inhibitors in major depression. J Clin Psychiatry 60(4):256–259, 1999 10221288

Pack QR, Mansour M, Barboza JS, et al: An early appointment to outpatient car-diac rehabilitation at hospital discharge improves attendance at orientation: a randomized, single-blind, controlled trial. Circulation 127(3):349–355, 2013 23250992

Papakostas GI, Petersen TJ, Nierenberg AA, et al: Ziprasidone augmentation of selective serotonin reuptake inhibitors (SSRIs) for SSRI-resistant major de-pressive disorder. J Clin Psychiatry 65(2):217–221, 2004 15003076

Papakostas GI, Shelton RC, Smith J, et al: Augmentation of antidepressants with atypical antipsychotic medications for treatment-resistant major depressive disorder: a meta-analysis. J Clin Psychiatry 68(6):826–831, 2007 17592905

Patorno E, Huybrechts KF, Bateman BT, et al: Lithium use in pregnancy and the risk of cardiac malformations. N Engl J Med 376(23):2245–2254, 2017 28591541

Patsopoulos NA, Analatos AA, Ioannidis JP: Relative citation impact of various study designs in the health sciences. JAMA 293(19):2362–2366, 2005 15900006

Pio CSA, Chaves G, Davies P, et al: Interventions to promote patient utilization of cardiac rehabilitation: Cochrane systematic review and meta-analysis. J Clin Med 8(2):E189, 2019 30764517

Pitchot W, Ansseau M: Addition of olanzapine for treatment-resistant depression. Am J Psychiatry 158(10):1737–1738, 2001 11579017

Riley RD, Higgins JPT, Deeks JJ: Interpretation of random effects meta-analyses. BMJ 342:d549, 2011 21310794

Ritchie ML, Romanuk TN: A meta-analysis of probiotic efficacy for gastrointestinal diseases. PLoS One 7(4):e34938, 2012 22529959

Safer DJ, Zito JM: Number needed to harm: its limitations in psychotropic drug safety research. J Nerv Ment Dis 201(8):714–718, 2013 23896857

Schou M, Goldfield MD, Weinstein MR, et al: Lithium and pregnancy. I. Report from the Register of Lithium Babies. BMJ 2(5859):135–136, 1973 4266975

Seager MA, Huff KD, Barth VN, et al: Fluoxetine administration potentiates the effect of olanzapine on locus coeruleus neuronal activity. Biol Psychiatry 55(11):1103–1109, 2004 15158430

Shelton RC, Tollefson GD, Tohen M, et al: A novel augmentation strategy for treating resistant major depression. Am J Psychiatry 158(1):131–134, 2001 11136647

Shelton RC, Williamson DJ, Corya SA, et al: Olanzapine/fluoxetine combination for treatment-resistant depression: a controlled study of SSRI and nortriptyline resistance. J Clin Psychiatry 66(10):1289–1297, 2005 16259543

Shelton RC, Osuntokun O, Heinloth AN, et al: Therapeutic options for treatment-resistant depression. CNS Drugs 24(2):131–161, 2010 20088620

Shuster JJ, Jones LS, Salmon DA: Fixed vs random effects meta-analysis in rare event studies: the rosiglitazone link with myocardial infarction and cardiac death. Stat Med 26(24):4375–4385, 2007 17768699

Sivakumar H, Peyton PJ: Poor agreement in significant findings between meta-analyses and subsequent large randomized trials in perioperative medicine. Br J Anaesth 117(4):431–441, 2016 28077529

Sterne JAC, Davey Smith G: Sifting the evidence—what's wrong with significance tests? BMJ 322(7280):226–231, 2001 11159626

Strasak AM, Zaman Q, Marinell G, et al: The use of statistics in medical research: a comparison of the New England Journal of Medicine and Nature Medicine. Am Stat 61(1):47–55, 2007a

Strasak AM, Zaman Q, Pfeiffer KP, et al: Statistical errors in medical research—a review of common pitfalls. Swiss Med Wkly 137(3–4):44–49, 2007b 17299669

Sun X, Ioannidis JPA, Agoritsas T, et al: How to use a subgroup analysis: users' guide to the medical literature. JAMA 311(4):405–411, 2014 24449319

Suvarna V: Phase IV of drug development. Perspect Clin Res 1(2):57–60, 2010 21829783

Tanniou J, van der Tweel I, Teerenstra S, et al: Subgroup analyses in confirmatory clinical trials: time to be specific about their purposes. BMC Med Res Methodol 16:20, 2016 26891992

Thase ME, Entsuah AR, Rudolph RL: Remission rates during treatment with venlafaxine or selective serotonin reuptake inhibitors. Br J Psychiatry 178:234–241, 2001 11230034

Thase ME, Corya SA, Osuntokun O, et al: A randomized, double-blind comparison of olanzapine/fluoxetine combination, olanzapine, and fluoxetine in treatment-resistant major depressive disorder. J Clin Psychiatry 68(2):224–236, 2007 17335320

Trivedi MH, Thase ME, Osuntokun O, et al: An integrated analysis of olanzapine/fluoxetine combination in clinical trials of treatment-resistant depression. J Clin Psychiatry 70(3):387–396, 2009 19284928

Turner EH, Matthews AM, Linardatos E, et al: Selective publication of antidepressant trials and its influence on apparent efficacy. N Engl J Med 358(3):252–260, 2008 18199864

Varnfield M, Karunanithi M, Lee C-K, et al: Smartphone-based home care model improved use of cardiac rehabilitation in postmyocardial infarction patients: results from a randomised controlled trial. Heart 100(22):1770–1779, 2014 24973083

Wang R, Lagakos SW, Ware JH, et al: Statistics in medicine—reporting of subgroup analyses in clinical trials. N Engl J Med 357(21):2189–2194, 2007 18032770

Weinstein MR, Goldfield M: Cardiovascular malformations with lithium use during pregnancy. Am J Psychiatry 132(5):529–531, 1975 1119612

Weisler RH, Ahearn EP, Davidson JR, et al: Adjunctive use of olanzapine in mood disorders: five case reports. Ann Clin Psychiatry 9(4):259–262, 1997 9511951

Wen XJ, Wang LM, Liu ZL, et al: Meta-analysis on the efficacy and tolerability of the augmentation of antidepressants with atypical antipsychotics in patients with major depressive disorder. Braz J Med Biol Res 47(7):605–616, 2014 24919175

White IR, Carpenter J, Horton NJ: Including all individuals is not enough: lessons for intention-to-treat analysis. Clin Trials 9(4):396–407, 2012 22752633

World Health Organization: WHO statement on public disclosure of clinical trial results. International Clinical Trials Registry Platform, April 9, 2015. Available at: http://www.who.int/ictrp/results/reporting/en. Accessed September 23, 2019.

World Health Organization: WHO data set (version 1.3.1). International Clinical Trials Registry Platform, 2019. Available at: http://www.who.int/ictrp/network/trds/en. Accessed September 23, 2019.

World Medical Association: WMA Declaration of Helsinki: Ethical Principles for Medical Research Involving Human Subjects, July 9, 2018. Available at: https://www.wma.net/policies-post/wma-declaration-of-helsinki-ethical-principles-for-medical-research-involving-human-subjects. Accessed September 23, 2019.

Yu T, Hsu YJ, Fain KM, et al: Use of surrogate outcomes in US FDA drug approvals, 2003–2012: a survey. BMJ Open 5(11):e007960, 2015 26614616

Zarin DA, Tse T, Williams RJ, Carr S: Trial reporting in ClinicalTrials.gov—the final rule. N Engl J Med 375(20):1998–2004, 2016 27635471

Zhang W, Perry KW, Wong DT, et al: Synergistic effects of olanzapine and other antipsychotic agents in combination with fluoxetine on norepinephrine and dopamine release in rat prefrontal cortex. Neuropsychopharmacology 23(3):250–262, 2000 10942849

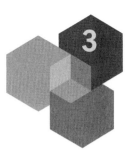

Thorough Assessment Techniques

So we can provide the best clinical care for our patients, each contact with them must focus on eliciting the most accurate and complete information possible. As computer scientists say, "garbage in, garbage out." Practitioners must be both *thorough* and *methodical* in their assessment prior to practicing psychopharmacology. Clinical judgments that are based on incorrect or incomplete information are doomed to fail. For example, simply asking patients if they are feeling well is never sufficient. Most will treat the initial contact and initial sentences with the provider as a social pleasantry, not an information-gathering exchange. Patients often say that they are doing "well" and then later describe torturous symptoms—but only if asked specifically. You may often need to ask them two or three times initially to tell you how they really are feeling and then ask very specific questions about every symptom and feeling about which you need more information. Your patients will quickly understand that this is a serious discussion and that although you do care how they feel, you need very specific information to be able to help them. If necessary, moving quickly into questions about sleep can be an important signal that the real interview has begun; most patients will respond readily.

Many patients, particularly those who have already been in psychotherapy, are unaccustomed to a detailed clinical interview. They may wish to go into depth about situations or feelings that they think will be helpful for you to know. Although this can help some patients in some situations, the role of the psychopharmacologist is not identical to that of the psychotherapist. It might be helpful to remember that you are likely the only person in their life eliciting this deeply important information; if you do not ask it, no one else will. You are helping patients by gathering this important information, not hurting them by not listening to all of their feelings. Therefore, you must remain cordially in control of the interview.

Interviewing patients with no family or others present is also quite helpful. Rarely, other considerations intervene, but if at all possible, the best assessment of a patient can be made without well-meaning others answering for the patient. If a patient cannot understand or provide certain information, the provider certainly needs to know this. If either the patient or others are concerned about the private interview, remind them that they have asked you to do your best evaluation and explain that this is how you think it may best be accomplished. You might agree for the others to join you once the evaluation is complete, if the patient agrees, or when the interview has reached the point where you actually need information from them. Most patients and their supporters should be willing to work with you in this way.

A few words may be helpful here about single sessions, in which the practitioner intends to combine good psychotherapy with good psychopharmacology. The paradigm of the good psychiatrist is that we are all doing this. Some patients even seek this. Although accomplishing both is not impossible in some cases, it is unlikely. Just as surgeons cannot work on two places on your body at the same time, the techniques and tasks of psychotherapy and those of psychopharmacology are not the same. Attempts to do both often result in neither being done well enough to benefit the patient. Asking the neurovegetative questions necessary to guide prescribing often takes the therapist away from psychotherapeutic responses, and vice versa. The best course is to separate the tasks into separate sessions, explaining the differences and rationale to the patient, at least until the practitioner is certain both are being accomplished (which, realistically, is very rare).

Physicians are often taught to perform physical examinations in medical school by always examining the body in exactly the same order, so as not to leave anything out. The same could be said for the clinical psychiatric interview. We do not all have to follow the same rigid order; however, we must all substantially gather the same information. You may find it helpful to clump the information you need into sections and then to naturally choose which sections to complete in which order so as to align them with the actual flow of your conversation with the patient. Each section must be covered and completed in detail, however. At times this may require cordially but clearly redirecting the patient. Time yourself in the session to make sure that you will be able to complete all the questions and elicit all the information you need before the interview is over.

Always remember that you are responsible for knowing what information is important and must be covered. Do not leave this up to patients; it is not their responsibility. For example, simply asking patients to rate themselves on scales from 1 to 10 is never sufficient. Actual rating scales have been highly standardized for clinical research. One can use standardized rating scales in a clinical practice, but remember that the clinician does the rating, not the patient. Similarly, asking patients to fill out written scales prior to the visit is not sufficient, because patients may approach the information very differently from how you approach it, including not sharing your definition of certain terms.

In research studies, a great deal of effort must be spent standardizing interrater reliability to obtain the most accurate data. Patients have not been trained in interrater reliability or in using standard scales. Some clinicians do not even clarify whether "10" is high or low. Well-standardized clinical scales are certainly not simple 1–10 scales; they essentially assign number values to each of the detailed questions you need to ask the patient. Peer-reviewed published reports also have indicated that nonpublished (non-peer-reviewed) scales can skew clinical outcome measurements (Marshall et al. 2000). As the professional, you must help your patients by knowing which information must be considered. The treatment you provide will be determined by the questions you ask and how well you elicit helpful answers.

Chief Complaint

Most initial evaluations will likely begin with the patient describing the reasons for the consultation. This usually involves current symptoms or problems being experienced, and it is reasonable in most circumstances to begin your evaluation with this information. Once the patient has explained and described his or her reasons for seeing you, move into the formal interview.

As part of the initial and ongoing assessment of your patients, you must obtain specific information about biological symptoms that have been reliably linked to psychiatric syndromes. Our diagnostic tool is very much a review of these symptoms in the clinical interview. The traditional term for these symptoms is *neurovegetative*, and understanding them is essential when deciding when medications should be prescribed and, if needed, which types of medications. Symptom review also is crucial for monitoring progress, remission, and recurrence. Patients' symptoms must be asked about, in full, at every contact. Eventually, your patients will expect the questions and be ready to answer completely. They will also develop improved self-monitoring skills that will aid the therapeutic process. A good journalist is trained to always answer the five questions: who, what, when, where, and why. The effective psychopharmacologist needs to have answers to *what* the symptom is, *when* it occurs, any *antecedents*, the *context* in which it occurs, any *change* from before, and *how* long it lasts (WWACCH, if you will).

If clinicians were allowed only one area of inquiry in the assessment of a patient, the most important would be sleep. By understanding a patient's sleep patterns, we obtain the most valuable data in diagnosis, prognosis, and treatment assessment. This is also a good place to begin asking about symptoms, because sleep is fairly objective and alerts the patient that we are going to be concerned about symptoms that are not always subjective (although we know sleep reports actually are). Spend enough time on this area to obtain clear answers, and you will be rewarded with helpful information. It is necessary to know what time a patient usually goes to bed. Patients often gravitate to extremes and outliers, but clarify for them that with all symptoms, you want the *most typical* case. What are the circumstances around bedtime? Have they been subjected to a lot of blue light from electronic screens? Is music playing or the television on? Do they read before bed? Does a bed partner or child/children sleep with them? Do they get up to breast or bottle feed? This gives a picture of how likely they are to have successful sleep without symptoms. Determine any further impediments to successful sleep, such as outside noise, a lack of curtains or shades, snoring partners, interruptions by children, elderly or ill relatives, and inadequate comfort, including mattress quality and room temperature (see Chapter 9).

Examining the present, how long does it *usually* take the patient to fall sleep? Is this a change from the past, and if so, when did the change occur? Taking more than 30 minutes to fall asleep is generally accepted as symptomatic. How long does the patient usually stay asleep? Is any awakening spontaneous or provoked? Either way, how long does it take the patient to return to sleep, if attempted? Once a patient has slept for at least 2 hours, waking up and remaining awake for more than 30 minutes before returning to sleep is symptomatic. Waking up more than 30 minutes too early for the day and not being able to return to sleep at all is also a symptom. The actual amount of sleep is less diagnostic, especially if the patient averages 6–9 hours of sleep per night. However, hypersomnia (oversleeping) is another important symptom. This would refer to persistence (over 1 month) of almost daily amounts of sleep longer than 9 hours, occurring any time of day or night. It need not be contiguous; ask about naps, clarifying whether they seem optional or mandatory, add them to the daily total, and ask how rested the patient feels after any sleep.

Make an important distinction between "tired" and "sleepy." Patients often use the word "tired" but mean many different things by it. At times, a patient may mean discouraged (e.g., "I'm so tired of this"), sleepy ("I wake up tired"), or having low energy ("I'm tired all the time"). Explain that by *tired* you mean having low energy, finding it difficult to move, and that by *sleepy* you mean unable to stay awake. These are different symptoms, and you need information about each to clarify diagnoses. This may need to be reiterated in subsequent sessions.

Understanding sleep, then, is crucial to many diagnoses and to side effect monitoring; as much time as necessary should be spent on it. Then explore appetite. Again, inquire directly about alterations in appetite or in the patient's weight and attempt to quantify changes in pounds, kilograms, or stone or in clothing (or belt) sizes. Was any weight change intended, or is the cause already understood? How long has this persisted? Note that both increases and decreases in weight and appetite are indicative in the differential diagnosis, so both must be explored. This may also be the time to ask about dysfunctional eating behaviors such as bingeing and purging, including quantification, and body dysmorphisms. Discussions about sleep and appetite will cover a great deal of what you need to know about neurovegetative symptoms, but other important areas to cover include memory and concentration, energy (as discussed earlier, sleepy vs. tired), motivation, and pleasure seeking, which can include sexual desire.

Memory evaluation is also included in the mental status examination (MSE) and is discussed later in the section "General Medical History and Review of Symptoms," but remember here that short-term memory, especially, is an important neurovegetative symptom in diagnosis and in assessment of treatment response. Memory is separated into immediate (seconds to minutes), short-term (within 3 days), and long-term recall (more than 3 days). Ask for the patient's global impression of each of these and then ask for specifics: Is the patient misplacing things too often? Forgetting to go places or missing appointments? Have others mentioned lapses in the patient's memory? Remember, true memory problems are difficult for patients to recall, and the patient also may be in denial about this symptom. A detailed oral history of a myriad of memory lapses is inconsistent with the actual symptom, however; more formal memory testing will be performed within the MSE.

Concentration also must be discussed. Clarify the term to ensure you and the patient are both referring to the ability to follow through on tasks or carry ideas to completion. Sometimes it might be helpful to ask if a patient can pay attention long enough to read a magazine article or book or even to watch television. Also, asking whether the person can pay attention while others speak to him or her is helpful.

Having already delineated energy terms (tired vs. sleepy), inquire also about excessive energy. Although this may be evident in the interview, ask whether the person can stay at a desk for 30 minutes or sit through a television show or a movie. Still differentiating *energy* from *motivation*, estimate the patient's interest in seeking pleasure. What did the patient enjoy previously, and has a change occurred? Has the patient recently become overly excited and interested in so many activities or hobbies that he or she cannot attend to them all? Does the patient create opportunities for fun or merely follow others and really not find enjoyment in it? Has the patient's interest in sexual pleasure changed—again, either an increase or a decrease? *Libido* is commonly used to refer to sexual desire. The term for a global lack of enthusiasm for finding enjoyment is *pervasive anhedonia*. *Mania* can correctly refer to excessive or overdetermined desires, but given the easy confusion with symptoms of psychosis or bipolar disorder, is best avoided here for clinical clarity. If a patient uses "mania," ask if it is the patient's own word choice or that of a professional and ask for other words to describe what the patient means.

Notice that these neurovegetative symptoms do not include mood or thoughts. Therefore, they are an important foil to misdiagnosis based on simply following one, two, or three symptoms. They are clearly objective and measurable. Less confusion is likely than when speaking of mood with a patient. Because many mental disorders involve distortions of reality, neurovegetative symptoms can help the clinician separate affective (mood) disorders from thought disorders in the differential diagnosis. They are an important foundation in diagnosis and in the monitoring of symptoms during treatment and should be asked about at each and every patient contact. Without this knowledge, the psychopharmacologist will have insufficient data with which to guide the use of medication.

Once the neurovegetative symptoms have been covered, other current symptoms may be explored or examined further, if not adequately covered in the patient's early statements before the full and formal MSE began. These may include moods, anxieties, hallucinations, delusions, anger, irritability, social withdrawal—anything pertinent to the patient's concern. Again, apply WWACCH as described earlier.

Anxiety is the most common presenting symptom in the community, even if it does not lead to a primary anxiety disorder diagnosis. Therefore, it is likely to come up in the chief complaint (Kessler et al. 2005). Use whatever words the patient finds useful: anxiety, nervousness, fear, stress, and so on. Many patients will state that they have "anxiety but not nervousness," or vice versa, so find the best way for them to talk about these feelings. Some patients may even use the word "dizziness" to indicate anxiety. This is also a time to inquire about the patient's strategies for taming that anxiety (e.g., alcohol, cannabis, avoidance).

Past Psychiatric History

More specific details about past mental health may now be explored. Some of this may have already been covered in the chief complaint, but now is the opportunity to explore it in greater detail. This is not part of a formal MSE; seek only history at this point. We are concerned not only with past diagnoses, again distinguishing between formal diagnoses given by professionals and patients' personal use of a term, but also with the onset of any relevant symptoms. Remember that symptoms from a syndrome that appear in childhood and adolescence may be different from routine symptoms that appear in adults. An excellent example is symptoms for depressive disorders: in children, these may manifest more as withdrawal and behavioral, somatic, and school problems than as subjective descriptions of dysphoric mood (Bhatia and Bhatia 2007; Herzog and Rathbun 1982). Be as specific as possible about the age of onset of any symptom, inquiring even into the patient's earliest memories of a symptom. Ask specifically if symptoms were present prior to the patient entering school or in elementary, middle, or high school or in college. Did any teachers or other adults in the patient's life express concerns, even if the concerns were not considered serious at the time? What, if any, evaluations were performed, and what type of professional performed them?

For example, was ADHD mentioned, suspected, or diagnosed? If so, was this by a parent, teacher, friend, pediatrician, primary care physician, psychologist, or psychiatrist? What tools, if any, were used for evaluation: psychoeducational testing, parent and teacher reports, neurological consultation, or clinical interview? Was treatment initiated, and what was the patient's response to the treatment? If treatment was changed or discontinued, why? How did the patient feel during and following the end of treatment? Patients may tell you that ADHD did not exist in their day, so although they may have had symptoms, no one was aware it was a medical issue. Point out that older terms used before ADHD included *minimal brain dysfunction* and *hyperactivity*; explore how the symptoms affected the patient's life and any limitations they imposed. Would the patient have been treated with medication if his or her parents had not disagreed or attempted alternative nonpharmacological treatments (Mattes 1983)? If the patient has no past psychiatric history, attempt to elicit the earliest onset of all symptoms determined in the chief complaint.

Ask specifically about any history of trauma patients may have experienced, direct and observed, because this carries important implications not only for diagnosis but also for treatment selection and outcome. Be alert to minimization and ask specifically about physical, sexual, and emotional abuse. Learn the ages these occurred and the details (which in some cases may be delayed into future sessions, should disclosure require a more solid therapeutic alliance). Inquire about any treatment the patients received for their trauma, including what form of counseling or psychotherapy, if any, and the results. Ask specifically about current and past posttraumatic symptoms such as flashbacks, nightmares, and easy startle response.

A "flashback" is not a simple recall of a trauma but is actually reliving the experience as though the patient were back in the original time and place, *while awake*. Although common shortly after a trauma outside normal everyday experience, it is uncommon for these to persist long term (Burkle 1996; Galea et al. 2005). Similarly, posttraumatic nightmares of the actual event usually abate within weeks of most traumas, and their persistence has important diagnostic implications. Sometimes, nonspecific nightmares also may occur. Ask directly whether your patient is easily startled, such as by another person greeting the patient or calling his or her name. Although current, these symptoms would likely be linked to past traumas and, if not covered in the chief complaint, should be explored here.

Take a detailed account of every psychiatric treatment your patient has been given, noting level of compliance and the effects, good and bad. Determine how long the treatments lasted, the reasons for stopping any of them, and how the patient felt subsequent to discontinuation. Try to elicit any dosages used. If any medications "quit working," explore what attempts were made to determine the cause. Carefully note how any treatments were combined, along with any resultant changes in response, and whether treatment was stopped abruptly or transitioned. Your knowledge of pharmacokinetics (see Chapter 6) will help you determine which treatments actually overlapped and which did not. Fluoxetine, which has a half-life of about 4 days, has an active metabolite, norfluoxetine, that has a half-life of 7–15 days, thus extending the drug's effective half-life (Altamura et al. 1994). This means that it takes 5–10 weeks of daily dosing to establish a steady-state serum level and a similar amount of time to exit the body once that level is achieved, after even rapid discontinuation. Trials of medication that take place within the first 2 months after abruptly stopping even a 1-month trial of fluoxetine would then actually have occurred in combination with fluoxetine. This might have implications for tolerability and outcome. Also inquire about any ongoing adverse events that may have been linked to treatment, such as tardive dyskinesia.

Ask about other somatic treatments such as electroconvulsive therapy, transcranial magnetic stimulation, and vagus nerve stimulation, obtaining similar details. Inquire about psychotherapies as well, because benefits from them must be calculated when assessing previous pharmacological treatments. If a patient does not know the type of psychotherapy used, which is likely, ask the patient to describe the setting, frequency, type of interaction, and the responses from the therapist, which should help decide this. Inquire about the patient's assessment of the benefit and also length of this treatment.

Family Psychiatric History

Elicit any information about family psychiatric history. Pertinent medical conditions relevant to your evaluation might include neurological and endocrinological disorders (discussed later). Psychiatrically, obtain all the information you can, asking the patient to obtain more from family members, if possible, considering the data in the manner discussed earlier. As always, do not assume that such familial diagnoses were necessarily accurate or that your patient necessarily has the same condition. As with evaluation of the patient, descriptions of family members' actual symptoms, especially longitudinally, are sometimes more helpful than unsubstantiated diagnoses. An awareness of whether any psychiatric problems have occurred in biological relatives is very helpful, however, as are responses to any treatments, including adverse events.

History of substance abuse is also important. Did a patient's mother use recreational substances during pregnancy, or did either a parent or caretaker have any mood or thought disorder during the formative stages of your patient's development? Ask specifically about a history of suicide, other self-harm, and violence in the family. All things being equal, failure of response to selective serotonin reuptake inhibitors in multiple biological relatives might indicate that an alternative mechanism is potentially superior for your patient. The sudden appearance of psychiatric symptoms in a late-middle-aged man with no past psychiatric or family psychiatric history behooves the evaluator to look especially carefully for underlying nonpsychiatric medical causes.

Mental Status Examination

A detailed MSE (Table 3–1) is the psychiatrist's tool of trade. It contains many, although not all, of the symptoms we need to make psychiatric diagnoses and is packaged so as to communicate them effectively with other physicians, especially other psychiatrists, and other mental health professionals. It may be performed during any stage of initial and subsequent assessment but is never sufficient alone for a thorough evaluation. The

TABLE 3–1.   Mental status examination

Appearance	Eye contact, clothing, grooming, motor activity
Speech	Volume, speed, prosody, delay
Orientation	Person, place, time, situation
Memory	Immediate, short, long term
Concentration	Length
Anxiety	Subjective
Mood	Subjective
Affect	Objective appearance of mood/anxiety and congruity
Thought process	Association, speed
Thought content	Hallucinations, illusions, delusions
Self-harm and violence	Suicidal or homicidal ideation, plan, and intent; lesser degrees
Insight	
Judgment	
Reliability	Including cooperation

structured nature of the MSE might make it easiest to complete near the end of the evaluation, once the more open-ended explorations have run their course, but each session will dictate its own timing.

Begin the MSE with an observation of the patient: include appropriateness of dress and degree of grooming. Is the patient dressed in such a way as to support the symptoms being described to you? If so, appearance can help you assess the degree of symptoms. A severely depressed patient with four children and a full-time job who lives an hour away from your office is likely to appear less groomed, given the greater effort it takes. An outlandishly dressed patient who has a conservative job might be another clue. Eye contact is important to record. Are the eyes downcast, darting around the room, or staring through you? We would expect someone to look directly at us most of the time, while looking away occasionally. This is also the time to assess speech: is it too slow or too fast? Does it flow at a reasonable and predictable pace (prosody)? A significant delay in starting responses to questions (speech latency) is common with mood disorders but might also occur if a patient is listening to an auditory hallucination prior to responding. Rapid speech that interrupts the examiner may accompany rapid thinking as well, but at this point, merely describe the speech.

Assess the sensorium for orientation to person (whether the patient knows his or her own name), place (location of the interview), time (including day of week, month, date of month, and year), and situation (patient's awareness of what is taking place in this conversation and the reasons for it). Insist on specific responses in a friendly but persistent manner before moving on. Patients with dementia may be likely to obfuscate as much as possible, assuring you that they know the information, without ever actually giving it to you. As noted, this part of the interview is particularly important to perform without family or others present who may answer for the patient.

If not already explored in the chief complaint, memory should be investigated here. The interview can then be moved beyond the subjective to more standardized memory testing by several well-known techniques: word recall, serial subtractions, and repetition of digits. For word recall, explain the test and then give the patient three or four random words, such as "apple," "bell," and "envelope." Have the patient repeat the words to you right away, then tell the patient you will ask about the words later. It is often helpful to write them down for your own recall and to note the time. Proceed with the interview; after 3 minutes, and again after 5 minutes, ask the patient to repeat the words back to you, offering no help at all until the test is completed. Do not indicate before then anything about the accuracy of responses.

Serial subtraction of numbers is usually attempted first by asking the patient to subtract 7 from 100 (equaling 93), 7 from the answer (86), 7 from that answer (79), and so on, until no answers remain. Write down every response. Stop the patient after 2 minutes. Successful efforts will complete the task within that time with no memory errors. Distinguish between *mathematical* and *memory* errors, because this is a memory test. A patient may answer 100, 93, **85, 77**, 70, 63, **55, 47**, 40, 33, **25, 17**, 10, 3. Note that although the highlighted answers are mathematically incorrect, they are still in order and relative position: the patient is not lost, she simply miscalculated. However, responses such as "100,... Subtract by what?... 93 [slowly]...86 [pause]...84, 77 [pause]...54, 46, 37..., 30..." before running out of time indicates, yes, arithmetical errors, but more importantly, loss of place—the patient cannot recall what the previous answer was, supporting memory symptoms. Do not help patients at all by reminding them of the task or their place until the 2-minute period is over. If subtracting 7 from 100 is overwhelming for the patient, try asking him or her to subtract 3 from 25 and proceed similarly.

Digit repetition is another commonly used screening test for immediate memory. Explain the test to the patient prior to starting and give an example: "I'm going to give you a series of numbers, and after I stop, I'd like to you repeat them in order. For example, if I say '1–2–3,' I'd like you

TABLE 3–2.   Random numbers for digit repetition

3–7–2–1–9–5–8–4–6–7–5–3–7–6–4–2–9–1–5–8–2–7–1–
6–4–3–9–2–4–1–9–7–6–3–5–2–9–1–7–4–9–6–2–4–1–7–
2–5–8–1–4–7–3–8–2–7–9–3–4–8–2–7–3–8–1–7–5–9–8–
5–2–4–1–3–7–4–6–1–5–3–8–6–4–9–1–5–7–2–8–4

to say '1–2–3.' I will add one new number each time." State a series of digits in a flat voice about 1 second apart, then ask the patient to repeat the digits, in order. Remind the patient to wait until you have stopped speaking before beginning, because otherwise you are likely to be interrupted. Begin with three digits, adding one each time until the patient cannot correctly respond, usually at six or seven digits. Using (so-called) random numbers is important because the numbers you make up at the time are likely to have a latent pattern that the patient will also discern, limiting the utility of this test for screening memory. Table 3–2 provides a list of random numbers, but you also can locate or generate these yourself with today's electronics. New numbers are used with each step. It is useful following the first error to repeat the task with the same number of new digits. Stop when the patient can correctly recall seven digits or misses a lower series twice.

Next, repeat the exact exercise but *in reverse*: "Now I'm going to give you a new series of numbers, and this time I want you to repeat them in reverse order, or backward. For example, if I say '1–2–3,' I want you to say '3–2–1.' Again, I'll add a number to the list each time." Explaining the directions in this detail, in advance, will save you a lot of time. A standard reverse digit repetition is four digits, measured the same way as the forward digits. It is best to not give the patient a running score while testing; if the patient asks, just be encouraging and supportive, without giving a grade.

If a patient becomes upset and embarrassed about a poor performance on these tests, reassure the patient that the purpose of your meeting is to identify any problems you might be able to help with, so you both certainly want those problems to show up in the assessment. It is surprising how many patients seek to show no disability at all, even during assessments for disability benefits. It may also be best to perform this part of the interview near the end, because a poor performance may reduce the patient's openness to further questioning.

Testing long-term memory may require a database that you are unlikely to possess. A patient might be asked to name his or her elementary school or a specific teacher, but unless the examiner knows the answer, the possibility of confabulation (unknowingly making up answers) is too great a risk. The same is true for asking about previous meals. Some professionals ask patients to name current government officials to assess orientation, but others might ask patients to name officials (such as U.S. presidents) in reverse order to test long-term memory. Although the patient may have recently read a book with this information, thus skewing the result, such a test is still likely to be somewhat helpful. Public databases therefore may be helpful, whereas relying on private ones may mislead the examiner.

Reviewing anxiety in the MSE assures that this information is covered, and although it is likely to have come up in the chief complaint, allows for further description and understanding. If these symptoms have been explored sufficiently in the chief complaint, fill in here with specific questions regarding phobias and phobic avoidance, specifically mentioning social anxiety, one of the most common psychiatric diagnoses (Kessler et al. 2005). Social anxiety can involve public speaking and social contacts, so inquire about both situations.

Next, the MSE covers mood and affect. This also might be evident from the chief complaint, because mood disorders are quite common, but in many forms of psychosis mood is dissociated from content, and specific questioning might have to occur. In a case of alexithymia (inability to identify subjective mood), some gentle suggestions might be made, although be sure not to lead the patient. New members of Alcoholics Anonymous are often prompted to begin with "happy, mad, sad, glad." Patients who are unaccustomed to examining themselves and describing mood may find a similar approach helpful. For the MSE, succinctly determine the subjective mood of a patient and then describe affect or what the mood looks like to you. Affects are examined for two main features: congruity with the subjective mood state and range. For example, if a patient describes the death of a parent and his or her sadness over this loss but is giggling at the same time, that is not congruent. We would say the patient has an *inappropriate affect*—an inappropriate match to the context and the subjective feeling. Similarly, someone happy about a job promotion or a new relationship who is not smiling and has a flat facial appearance or tears also has an inconsistent or inappropriate affect. The term *inappropriate* here refers to the degree of match of mood and affect, not a judgment of a patient's feeling or behavior.

Range of affect refers to the degree and broadness of the expression. We might expect someone to be calmly pleased by winning $2 in the lottery, but an overly ecstatic and unrealistic euphoria about the $2 win is too broad to be considered within expected range. Extreme anger, crying, shouting, praise, or criticism that does not empathetically feel justified to the examiner may be defined as *expansive*, and if it changes quickly from one extreme to another within a brief amount of time, such as the interview, it may be defined as *labile*.

After assessing mood and affect, assess thought processing and thought content. *Thought processing* refers to how thoughts are linked together, and *thought content* is what the actual thoughts are. Examples of thought processing abnormalities include circumstantiality, rapid (or racing) thoughts, loose associations, and tangentiality. *Circumstantiality*, common in psychosis and dementia, describes patients going into excessively minute detail about past events such that you are repeatedly tempted to answer for them or ask them to get to the point, because it never seems they will arrive. If present, this will most likely be repeated throughout the interview. Once determined, gentle prodding and redirection will likely be necessary to complete the assessment.

Loose associations, tangentiality, and flight of ideas occur along a continuum, the last being the most extreme form. We expect thoughts to be somewhat connected: if someone mentions going to the mailbox yesterday, we might expect that the next statement will refer to that same action. If it does not, and the next statement is completely out of context, that would demonstrate *flight of ideas:* "I was at the mailbox. My car is blue. I have to eat. What is your name? My daughter is sick." An extreme form of this is called "word salad" because the listener can make no logical connections among random words, such as "bank, lettuce, airplane, purse." When thoughts are *tangential,* a logical connection exists among the thoughts, but they do not progress to the original logical conclusion: "I went to my doctor about my mood; they have a new receptionist. She reminds me of an actress, the one in that movie everyone talks about. I love movies, but recently I've been watching so much TV. Don't you just love the new shows?" *Loose associations* are a milder form of this absence of logical flow of ideas: a connection can be made and the patient has more direction, but he or she is not getting quickly to the point.

Racing thoughts is perhaps one of the most misunderstood terms in all of psychiatric terminology, behind *schizophrenia* and *split personality*. It has become such a nonspecific term that patients have co-opted it to mean almost anything. The alternative term, *rapid thinking,* may be more helpful in clarifying what the patient is describing. This is a subjective description that the patient must tell you about, because you cannot determine it unilaterally. Rapid speech may require rapid thinking, but patients with rapid speech often will not be aware of what they are going to say in advance: "My mouth is going faster than my thoughts" is a common description. At the same time, patients presenting with prominent *speech latency*, or delay in initiating speech, may have underlying extremely rapid thoughts, and they are delayed because they are waiting for a place to jump in. The only way to know is to ask; it is helpful to clarify this definitively because it is an important diagnostic distinction to make. Ask the patient if he or she can complete one thought before the next one interrupts. This should help both of you agree on the correct term. Again, this is a subjective symptom; do not substitute your own observation of the patient's speech.

The ability to abstract is another measure of thought processing; this is traditionally tested by having patients interpret proverbs or wise sayings. The usefulness of this testing, however, is limited by several factors. Below-average intelligence and low levels of education will mostly likely lead to literal interpretations of proverbs (Nippold et al. 1997; Sponheim et al. 2003), and cultural familiarity may lead to misapplication or rote memorization of an abstract meaning rather than evidencing the patient's true abstraction ability (Chakrabarty et al. 2014; Cunningham et al. 1987). Therefore, although using proverbs is standard practice, interpretation should only be made in careful context. In our multicultural society, the examiner must be certain of the intended latent meaning and understand what any other abstracted meaning may look like. Other clues about the patient's ability to abstract may appear in the body of the interview, for example, when initially asked what brought the patient to see the provider, he or she may respond "the bus." This is often a clear example of lack of abstraction.

Once thought processing has been understood and described, thought content is assessed. Content abnormalities occur only while the patient is awake and include *perceptual illusions, hallucinations*, and *delusions*, including paranoia. Any symptoms present while the patient is asleep are not counted. Illusions and hallucinations that occur only while a patient is falling asleep (*hypnagogic*) and while or just after awakening (*hypnopompic*) are in most circumstances also not considered symptoms.

An *illusion* in psychiatric context is a distortion of an actual sensory stimulus: the patient may perceive a chair as an animal, but the chair really exists. Sounds, touches, and smells may also be distorted into illusions; be sure to inquire about all four areas (e.g., "Do you ever hear sounds that others hear differently? Can you give me an example?"). *Hallucinations* are perceptual disturbances that occur in the absence of any sensory stimulus; for example, the patient sees a nonexistent animal when nothing is visible in the indicated space, hears voices when no sounds are being made, or notices a smell when none is present. If hallucinations are occurring during the examination, this is easier to assess, but if the patient is describing them at some other time, try to determine the accuracy of the lack of stimulus, either through the nature of the event, the circumstances, or corroboration.

Remember that hallucinations, like illusions, are not just visual and auditory: they are also tactile and olfactory. Sometimes the hallucinations are combined: seeing, hearing, and feeling touched by a dead relative while awake, for example (unless culturally sanctioned, in which case we do not necessarily define this as a thought content abnormality [Pellegrini and Putman 1984]). Each symptom carries important diagnostic implications, so asking about all four areas is crucial. We tend to view auditory hallucinations as being more associated with primary psychiatric diagnoses and olfactory, tactile, and visual hallucinations as being more associated with nonpsychiatric neurological diagnoses, although any hallucinations may occur in either case, especially in acute delirium. Patients will not always volunteer or even think of each symptom, so the clinician must inquire: "Do you ever feel like something is touching you when it is not?"

Delusional thoughts are not sensory perceptions but ideas that do not fit within the generally accepted view of reality. They are also neither religious or political views nor personal opinions. Delusions contradict generally accepted facts. An event did or did not happen. A person is or is not a physician. As with other MSE areas, data that help determine whether the symptom is present are essential, so corroboration may be necessary. *Paranoia*, one type of delusion, is a patient's feeling that someone or something is harmful to them, beyond the usual risks. This may include people or organizations spying on them in some manner and intending harm, either physical or by sabotaging goals. There are degrees of delusion: patients with *ideas of reference* think that others are probably talking about them, whereas patients with *delusions of reference* insist that this is true.

Delusions have often been further subcategorized in the belief that this is helpful diagnostically, such as distinguishing between mania and schizophrenia. Some clinicians make a distinction between delusional thoughts and bizarre ideations: whereas any paranoid thought might qualify for the former ("People are following me"), a particularly unusual one might describe the latter: "Martians are putting fillings in my teeth to communicate with the Queen of England." Currently, this emphasis seems less clinically valid and helpful (Mojtabai and Nicholson 1995), although clarifying whether delusions are present and understanding their details may help protect the safety of the patient and others.

Suicidal ideation must be assessed at each and every session, even if it seems ridiculous. New providers are often reluctant to bring up suicide for fear of putting the idea into patients' heads. Conversely, not only will many patients expect to be asked, those harboring such thoughts are often relieved to be able to discuss the topic, because it is such a weighty issue with family and friends. Practitioners are being not only thorough but also kind and therapeutic by asking. Long-term patients who have come to expect the question at every session will appreciate the ongoing thoroughness and concern. Note that not asking about suicidal thoughts was an automatic reason for failing the American Board of Psychiatry and Neurology Part II Examination for certification in general psychiatry. It is that important.

Again, with practice, the question can be directly applied at any part of the interview, certainly when pertinent to the chief complaint or past psychiatric history, but even as part of the structured MSE when the patient shows little indication of ideation being present. Never assume. "Have you ever had any thoughts of harming yourself in any way?" inquires about self-harm in general but still may not be specific enough. Patients may deny this, then say "No, but I've thought of killing myself." Again, do not put the responsibility for knowing what to cover on your patients. Ask them specifically about thoughts of suicide in the present and past; any attempts of self-harm, with details; and whether lethality was intended. If a patient has attempted suicide in the past, learn the mechanism and other details, whether any permanent medical injuries or problems resulted, and how the patient felt about not succeeding (Henriques et al. 2005). Appreciating current suicidal risk not only is essential in our therapeutic alliance but also gives the psychopharmacologist ideas about the safety of the prescriptions the patient may receive.

Whereas traditional attempts to assess the probability of suicide from suicidal ideation focused on the lethality and immediacy of the method (gunshots or jumping from a bridge indicates high probability, overdose or cutting oneself indicates low probability), the full context must be considered (Brown et al. 2004). A woman who runs her gasoline-powered car in her closed garage 20 minutes before her family is expected home represents a different risk from someone making the same attempt 30 minutes after the family *leaves* home for school and work. As with evaluating research data, clinicians must use their entire resource of knowledge, experience, and judgment to assess lethality. Also, remember during assessment that anxiety, agitation, impulsivity, and aggressiveness are better correlated with suicide than is depressed mood, so all should be thoroughly assessed (Simon et al. 2001). When interviewing young patients, questions of encounters with bullying are also important and should be part of the assessment. The risk of suicide in youth related to bullying is relatively high according to the Centers for Disease Control and Prevention (2014).

Recent studies have also proposed several questions to be particularly helpful in assessing lethality. In youth, positive responses to 1) currently thinking they would be better off dead, 2) wishing to die, and 3) suicidal ideation, along with 4) a past suicide attempt have been highly correlated

with suicide (Horowitz et al. 2012). Simply having thoughts of being better off dead or self-harming indicates an elevated risk for suicide attempts
and death from suicide, but if the patient also reports having these
thoughts more than half of the days or daily, the risk for attempts has been
found to increase 91% for each level of frequency (Simon et al. 2013). If
a patient answers affirmatively that he or she would be better off dead,
this is associated with higher risk. It appears helpful, then, to specifically
ask these questions at every encounter.

Self-harm should be investigated separately from suicide. Ask if patients
have ever harmed themselves in a nonlethal way, or without lethal intent,
and inquire as to what was done, when this occurred, and how recently. Explore how the patients felt after the self-harm act and any methods they employ for reducing this behavior. Has this been a focus in psychotherapy?
Also ask about violent ideation and past violence, remembering that discussing homicidal ideation, intent, and behavior may not include lower levels of violence. "Have you ever wanted to harm anyone in any way?"
Always ask if a specific victim is intended and assess for duty to warn.

Complete the MSE by making a general assessment about the final
triad: insight, judgment, and reliability. These are rather subjective assessments and should be based on as much objective data as possible. *Insight*
refers to the patient's awareness of the situation: that this is an assessment
for a possible medical issue and that he or she may have a problem. Patients with paranoid delusions may be aware that their thoughts are not
necessarily completely true and that they need help. Adequate insight is
usually necessary to allow the formation of a therapeutic alliance with
your patient, so its assessment is critical before moving into treatment
planning. Legal implications for informed consent make insight important
as well. Your interaction with your patient should give you a good idea
about the degree of insight present, although it is essential to monitor this
throughout treatment.

Judgment should also be somewhat clear from a detailed history, but
there are traditional ways to objectify it. Describing a scenario in which
the patient might find a stamped letter ready to mail or a wallet on the
ground and asking how the patient would respond might be helpful: certainly, most have learned the correct answers. This might lead more to a
game of "What am I thinking?" than to a true assessment of judgment,
however. So again, subjective assessment from the historical details is
likely a better path.

Reliability is your measure of how likely the information the patient
has given you is honest and correct. If this is not obvious, and cannot be
corroborated by others, it may just be a guess, but again it has implica-

tions for forming a therapeutic alliance. The degree of a patient's cooperativeness, although not always included in an MSE, is often helpful not only to assess but also to document.

General Medical History and Review of Symptoms

No competent psychiatric evaluation can be completed without a thorough general medical history and review of symptoms (Table 3–3). Psychiatrists must know general medicine *and* psychiatry; we cannot forgo the former because we practice the latter. The same is also true for any practitioner of psychopharmacology. Acute intermittent porphyria and thyrotoxicosis are rare causes of acute psychosis (Ugwu et al. 2016). Almost 10% of dementias may be medically reversible (Clarfield 2003). Antidepressant efficacy may be influenced by an underlying thyroid condition (Berent et al. 2014). Although statins are being evaluated to determine whether they can improve cognition in some patients, they also have a risk of causing reversible impaired memory and concentration in others (Schultz et al. 2018).

Determine when and by whom the patient's most recent physical examination was performed and obtain a copy of the results, if possible. If not recent enough, consider referral for an examination and obtain that assessment, if you do not perform these yourself.

We cannot assume that a referring physician took the time or had the knowledge to inquire about a patient's complete medical situation. We also cannot assume that patients were forthcoming with their long-term primary care physician, perhaps out of fear of embarrassment. It is not at all unusual for a patient referred for an ADHD evaluation to not disclose frequent cannabis use to the primary care physician and yet, months into abstinence, have his or her concentration return to normal.

Therefore, in addition to the chief complaint, past psychiatric history, family psychiatric history, and MSE, the competent psychopharmacologist *must* complete a full medical history and medical review of symptoms. The review may be integrated into the medical history easily by asking about specific symptoms as you inquire about general areas. The medical history and review of symptoms may be abbreviated in subsequent interviews, as indicated, but must be fully completed during the initial assessment. With practice, you should be able to cover this with most patients in far less than 10 minutes.

Begin by measuring the weight and blood pressure of every new patient. Remeasure the patient's weight at each visit, unless you have a clinical reason not to (as with some patients with eating disorders). Even in

TABLE 3–3.   **General medical history and review of symptoms**

Appearance	Blood pressure and weight
Birth and development	Perinatal complications, delays, learning disorders
Past medical problems	Including injures (especially to head), surgeries, cancers, infections
Allergies	Medication and food
Current medications	Prescription and over the counter, including those used as needed
Substance use	Alcohol, nicotine, caffeine, legal and illegal drugs
Neurological	Loss of consciousness, cerebrovascular accident, seizures, headaches, memory, motor, sensory, balance, gait, tremor, vision, hearing, olfaction
Endocrinological	Diabetes mellitus, hypoglycemia, thyroid, parathyroid hormone
Sexual	Desire, arousal, tumescence, ejaculation, orgasm, activity, sexually transmitted diseases
Menstruation and pregnancy	Menarche, gravida/para/abortus, last menstrual period, contraception, plans
Cardiovascular	Including heart block and arrhythmias, deep vein thrombosis
Respiratory	Including asthma, chronic obstructive pulmonary disease, cough
Gastrointestinal	Swallowing, nausea, diarrhea, constipation, hepatic
Orthopedic	Fractures, mineralization
Hematological	Anemia, bleeding

these cases, weight might be measured with the patient looking away from the scale. Never consider prescribing stimulants to a patient without first assessing the patient's blood pressure yourself, because the most common cardiovascular side effects of stimulants in adults are elevated blood pressure and pulse, which are often asymptomatic (Hammerness et al. 2011). Many medical staff are not effectively trained and careful enough that you can trust your patient's safety with the values they record. Also, electronic measurement is not always reliable. Finger and wrist measurements are largely inaccurate, and although upper-arm cuff machines may give valid readings, only a small number of manufacturers' products have actually been certified as doing so (Parati et al. 2008). Unless you are certain of a staff member's skill and the accurate calibration of any electronic sphygmomanometer, use a calibrated analog version. Recheck the blood pressure at each visit of any patient receiving a stimulant, and in cases in which elevated or low blood pressure may be side effects or comorbid conditions, add orthostatic measurements as indicated. A patient with no history of hypertension may demonstrate a blood pressure of 180/100 upon initial screening. Prescribing a stimulant to that patient risks provoking a cerebrovascular accident.

Proceed to a history of the patient's own birth and delivery. Were there complications in the peripartum period? Get as much information as possible; occasionally the patient may need to inquire of family for additional details. The same is true for developmental history. You can even ask if the patient seemed to walk and talk at the "right" ages. Did the patient receive speech therapy, for example, and if so, why? Was it helpful?

Ask specifically about any hints or diagnoses of learning disorders, helping patients to understand that these are not directly connected with intelligence and are far from rare. Again, if anyone suggested ADHD or hyperactivity, who was it, how were the problems manifested, at what ages, what assessments were done, what type of professional performed the assessments or treated the patient, and what appeared to be the outcome?

Of course, ask about all past and current medical problems prior to the review of symptoms, again eliciting as many details as possible, including treatments, lack of treatments, failures, successes, and compliance. This can be particularly important when we later attempt to assess the efficacy of past psychiatric treatments. For example, antidepressants that "quit working" may have done so due to transient but concomitant hypothyroid conditions.

Ask about all allergies (food, environmental, and pharmaceutical), with details. Try to separate actual allergic reactions from side effects and other adverse events. Patients may often report nausea as an allergy. True allergies usually involve a rash, swelling (edema), respiratory difficulties (dyspnea), or joint pains (arthralgias). Reassure the patient that you have little to no intention of prescribing this medication for them, but you must distinguish the actual medical processes involved. Determine if any treatment for the adverse event was necessary and whether the patient has had any reexposure to the drug, with the result. You will then need to elicit a complete list of current medications being taken for all conditions and reasons, including all supplements, again ascertaining current compliance. Be sure to include medications taken only occasionally but still available. Of particular importance to psychiatric evaluation are stimulants such as decongestants (notably pseudoephedrine) and over-the-counter cough syrups (dextromethorphan or pseudoephedrine), as discussed in Chapter 9. Ask whether use of any of these has resulted in adverse symptoms and record these in detail (e.g., psychosis with dextromethorphan). Patients may not come prepared with this important information, even if they are seeking a second psychopharmacological opinion, but final assessment must be delayed until this information is available. Under no circumstance should you accept a patient's guess.

Take a detailed account of the use of all alcohol, being careful to obtain actual amounts and not just the proverbial "glass of wine with dinner," and determine when the patient started to drink alcohol as well as what the patient drinks and how it affects him or her, including the day after. The same is true for nicotine (all forms, including vaping and clove and e-cigarettes) and all illegal and recreational drugs. Determine not only what substances have been used but also how much, how often, and how the patient felt while taking them and after use. Clarify the ages at which these substances were used, because that may be a clue as to how development might have been affected (Lydon et al. 2014). Ask every question rather than allowing patients to offer you their own summary and conclusions about whether it was helpful, harmful, or a problem. Obtain details about any past and current treatments for substance abuse problems. Never equate legal use with problem-free use, and remember to inquire about cannabis in food. Occasionally, a family member may have purchased an edible cannabis item and shared it without fully informing the patient; patients should also be alerted to this possibility by your question.

Also inquire about use of caffeine, and remember that our society consumes it in many forms, such as coffee, tea, soft drinks, and all chocolate, including many forms of commercially produced white chocolate. Decaffeinated products still contain caffeine: the average decaf coffee contains about 10% of the original amount of caffeine, and a darker roast decaf, such as French or espresso, contains less, although individual servings might vary greatly (McCusker et al. 2006). This will have implications not only for diagnosis but also for successful treatment outcomes, as covered in Chapter 9. Again, be sure to elicit specific amounts of each source consumed and the frequency.

One of the most important medical areas to inquire about is any injury to the head or brain. For many reasons, this can also be a most difficult area to discuss. Patients may often equate head injury with "brain damage," which they stigmatize. We know that injuries to the brain are often associated with neurological and psychiatric symptoms that may alter mental status as well as complicate the safety of treatments we may offer. It is essential to investigate these possibilities until the information is complete and clear. Again, this may require patients to inquire of family or to help obtain medical records of past assessments and treatments. Adults who experienced physical trauma as a child may have been "protected" by family who withheld important details from them but are willing to disclose them now to aid in assessment.

When assessing insults to the head, be sure to carefully address semantics. We need to know if the patient has sustained any "bumps" to the head, even if he or she saw them as insignificant. This includes accidents and sports as well as everyday life events such as bumping the head on a shelf or trunk. In a motor vehicle accident, was an airbag deployed? Was the cyclist wearing a helmet during the fall? Inquire as to what sports were played at what ages, to what level of competition, and whether the sport put the head at risk (e.g., boxing, rugby, lacrosse, American and Canadian football, and "headers" in soccer[1]). Details of actual experiences and job duties during military service and employment also may provide clues.

Granted, many events will actually prove to be insignificant and require no additional investigation, but clarifying this is difficult initially. A patient may fully deny any bumps to the head, twice, only to answer when asked about loss of consciousness, "Oh, yeah, I had a concussion and got knocked out, but it wasn't a problem." Fortunately, society is becoming increasingly aware of traumatic brain injury, so we can hope that growing appreciation for this important clinical information will aid you in your assessments and treatments.

Should an insult to the head be elicited, obtain as much information as possible, including whether assessments were done in the emergency department, where a nonenhanced CT scan is a commonly used tool; by emergency medical services personnel or at any other location such as a physician's office; or by a team doctor or trainer on the sidelines or in the locker room. Try to clarify what level of professional did the assessment(s) and whether neurology was consulted. How long after the incident did the assessment(s) take place, including any imaging? A CT in the emergency department may show nothing notable, whereas an MRI with contrast

---

[1]Current data show that a properly performed header may not be what leads to long-term brain injury but rather that other closed head injuries acquired while attempting to perform this feat, as well as the play in general, are to blame (Bunc et al. 2017).

performed 3 weeks later may show scarring once inflammation processes have had time to alter tissue. If possible, obtain copies of any assessments and imaging from the appropriate facility, the patient, or even the patient's family. Attempt to clarify whether the patient noticed any transient or persistent alterations after the insult.

To patients, this line of questioning may appear as excessive interest in an area they deem inessential, yet failing to provide this information may lead to catastrophic consequences for them. As an example, one patient steadfastly denied any closed head injury, only to suffer a seizure after 1 week on a selective serotonin reuptake inhibitor. This led to imaging, the discovery of a scar in the temporal area, and the patient's eventual disclosure of a prior closed head injury from a motor vehicle accident. State-mandated interruption of driving for the patient held consequences for her employment. The provider, having diligently inquired about closed head injury and been misinformed, was not at risk, but the results were devastating for the patient, when they could have been averted with proper disclosure. As in this case, the information may still not be forthcoming, but providers must persist in inquiry.

Similar to reviewing closed head injury, any alteration or interruption of consciousness should be queried and explored. Determine if the patient experienced actual loss of consciousness or came close. Explore antecedents, possible causes, and descriptions. Ask if the event was observed, and obtain a physical description. Determine the length of any loss of consciousness and the sequelae, such as postictal depression or motor weakness. Ask about any loss of bladder or stool control, as might occur during a seizure. Specifically ask if the patient has ever had or been diagnosed as having a seizure, describing the various types if necessary. Learn how many times a seizure might have occurred and all the surrounding details. Inquire as to the type of assessment done (if any) and the type of professional performing it. Was electroencephalography performed, and if so, when? How many? Were they sleep deprived, and were lights flashed in the patient's eyes or electrodes put in the patient's nose? How long did the electroencephalogram last, particularly now that 24- and 72-hour studies are more common? Was imaging performed? If so, what type, and was contrast used? Find out what the patient was told about the results and obtain them if possible. Inadequate evaluations and conclusions about loss of consciousness and even diagnosed seizures are rife within medicine, so the psychiatrist might be the most interested provider; we are often left to treat patients when everyone else has passed them on.

Headaches are frequent human complaints and show up as one of the most common adverse events in clinical trials. Discussing your patient's experience with headaches at the first visit, prior to treatment, is important. Have the patient describe the actual symptoms, not diagnoses. Even medical professionals use the term *tension headaches* to mean many different things, and laypeople have the same problem with the term *migraine*. Should a patient use a diagnostic term for headache, ask if this is the patient's word or if a physician used the term as a diagnosis. In addition to eliciting descriptions of the events and understanding the frequency, severity, antecedents, and successful and unsuccessful treatments for the headaches, be sure to ask about auras so that these can be distinguished from other hallucinations. You will likely have to decide for yourself if what the patient is describing is consistent with migraine.

Continue the neurological history by asking about any other diagnoses, including memory, motor, or sensory problems, themselves also possible clues to unmentioned cerebrovascular accident. Memory will, of course, be assessed in the MSE and in the chief complaint (discussed earlier), but a discussion of any history of memory problems should also take place in the medical history. Any actual memory problems may require supplemental information from other sources, but you must determine what memory and awareness the patient retains on this topic, along with any medical explanations or investigations of which he or she is aware. Again, true cases of dementia may minimize difficulties in these areas, but this is part of the process in distinguishing dementia from pseudodementia. The names and definitions of memory types vary widely throughout the literature, and no specific agreement on nomenclature remains (Cowan 2008). As discussed, it can be clinically useful for the sake of office evaluation to use three categories—immediate (usually only 20–30 seconds, certainly less than 1 hour), short-term (1–3 days), and long-term recall—and to explore both short-term and long-term memory problems using these criteria (e.g., "Do you have trouble remembering things for more than 3 days?"). It is useful to ask about specific memory functions such as misplacing items too often, forgetting to go places, missing appointments, and delays in recall, such as for names. Immediate recall should be evident during the interview and with the formal testing in the MSE. Exploring memory function is important in both diagnosis and adverse event monitoring, although it may not be a chief complaint to your patient.

Some practitioners, especially those in primary care, favor the Mini-Mental State Examination (MMSE; Folstein et al. 1975) because it is easy for the average provider to use. It covers some information from the formal MSE and tests for language, praxis, and copying figures. Various scores on the MMSE have been proposed as consistent with dementia, although false findings occur with almost all scores. The MMSE is one useful tool, but it cannot replace a comprehensive clinical evaluation (Creavin et al. 2016). Similarly, the clock drawing test, during which patients are asked to draw a clock face with a specific time, has been used since 1915 for cognitive screening (Hazan et al. 2018). As with the MMSE, various rating scales have been developed, but analysis has shown that using both quantitative/semiquantitative and qualitative interpretation gives the best diagnostic value (Spenciere et al. 2017).

Completing the neurological history with assessment of balance and gait is very important diagnostically, as well as for monitoring side effects. The same is true for tremor. Some of our medications affect cerebellar function, and baseline assessment is essential to be aware of side effects when they occur. Inquire about falls, stumbling, and dropping things too often. Take a careful history of any possible tardive, withdrawal, or other dyskinesias and record the responses or changes to treatment they triggered. Tremor is one of the most disconcerting physical problems psychiatric patients may experience. Tremors not only affect function, such as handwriting and eating, but are also quite visible to everyone. Many observers do not seem able to help themselves from commenting, which upsets many patients. Because patients will likely want every effort made to minimize tremors being induced or worsened by treatment, this is best managed by having a clear and agreed-upon baseline prior to treatment. Otherwise, patients may discontinue an effective, safe, and actually well-tolerated treatment in the misbelief that it has worsened a tremor.

After the nervous system, the next most important area to explore is the endocrine system. Myriad endocrinological disorders lead to psychiatric symptoms or interfere with our treatments, so no stone should be left unturned. Ask about sweating, nocturia, weight changes, and hair changes and ask specifically about diabetes or blood sugar problems, including hypoglycemia. Hypoglycemia has been reported to be far rarer than patients self-diagnose, so always ask if this diagnosis was made by a medical provider using a glucose tolerance test (Lev-Ran and Anderson 1981). Another helpful clue is whether the patient was prescribed or actually complies with a hypoglycemic diet.

Inquire about sexual health, including desire, arousal, and orgasm, noting any temporal changes. Explore menstruation with female patients, including any changes and any psychiatric symptoms that may change during a cycle. Ask about menarche, because this can provide important diagnostic information for psychiatry, as well as menopause and "perimenopause" and any treatment (including previous); obtain a full picture of any medications used and responses, physical and mental. Take a full pregnancy history and specifically ask about any mental health changes and treatments in the peripartum and postpartum periods up to 2 years after delivery. Ask about birth control methods and obtain the type and dosages of any contraceptive used, because progesterone in particular may affect mood stability (Skovlund et al. 2016). Additionally, some of our treatments may interact with oral contraceptives (Dutton and Foldvary-Schaefer 2008). Specifically, although many anticonvulsants may lower levels of estrogen, making oral contraceptives with estrogen ineffective, lamotrigine levels are lowered by the presence of some oral contraceptives (Sabers et al. 2003). Starting, stopping, or changing oral contraceptives has implications for pharmacotherapy, even beyond fetal safety, and must be monitored each visit. Always note and document the current method of birth control, even if it is not an oral contraceptive, and the patient's last (most recent) menstrual period.

With males, ask about changes in muscle mass and strength, weight, tumescence, and ejaculation, because this can be helpful diagnostically and help monitor pharmacological outcomes. A patient who indicates he has morning erections is less likely to be experiencing low testosterone or erectile dysfunction from pharmacotherapy. When reviewing any measurement of testosterone, measure the free, not just total, testosterone and ensure that the measurement is drawn between 8:00 and 10:00 in the morning due to standardization in the face of the diurnal variation (Winters 2016). Salivary measurements, although used in research (and sold at too many pharmacies), are not recommended for clinical practice (Wood 2009). The determination of testosterone may not have a direct impact on psychiatric diagnosis, because high levels are actually rare, but it can help determine side effects such as erectile dysfunction.

One of the most important endocrine problems to determine in psychiatry involves the thyroid; fortunately, we now have many tests to aid us in assessing this. Essentially, we are most interested in low thyroid function (hypothyroidism), high thyroid function (hyperthyroidism), and thyroiditis (often called Hashimoto's disease). Some patients may confuse the terminology, so be sure to clarify that by "hyperthyroidism" they actually mean high thyroid function, and so on. Again, do not accept the patient's guess; obtain the data. Find out when dysfunctional thyroid states were present, because this could have a definite impact not only on symptoms but also on treatment outcomes. Thyroid hormones have been found to alter serotonergic and noradrenergic function, affecting affective disorder symptoms and the role of antidepressants (Mason et al. 1987; Whybrow and Prange 1981). Any dysfunctional thyroid state may possibly affect the results of an antidepressant trial or attempts at remission, and this should always be considered (Dayan and Panicker 2013; Esposito et al. 1997).

Many patients have either been screened with a simple T_4 test or T_3 resin uptake test rather than the helpful thyroid-stimulating hormone (TSH) measurement, and most have never been tested for thyroid antibodies, particularly antithyroglobulin and antithyroid peroxidase. As a result, undiagnosed patients experience severe thyroiditis, again with implications for psychiatric diagnosis and treatment. In addition to asking about lab work, ask about findings of nodules or cysts on physical examinations or from ultrasounds of the thyroid. A patient with thyroiditis may be euthyroid, hypothyroid, or hyperthyroid at any given time, so frequent monitoring of status is essential for the psychiatrist, not just the endocrinologist.

Healthy TSH range has changed significantly in the past four decades, but, unfortunately, many practitioners in every specialty remain unaware. We tend to think, as we were taught, of noneuthyroid states as extreme caricatures: anxious, lean, agitated patients with exophthalmos have hyperthyroidism, whereas obese, sluggish, froggy-throated patients have hypothyroidism. These may have been common presentations 50 years ago, before TSH became a useful tool for diagnosing mild and "subclinical" cases prior to patients reaching these extremes, but now they are actually rare. Although we certainly would not want to make a diagnosis based entirely on laboratory findings, ignoring physical and clinical assessment, we must still not ignore any abnormal laboratory findings, given the implications for our psychiatric patients.

Prior to readily available and helpful lab tests, primary care physicians were known to commonly and empirically prescribe T_4 to their patients for sluggishness—what we today might diagnose as a depressive disorder and what might have been, in many cases, hypothyroidism. Some patients improved. In the 1980s, measurement of TSH improved, and standardization of its interpretation proceeded. By the middle of that decade, a value of >10 mU/L was proposed as the new cutoff for hypothyroidism, a figure lower than that previously considered. Remember that by measuring TSH, we are measuring the signal from the pituitary gland to the thyroid, telling it to make more T_4: it is a reverse signal. High TSH means low thyroid function and low TSH indicates high thyroid function. So, a TSH of 11 mU/L was consistent with hypothyroidism, whereas a value of 9 mU/L was not. The science improved further, and by the early 1990s, a value of about 4.6 mU/L was the standard cutoff in most labs, followed by a growing recognition that individuals possess genetically determined average set points that are not always in concert with the "standard norms" (Andersen et al. 2002). Since then, the literature has supported an upper value of 2.5 mU/L as the most helpful cutoff in screening patients for hypothyroidism and for monitoring treatment (Biondi 2013).

This information is essential to understand and to use in psychiatric practice. A patient should not be considered euthyroid for the purposes of psychiatric treatment with sustained TSH values >2.5 mU/L (Talaei et al. 2017). TSH is a homeostatic (autoregulatory) mechanism, so it may show normal and transient physiological variations, but average values should remain 0.3–2.5 mU/L with most labs. A value <0.3 mU/L is consistent with hyperthyroidism. Again, without measuring thyroid antibodies at least every few years, we cannot assume a patient's TSH will remain in the euthyroid range, and it may vary substantially with thyroiditis, with implications for our diagnoses and treatments. Testing for at least a third-generation TSH, antithyroid peroxidase antibodies, and antithyroglobulin antibodies is essential (Åsvold et al. 2012; Walsh et al. 2010).

Should a patient have a TSH value too high or too low after two or three repeated measurements, or any notable antibodies, he or she should be referred to endocrinology for further evaluation and treatment; psychiatric treatment cannot be definitive until euthyroid status is achieved. Given the not insignificant risks of thyroid hormone replacement therapy (e.g., for cardiac function and osteoporosis), endocrine consultation and cooperative treatment with a knowledgeable specialist who is accustomed to evaluating psychiatric patients for endocrine abnormalities is recommended. It may yet fall to the psychiatrist to monitor the patient's TSH, however, because many clinicians remain laissez-faire about its importance. Trials of an antidepressant when the patient is not euthyroid (according to contemporary definitions) will be uninterpretable. Similarly, when a patient doing well on an antidepressant loses the benefit, measuring the TSH and thyroid antibodies is one of the first and most important steps in determining the cause of the relapse, even if it has been thoroughly evaluated in the past.

In addition to the thyroid, the parathyroid should also be investigated. Asking about kidney stones can be a helpful clue, because parathyroid hormone (PTH) imbalances often lead to these. Abnormal primary parathyroid function may carry associated symptoms of depression and anxiety and increased risk for suicide that often ameliorate with surgical intervention (Weber et al. 2013). Laboratory testing should include standard renal function tests, a PTH assay, and serum calcium, phosphorus, and vitamin D levels so that parathyroid gland problems may be identified. Such problems are classified as *primary* (high serum calcium and PTH, often with low serum phosphorus) or *secondary* (high PTH, low calcium; commonly caused by vitamin D deficiency or chronic renal failure, which may also lead to high phosphorus levels). Vitamin D deficiency and supplementation is discussed in Chapter 8.

Continuing the full medical assessment, ask about vision and hearing, exploring any impairments or conditions, plus treatments for them, as you would the conditions already discussed (e.g., pituitary tumors may present as narrowing visual fields). Also ask specifically about olfaction (smell)—not only difficulties with it (perhaps another sign of trauma or tumor) but also whether a patient notices smells that do not turn out to be objectively present. Olfactory hallucinations, as noted earlier, should always be asked about in subsequent visits during the MSE; they are usually consistent with neurological disorder, including tumors and seizures. One patient, a young woman in her early 20s, once answered affirmatively to such questioning, although she had come for assessment of mood. She was almost amused to offer that she actually did smell coffee when none had been brewed. This single symptom led to further evaluation and, sadly, an additional diagnosis of multiple sclerosis.

Take a full cardiac and vascular history for judging safety of treatment as well as considering thromboses as sources of cerebrovascular accident. Explore the respiratory system by asking about any breathing problems, primary or secondary, and ask specifically about asthma, emphysema, and environmental allergies. Patients with chronic obstructive pulmonary disease often experience high levels of anxiety (Willgoss and Yohannes 2013). Swallowing problems may indicate an enlarged thyroid, whereas a drop in voice pitch may accompany hypothyroidism. The gastrointestinal system should also be thoroughly reviewed, particularly considering how important the liver is in the metabolism of most medications we might prescribe. Knowledge of any hepatic problems is essential prior to prescribing, because alternative dosages or medications may have to be considered. For example, long-acting versions of valproic acid might not be the best treatment to start with when a patient has hepatitis. Additionally, pretreatment assessment of gastric and bowel function is important for distinguishing ongoing problems from side effects of a new medication. The anticholinergic side effects of many psychotropic drugs will often lead to constipation, and nausea is a common side effect.

Similarly, renal function should be discussed, again asking about kidney stones as well as any renal function impairments that might indicate need to alter dosages or treatments. Prescribing lithium to a patient with renal impairment would certainly be risky, and given that gabapentin is entirely excreted though the kidney, dosages might have to be significantly adjusted in these cases, if used at all. We expect to check renal function prior to prescribing lithium, but many providers might not do so before giving gabapentin. This information is necessary in advance of treatment.

Inquiring about orthopedic problems or injuries may not only give clues as to endocrine status but also serve as an additional check on injuries received. Brain injury may occur when another part of the body has actually taken the hit.

Complete the history by clarifying any cancers, infections, anemia, and other problems not already mentioned. Obtain all of this information up front, not after something goes wrong. Remember every clinical clue you can from your training that might bear any significance upon psychiatric diagnosis or treatment and apply it to each and every assessment. The patient examples described here are real ones that occurred in actual office treatment. One hundred "no" responses never preclude that answer 101 might be an important "yes."

Laboratory and Imaging Assessments

Certain laboratory tests have already been suggested: TSH, antithyroid peroxidase antibody, antithyroglobulin antibody, PTH, serum calcium, serum phosphorus, vitamin D, and, under some conditions, total and free testosterone. Certainly, serum levels of any psychotropic medications the patient is currently receiving that have valid links with clinical outcome (e.g., valproic acid does, fluoxetine does not) should be obtained if not recently done (Table 3–4). An electrolyte panel with serum creatinine and liver enzymes may prove useful, again depending on the pharmacological interventions being employed or considered. More is discussed in Chapter 12.

During the initial assessment, order those tests necessary to bring current monitoring up to date and to screen for general medical problems that will complicate safety or efficacy. If any closed head injury or potential for seizure is suggested, obtain a sleep-deprived electroencephalogram, read by an experienced neurologist who knows you want a full report of any and all abnormalities, not just a yes or no on whether the patient had a seizure during the scan. Longer studies do not seem to produce any more useful information than well-performed and interpreted routine electroencephalograms. Ask for the full written assessment, if you are not trained to review it yourself. Remember, a normal or unremarkable electroencephalogram never rules anything out, and one abnormal study means an abnormality is probable, even if several other studies are "normal." We do not wish to be deceived by sampling error, because we are looking for risk of electrical instability, which is not likely to be demonstrated constantly. If the need for further imaging is suggested, obtain it. Remember that it often takes 2–3 weeks after a closed head injury for inflammatory changes

TABLE 3–4. Laboratory studies and ranges

Serum level	Accepted range
Sodium	125–135 mmol/L
Phosphorus	2.5–4.5 mg/dL
Calcium (>age 40 years)	9.0–10.0 mg/dL
Calcium (<age 40 years)	9.0–10.7 mg/dL
Vitamin D (as total 25[OH]D; see Chapter 8)	<20 ng/mL (50 nmol/L) = deficiency; 20–29 ng/mL (52.5–72.5 nmol/L) = insufficiency; >50 ng/mL (125 nmol/L) = toxicity
Thyroid stimulating hormone	0.3–2.5 mU/L
Parathyroid hormone	10–65 pg/mL
Lithium	0.5–1.2 mEq/L; 0.8–1.2 mEq/L often ideal
Valproate (Depakote)	50–125 μg/mL; 85–125 μg/mL often ideal
Carbamazepine	8–12 μg/mL

to be demonstrated in imaging. Under most cases, obtain the CT or MRI of the brain with contrast unless renal function or allergy prohibits. This makes it more likely you will see any neoplasms.

Summary

Psychiatric and psychopharmacological assessment must include a complete psychiatric history (chief complaint, past psychiatric history, family psychiatric history, MSE) *plus* a complete general medical history and review of symptoms, followed by indicated laboratory and diagnostic tests. Again, the key words for patient assessment, at every visit, are *thorough* and *methodical*. Although the instructions described here may appear overwhelming at first, practice will make them easily mastered and routine; success with them will only reinforce how crucial they are to effective psychopharmacological practice. Psychiatry is a branch of medicine; we are practicing actual holistic medicine as we consider every aspect of a patient's health to learn how we can best improve the symptoms brought to us. We can only know how to help patients safely, completely, and as rapidly as possible by performing this thorough assessment. Making it methodical and routine ensures it will always be used.

Key Points

- Psychopharmacologists are likely to ask questions no other pro- vider will. A routinely thorough and methodical assessment is es- sential.

- A thorough medical history and review of symptoms is as import- ant as a psychiatric history.

- Never guess about important answers. Obtain the data.

- As specialists, psychopharmacologists must know the accept- able laboratory values for their patient population.

- Minor head injures may have significant consequences and should be thoroughly explored.

- Always ask about self-harm and suicidal and violent ideation.

Self-Assessment

1. Which of the following symptoms are examples of abnormal sleep? (Choose all that apply)

   A. Hypersomnia
   B. Taking more than 30 minutes to fall asleep
   C. Waking up after 2 hours of sleep and taking more than 30 minutes to return to sleep
   D. Waking and staying up more than 30 minutes earlier than planned

2. Serial subtraction of 7s or 3s during the mental status examination or Mini-Mental State Examination measures

   A. Mathematical ability
   B. Immediate memory
   C. Long-term memory
   D. Intelligence

3. Rapid thinking

   A. May be expressed as rapid speech
   B. May be determined by observation
   C. May be expressed as speech latency
   D. A and C

4. Head injuries (choose all that apply)

A. Are often minimized by patients
B. Cannot be assessed by a description of the event
C. Often require repeated questioning to explore
D. May lead to serious consequences for patients if not diagnosed prior to treatment

5. Contemporary standards find a thyroid-stimulating hormone level consistently in the range of 2.7–3.2 mU/L to be

A. Consistent with hypothyroidism
B. Consistent with euthyroid state
C. Consistent with hyperthyroidism
D. Diagnostic of thyroiditis

Discussion Topics

1. An 82-year-old woman is brought for evaluation of memory by her daughter and granddaughter, both of whom are quite solicitous regarding her. In their concern, they prompt and often answer for her. Your suggestion that they allow you to, at least initially, examine the patient alone is met with anxious resistance. How might you proceed with the family and the patient?

2. A 36-year-old male patient is being evaluated for depressed mood. He is abrupt with your attempts to take a thorough medical history and refuses to answer questions about sexual health or function. How might you work through his resistance and build a therapeutic alliance while maintaining your thoroughness?

Additional Reading

El-Hay A, Ahmed M: Essentials of Psychiatric Assessment. New York, Routledge, 2018
Hage MP, Azar ST: The link between thyroid function and depression. J Thyroid Res 2012:590648, 2012
Poole R, Higgo R: Psychiatric Interviewing and Assessment. Cambridge, UK, Cambridge University Press, 2006
Simon RI, Hales RE: The American Psychiatric Publishing Textbook of Suicide Assessment and Management, 2nd Edition. Washington, DC, American Psychiatric Publishing, 2012
Zollman FS (ed): Manual of Traumatic Brain Injury: Assessment and Management, 2nd Edition. New York, Demos Medical Publishing, 2016

References

Altamura AC, Moro AR, Percudani M: Clinical pharmacokinetics of fluoxetine. Clin Pharmacokinet 26(3):201–214, 1994 8194283

Andersen S, Pedersen KM, Bruun NH, et al: Narrow individual variations in serum T(4) and T(3) in normal subjects: a clue to the understanding of subclinical thyroid disease. J Clin Endocrinol Metab 87(3):1068–1072, 2002 11889165

Åsvold BO, Vatten LJ, Midthjell K, et al: Serum TSH within the reference range as a predictor of future hypothyroidism and hyperthyroidism: 11-year follow-up of the HUNT Study in Norway. J Clin Endocrinol Metab 97(1):93–99, 2012 22049180

Berent D, Zboralski K, Orzechowska A, et al: Thyroid hormones association with depression severity and clinical outcome in patients with major depressive disorder. Mol Biol Rep 41(4):2419–2425, 2014 24443228

Bhatia SK, Bhatia SC: Childhood and adolescent depression. Am Fam Physician 75(1):73–80, 2007 17225707

Biondi B: The normal TSH reference range: what has changed in the last decade? J Clin Endocrinol Metab 98(9):3584–3587, 2013 24014812

Brown GK, Henriques GR, Sosdjan D, et al: Suicide intent and accurate expectations of lethality: predictors of medical lethality of suicide attempts. J Consult Clin Psychol 72(6):1170–1174, 2004 15612863

Bunc G, Ravnik J, Velnar T: May heading in soccer result in traumatic brain injury? A review of literature. Med Arch 71(5):356–359, 2017 29284906

Burkle FM Jr: Acute-phase mental health consequences of disasters: implications for triage and emergency medical services. Ann Emerg Med 28(2):119–128, 1996 8759574

Centers for Disease Control and Prevention: The Relationship Between Bullying and Suicide: What We Know and What It Means for Schools. Atlanta, GA, Centers for Disease Control and Prevention, 2014

Chakrabarty M, Sarkar S, Chatterjee A, et al: Metaphor comprehension deficit in schizophrenia with reference to the hypothesis of abnormal lateralization and right hemisphere dysfunction. Lang Sci 44:1–14, 2014

Clarfield AM: The decreasing prevalence of reversible dementias: an updated meta-analysis. Arch Intern Med 163(18):2219–2229, 2003 14557220

Cowan N: What are the differences between long-term, short-term, and working memory? Prog Brain Res 169:323–338, 2008 18394484

Creavin ST, Wisniewski S, Noel-Storr AH, et al: Mini-Mental State Examination (MMSE) for the detection of dementia in clinically unevaluated people aged 65 and over in community and primary care populations. Cochrane Database Syst Rev (1):CD011145, 2016 26760674

Cunningham DM, Ridley SE, Campbell A: Relationship between proverb familiarity and proverb interpretation: implications for clinical practice. Psychol Rep 60(3 pt 1):895–898, 1987 3615732

Dayan CM, Panicker V: Hypothyroidism and depression. Eur Thyroid J 2(3):168–179, 2013 24847450

Dutton C, Foldvary-Schaefer N: Contraception in women with epilepsy: pharmacokinetic interactions, contraceptive options, and management. Int Rev Neurobiol 83:113–134, 2008 18929078

Esposito S, Prange AJ Jr, Golden RN: The thyroid axis and mood disorders: overview and future prospects. Psychopharmacol Bull 33(2):205–217, 1997 9230632

Folstein MF, Folstein SE, Mchugh PR: "Mini-mental state." A practical method for grading the cognitive state of patients for the clinician. J Psychiatr Res 12(3):189–198, 1975 1202204

Galea S, Nandi A, Vlahov D: The epidemiology of post-traumatic stress disorder after disasters. Epidemiol Rev 27(1):78–91, 2005 15958429

Hammerness PG, Surman CB, Chilton A: Adult attention-deficit/hyperactivity disorder treatment and cardiovascular implications. Curr Psychiatry Rep 13(5):357–363, 2011 21698412

Hazan E, Frankenburg F, Brenkel M, et al: The test of time: a history of clock drawing. Int J Geriatr Psychiatry 33(1):e22–e30, 2018 28556262

Henriques G, Wenzel A, Brown GK, et al: Suicide attempters' reaction to survival as a risk factor for eventual suicide. Am J Psychiatry 162(11):2180–2182, 2005 16263863

Herzog DB, Rathbun JM: Childhood depression. Developmental considerations. Am J Dis Child 136(2):115–120, 1982 7064924

Horowitz LM, Bridge JA, Teach SJ, et al: Ask Suicide-Screening Questions (ASQ): a brief instrument for the pediatric emergency department. Arch Pediatr Adolesc Med 166(12):1170–1176, 2012 23027429

Kessler RC, Berglund P, Demler O, et al: Lifetime prevalence and age-of-onset distributions of DSM-IV disorders in the National Comorbidity Survey Replication. Arch Gen Psychiatry 62(6):593–602, 2005 15939837

Lev-Ran A, Anderson RW: The diagnosis of postprandial hypoglycemia. Diabetes 30(12):996–999, 1981 7308588

Lydon DM, Wilson SJ, Child A, et al: Adolescent brain maturation and smoking: what we know and where we're headed. Neurosci Biobehav Rev 45:323–342, 2014 25025658

Marshall M, Lockwood A, Bradley C, et al: Unpublished rating scales: a major source of bias in randomised controlled trials of treatments for schizophrenia. Br J Psychiatry 176:249–252, 2000 10755072

Mason GA, Bondy SC, Nemeroff CB, et al: The effects of thyroid state on beta-adrenergic and serotonergic receptors in rat brain. Psychoneuroendocrinology 12(4):261–270, 1987 2821568

Mattes JA: The Feingold diet: a current reappraisal. J Learn Disabil 16(6):319–323, 1983 6886552

McCusker RR, Fuehrlein B, Goldberger BA, et al: Caffeine content of decaffeinated coffee. J Anal Toxicol 30(8):611–613, 2006 17132260

Mojtabai R, Nicholson RA: Interrater reliability of ratings of delusions and bizarre delusions. Am J Psychiatry 152(12):1804–1806, 1995 8526250

Nippold MA, Uhden LD, Schwarz IE: Proverb explanation through the lifespan: a developmental study of adolescents and adults. J Speech Lang Hear Res 40(2):245–253, 1997 9130197

Parati G, Stergiou GS, Asmar R, et al: European Society of Hypertension guidelines for blood pressure monitoring at home: a summary report of the Second International Consensus Conference on Home Blood Pressure Monitoring. J Hypertens 26(8):1505–1526, 2008 18622223

Pellegrini AJ, Putman P 3rd: The amytal interview in the diagnosis of late onset psychosis with cultural features presenting as catatonic stupor. J Nerv Ment Dis 172(8):502–504, 1984 6747622

Sabers A, Öhman I, Christensen J, et al: Oral contraceptives reduce lamotrigine plasma levels. Neurology 61(4):570–571, 2003 12939444

Schultz BG, Patten DK, Berlau DJ: The role of statins in both cognitive impairment and protection against dementia: a tale of two mechanisms. Transl Neurodegener 7:5, 2018 29507718

Simon GE, Rutter CM, Peterson D, et al: Does response on the PHQ-9 Depression Questionnaire predict subsequent suicide attempt or suicide death? Psychiatr Serv 64(12):1195–1202, 2013 24036589

Simon OR, Swann AC, Powell KE, et al: Characteristics of impulsive suicide attempts and attempters. Suicide Life Threat Behav 32(1 suppl):49–59, 2001 11924695

Skovlund CW, Mørch LS, Kessing LV, et al: Association of hormonal contraception with depression. JAMA Psychiatry 73(11):1154–1162, 2016 27680324

Spenciere B, Alves H, Charchat-Fichman H: Scoring systems for the clock drawing test: a historical review. Dement Neuropsychol 11(1):6–14, 2017 29213488

Sponheim SR, Surerus-Johnson C, Leskela J, et al: Proverb interpretation in schizophrenia: the significance of symptomatology and cognitive processes. Schizophr Res 65(2–3):117–123, 2003 14630304

Talaei A, Rafee N, Rafei F, et al: TSH cut off point based on depression in hypothyroid patients. BMC Psychiatry 17(1):327, 2017 28882111

Ugwu ET, Maluze J, Onyebueke GC: Graves' thyrotoxicosis presenting as schizophreniform psychosis: a case report and literature review. Int J Endocrinol Metab 15(1):e41977, 2016 28835762

Walsh JP, Bremner AP, Feddema P, et al: Thyrotropin and thyroid antibodies as predictors of hypothyroidism: a 13-year, longitudinal study of a community-based cohort using current immunoassay techniques. J Clin Endocrinol Metab 95(3):1095–1104, 2010 20097710

Weber T, Eberle J, Messelhäuser U, et al: Parathyroidectomy, elevated depression scores, and suicidal ideation in patients with primary hyperparathyroidism: results of a prospective multicenter study. JAMA Surg 148(2):109–115, 2013 23560281

Whybrow PC, Prange AJ Jr: A hypothesis of thyroid-catecholamine-receptor interaction. Its relevance to affective illness. Arch Gen Psychiatry 38(1):106–113, 1981 6257196

Willgoss TG, Yohannes AM: Anxiety disorders in patients with COPD: a systematic review. Respir Care 58(5):858–866, 2013 22906542

Winters SJ: Laboratory assessment of testicular function, in Endotext [internet]. Edited by De Groot LJ, Chrousos G, Dungan K, et al. MDText.com, 2016. Available at: https://www.ncbi.nlm.nih.gov/books/NBK279145. Accessed September 25, 2019.

Wood P: Salivary steroid assays—research or routine? Ann Clin Biochem 46(pt 3):183–196, 2009 19176642

Rational and Methodical Treatment Planning

4

You have studied and discussed the literature, using your best analytical tools, to form the finest bias-free knowledge base you can. Your assessment of your patient is as complete and thorough as possible, based on adequate time and a methodical approach: your algorithm is functioning. You have also created an initial working therapeutic alliance with your patient to get to this point. That alliance will now have to be matured to the next level: looking together at solutions to the patient's problems that you both can accept.

The patient evaluation must be transformed into useful groupings, syndromes, that can be used to predict the outcome of a natural state or the response to treatments. You could consider symptoms and other diagnostic data as *signals* we are seeking to clarify out of *noise* (large amounts of data, relevant and irrelevant). Proper assessment of the signals would include accurate diagnosis. Treatment should target the entire syndrome, not individual symptoms. Because syndromes are composed of symptoms, attempting to treat each symptom separately would lead to confounding effects, interactions, and side effects that are usually quite dysfunctional for a patient.

Lest you doubt how often this occurs, think of treating major depression, which contains about 8–10 symptoms in an average patient, such as insomnia, anergy, appetite change, pervasive anhedonia, depressed mood, irritability, poor concentration, poor short-term memory, anxiety, and suicidal thoughts. Although many antidepressants have been found to reverse almost all of these symptoms as a single treatment within 3–6 weeks, how many patients are also prescribed antianxiety medication, stimulants for concentration or energy, and a soporific at the same time as the antidepressant? At best, these additional medications are unnecessary and expensive. At worst, they work against recovery from the primary syndrome being treated (benzodiazepines and stimulants may both worsen mood) and may produce unnecessary side effects that themselves must be treated with additional medications. We want to avoid taking our patients off caffeine and alcohol to allow treatment success (see Chapter 9) and then giving them our own stimulants and sedatives that can complicate successful treatment.

Use Occam's razor ("the simplest explanation is best") and focus on making the most accurate and fewest number of diagnoses you can make. A new patient might, for example, actually have bipolar disorder plus ADHD; when a primary DSM-5 (American Psychiatric Association 2013) diagnosis contains the symptoms that largely represent a secondary diagnosis, hold off on the second diagnosis until you can see whether treatment for the primary condition eliminates these symptoms. ADHD, in addition to being based on clinical history and description, is also a diagnosis of exclusion: if diagnostic criteria persist when all other possible causes have been removed, and fit the natural history of the diagnosis, then the second diagnosis might be valid. Not every patient who cannot concentrate has ADHD—the incidence of the diagnosis is around 5% (Polanczyk et al. 2007), but the incidence is higher for the symptom—the inability to concentrate—which occurs in a myriad of psychiatric and nonpsychiatric medical conditions.

Avoid the temptation to treat each individual symptom with a separate medication; treat a syndrome with the fewest number of medications that are likely to reverse symptoms according to randomized controlled trials (RCTs) and allow time for the complete response you are seeking. If we know that it will take the average antidepressant 3–6 weeks, and sometimes 8 weeks or longer, to lead to a complete response while treating major depression, altering the treatment plan purely for a lack of efficacy at week 2 is irrational—and we are rational psychopharmacologists.

Helping your patients understand the value of centralizing treatment to the fewest number of agents possible and supporting them while waiting the expected amount of time for a response before considering changing the treatment plan is essential in managing your therapeutic alliance. Explaining the expected time to response of each treatment during the initial discussion of treatment options is also crucial. Otherwise, your patients may feel you are making excuses for disappointing treatment results rather than truly understanding the landscape prior to prescription.

The task is to link patient complaints with tools found in RCTs to be effective in removing them, viewed singularly or with valid meta-analysis (see Chapter 2). Again, we use the data from the outcome of clinical trials, not the theories behind them, to choose clinical treatments (see Chapter 5). If a medication has been found to treat insomnia, it could be a tool, regardless of its mechanism of action. If no data support a medication for the treatment of a particular syndrome, that medication should not be considered, even if others with similar mechanism of action have been found effective: efficacy within classes does vary (Cipriani et al. 2009, 2018). Remember, the absence of data is *the absence of data*, not necessarily a negative or positive result. Class indications are insufficiently reliable; only individual indications to treat syndromes are to be trusted. Eschew clinical gossip and unsupported extrapolations.

Probabilities in Treatment

The practice of clinical psychopharmacology, at best, is actually based on probability: the probability your diagnosis is correct, the probability that the RCT data will apply to your patient, and the probability that any one patient might respond to any one treatment. We all know that 100% probability never occurs in medicine (see Chapter 2). John Maynard Keynes (1921; another name you probably did not expect to see in a psychopharmacology text) usefully described *probability* as measuring "the degree of belief which it is rational to entertain in given conditions...this theory tells us what further rational beliefs, certain or probable, can be derived by valid argument from our direct knowledge" (p. 3).

As explored in Chapter 2, probability is best handled with—in fact *is*—a branch of statistics. Unfortunately, the human brain did not evolve to conceive of statistics. It evolved to keep us alive and to pass down our genes. The human mind abhors the uncertainty inherent in probability and will often unconsciously attempt to avoid it, even irrationally. Any treatment plan must be developed with the understanding that uncertainty remains, although described by the probability you can give the patient. By understanding and accepting probabilities, clinicians and their patients can use RCT-based data to help guide treatment selection.

Because the human brain is not wired for statistics, we attempt to overlay statistical concepts upon it. Even for the practitioner, this is actually difficult to keep in perspective, so you can understand the difficulties your patients are having. Keeping it simple for both of you is usually the best plan. Never promise that a treatment will work, but share your expected probability of success for each treatment option with the patient. For example, when treating major depression, you might say that the chance that the first antidepressant chosen will reverse symptoms in 3–6 weeks is more than 54%, all things being equal, or that the chance the patient will develop nausea as a side effect in the first week is 5%.

Intellectually, most patients will understand that 54% is a little better than average and 5% is a low number. Recall emotional bias, however (discussed in Chapter 1); many of us react to these data more emotionally than cognitively. As humans evolved, we could not survive with a 65% chance that the long thing on the trail was a stick and not a snake: it either had to be or not. Emotionally, while considering numbers between 1% and 99%, most humans will actually evaluate the risk or opportunity as 50/50—50% chance yes and 50% chance no—even when discussing the actual numbers. Be prepared, then, for human emotional reactions to your beautiful statistics—our brains are just doing what they developed to do.

An excellent clinical practice example involves the finding that adding one or more atypical antipsychotics could reverse treatment-resistant depression in patients treated with fluoxetine and some other selective serotonin reuptake inhibitors (SSRIs; see Chapter 2). A 27% chance of improvement has been found, most commonly seen within a few weeks; long trials are not necessary (Thase et al. 2007). Patients treated with antipsychotic medications are, we hope, accustomed to hearing about the risks of tardive dyskinesia as a side effect (see Chapter 11). Many patients with major depression, however, have never heard of this condition and are often horrified when they learn of the small risk an atypical antipsychotic presents for developing permanent tardive dyskinesia—less than 1% annually (Woods et al. 2010). When we consider that the trial, if unsuccessful, will be for only a few weeks, that risk may be even lower. Mathematically, this is a very, very small risk, especially compared with the much higher risks of suicide, morbidity, and loss of economic outcome while continuing to suffer from treatment-resistant depression. Emotionally, when you consider that tardive dyskinesia is still considered permanent, even with the newest treatments (Solmi et al. 2018), the risk is more like 50/50—it either will or will not happen. However, very few patients and families will agree to even a 1-week trial of an antipsychotic as a result, even though they understand the situation intellectually.

When attempting to navigate patients through these unnatural approximations of uncertainty, certain approaches might help. First, state the percentage involved, but then rephrase it in terms of 100: "There is a 2% chance of developing this side effect. In other words, it should happen 2 out of 100 times." This refocuses you, the patient, and any family involved on the actual probability rather than just on the phrase describing what the risk is, thus giving an enhanced perspective. Second, reverse the numbers: "There is a 10% chance of developing this side effect; it should occur in

10 of every 100 people. That also means there is a 90% chance it will not happen—90 people out of 100 should not experience this effect." This will not eliminate the emotional bias, but it will help cognition to balance the bias so the patient has the best appreciation of the opportunity and the risk.

Choosing the best treatment plan, then, involves layering probabilities: the highest probability of desired outcomes along with the lowest probability of undesirable outcomes. Bayesian inference was introduced in Chapter 1: modeling based on initial assumptions (prior probability, or priors) and then corrected based on continued observation (posterior probability). Prior assumptions have a very strong influence over our interpretation of data. We all have a few favorite theories, usually simple ones, analogous to other known information in observable scales. Because the interpretation of data through arbitrary definitions of significance in null-hypothesis testing (*P* tests) has limits, and so much noise and information can be gleaned, priors give direction and a method for sorting probability into rationality (see Chapters 1 and 2 in this book as well as Chapter 10 in Ellenberg 2014). With Bayesian logic, improbable remains improbable, low risk remains low risk, unless a wealth of data indicate otherwise; new data are always examined in the context of previous knowledge. We also observe this in frequentism (see Chapter 1). Although, as also noted in Chapter 1, this can slow scientific revolutions, it also guards against spurious and impulsive dead ends. That is why we seek the preponderance of data in layering and amending probabilities for treatment planning.

Discuss this method with your patients so that they understand how you are thinking through the options. This approach will help them participate in treatment planning, give their well-informed consent, and share ownership of the plan and will lead not only to shared responsibility but also to improved compliance. It also prepares them to accept that additional treatments may need to be attempted if the first or second is not satisfactory. If our initial expectation that a patient will respond to an antipsychotic medication fails, we do not blindly and mechanically repeat essentially the same treatment for the same diagnosis; we reevaluate our model and expectations in view of the failed outcome (see Chapter 12). Again, turning to Keynes (1921, p. 7): "the probability of a theory turns upon the evidence by which it is supported; and it is common to assert that an opinion was probable on the evidence at first to hand, but on further information was untenable."

We should make treatment decisions based on RCT outcomes rather than mechanism of action, but the mechanism of action, if known, might be considered when changing treatment plans. For example, some nonspecialists consider all antidepressants to be interchangeable. A patient might present to you for the treatment of major depression, having been given failed, yet adequate, trials of first fluoxetine, then sertraline, next citalopram, followed by escitalopram (even though these last two are the same active ingredient)—this despite each SSRI having been shown in RCTs to treat major depression better than placebo. Although it is possible that a patient would respond to one SSRI after failing to respond to another, the odds are small with the first change. However, by changing the treatment category according to mechanism of action, we now can employ two alternative strategies that have also been found by RCTs to treat major depression. Assuming the accuracy of the original diagnosis, a change to either a serotonin-norepinephrine reuptake inhibitor (SNRI) or bupropion may yield a higher chance of response. RCTs show that this change may offer somewhere between a small and a significant advantage, yet most agree that for an individual patient it could mean the difference between response and resistance to treatment. All things being equal, then, change the approach using equally valid, but mechanistically different, treatment options if results are not as expected (Connolly and Thase 2011; de Sousa et al. 2015; Papakostas et al. 2008). You may be treating an outlier.

Determine Optimal Treatment Dosage

Choosing the correct dosage for a response is essential. Dosages recommended by the FDA for marketing are based on the pivotal studies submitted for approval. They are, therefore, dependent upon the choices made by the researchers who performed the studies and may or may not match the needs of individual patients. As discussed in Chapter 2, studies using active comparators may also not use realistic enough dosages to result in adequate responses. The FDA provides safety ranges for dosages, although again these may be conservative, based on study designs sponsored by pharmaceutical companies to show efficacy with few side effects and low patient dropout. Scan the literature for separate studies, not necessarily submitted to the FDA, for information on efficacy, dosing, safety, toxicity, and tolerability and seek any postmarketing data available. The *Physicians' Desk Reference,* as you probably know, is a collection of the medication guides (also known as package inserts) provided to patients and practitioners as required by the FDA. Explain to patients that these basic data represent only a starting place and hardly contain the most complete and current data that we need to consider prescription choices.

Sometimes clinical direction is given only by the weight-based dosage of a medication, such as with fluoxetine (Amsterdam et al. 1997); other times it will be guided by an effective and safe serum level, such as with lithium or nortriptyline. Lithium has a linear response curve, whereas nortriptyline appears to have a nonlinear, authentic therapeutic window: serum levels below and above a narrow range are not expected to be effective for most patients (Vandel et al. 1978; Ziegler et al. 1976).

Personalize Treatment and Educate Patients

Many people attempt to pressure clinicians into adopting a standard first, second, and third approach to treatment, such as for antidepressants. This strategy models the use of antibiotics, also based on probabilities, until sensitivities can be determined. However, antibiotics represent vastly simpler decision making than the multifaceted issues involved in mental health treatment. No standard order has been established for trying medications, and each treatment plan must be individualized as much as possible to enhance the chances of success. For example, we may determine we have a 54% chance of success in treating major depression with any of the antidepressants shown in RCTs to be superior to placebo. Based on cost and side effect profile, you and your patient may consider venlafaxine hydrochloride as a reasonable choice for an initial trial, especially because it may have the highest chance of working compared with SSRIs and other SNRIs (Bauer et al. 2009; Einarson et al. 1999; Thase et al. 2001). However, what if your patient reports a twin sibling who received venlafaxine hydrochloride for major depression and did not respond, although she *did* respond to the SSRI sertraline? Layering probabilities, beginning treatment with a trial of sertraline instead would be prudent to consider. There goes a standard first choice. This simple example illustrates how rigid prescribing practices will often be tweaked by exigencies, so go ahead and begin with seeking personalized rather than *one-size-fits-all* treatment plans.

List and discuss all of the treatment opportunities, or at least a fair number, with your patient. When treating psychosis, ambivalence is often a symptom; after discussing many options you might have to narrow it down and make a specific suggestion. The patient should be told, however, whenever many options are available, and ordering the options in descending chance of positive outcome or medical necessity is helpful (e.g., we are unlikely to rank lithium as a first treatment in a patient with kidney disease). Discuss the pros and cons of every option, using the techniques discussed in this chapter. Never shy away from or minimize the risk of side effects, just state them as accurately as you can. Pause and invite as many questions as patients want to ask. If they cannot make a decision in a single visit, explore the reasons and attempt to help them meet the criteria for making one. Do they need more family support, more information, or to see for themselves online if any other options are available? Also support second opinions on diagnosis or treatment plan as essential to the healthy practice of medicine, but only if provided by another professional trained in psychopharmacology (see Chapter 12).

Patients educating themselves as much as possible with valid information is wonderful for the therapeutic alliance and therapeutic outcome. Ask if they would like you to suggest sources and be prepared to do so. Many such sources will be websites, so keep track of those you suggest to ensure the information remains accurate, balanced, and helpful. Inform patients that although you have never known the source to give incorrect information, it could happen tomorrow, and encourage them to discuss what they find there with you. Encourage responsibly curated sources and, if not actually discouraging chat-room or comment-type discussions, put them in perspective. Someone out there is sure to say anything about everything, so stress that random internet comments are not always accurate and should be discussed in session before any treatment decisions or changes are made. Read any written materials you suggest, and prepare yourself to discuss them. This will give your patients greater confidence in your care.

Summary

Treatment planning targets syndromes, not individual symptoms. Adding unnecessary medications to treat isolated symptoms contained within an addressed syndrome may only confound results. Make the smallest number of accurate diagnoses possible that fit the data and fulfill DSM-5 criteria. Discuss the expected time to response for each treatment option and allow this amount of time before considering a change in treatment due to lack of efficacy. Treatment options are based on the outcomes of RCTs and valid meta-analyses—mechanism of action may only be considered when changing from an ineffective treatment.

Statistics are unnatural to the human brain, and we use probabilities to inform the order of treatments to be tried. Use numbers on a 100-point scale to discuss probabilities, and give the obverse as well (3 out of 100 vs. 97 out of 100). Bayesian logic, using prior assumptions corrected with outcome data, is an effective method for modeling diagnosis and treatment planning. Dosages based on weight or serum levels are determined by the totality of responsible data in the literature, not just medication guides. Treatment plans are highly individualized and preclude a standard order of treatment options. Support patient education by remaining familiar with reputable sources to recommend.

Key Points

- Group symptoms into syndromes.
- A treatment should target the entire syndrome, not individual symptoms.
- Use data from the outcome of randomized controlled trials and valid meta-analyses, not the theories behind them, to choose clinical treatments.
- Class indications are not sufficiently reliable; use individual indications.
- Probability is used to estimate the uncertainty of treatment outcomes and to order treatment options.
- Irrational responses to statistical data are common from practitioners and patients.
- Prior knowledge informs the interpretation of new data.
- List all treatment options and the expected time to response of each during the initial discussion of treatment options.
- Individualized treatment plans should replace any standing order of treatments.
- Dosages should be based on the preponderance of data from randomized controlled trials and postmarketing analysis.

Self-Assessment

1. Which two of the following are usually helpful?

   A. Making the fewest number of diagnoses that can still explain the data
   B. Prescribing medications to treat individual symptoms while separately treating the underlying condition
   C. Explaining all possible treatments during treatment planning
   D. Using a standard order of treatment options

2. Probability theory can help in treatment planning by

   A. Providing a rational basis for belief, given available data
   B. Comparing treatment options based on outcomes from randomized controlled trials
   C. Using prior assumptions to help evaluate new data
   D. All of the above

3. Dosages should be based on

   A. The medication guides mandated by the FDA and published in
      the *Physicians' Desk Reference*
   B. Only those used in pivotal studies
   C. The preponderance of data from randomized controlled trials
      and postmarketing analysis
   D. What is standard in your community

4. Which of the following statements is true?

   A. Mechanism of action alone is a rational foundation for initial
      treatment planning.
   B. Mechanism of action might be used effectively when changing
      treatment plans.
   C. After initial failure, choosing a second treatment with the same
      mechanism of action is the best strategy.
   D. A treatment may not be used unless its mechanism of action is
      fully understood.

5. Which of the following should always be discussed during initial
   treatment planning? (Choose all that apply)

   A. All reasonable treatment options
   B. Expected time to efficacy for each proposed treatment
   C. Possible side effects and adverse events
   D. Treatment options in ascending order of medical necessity

Discussion Topics

1. During initial assessment, you learn that a patient meets criteria for
   major depression, but she reports failure to respond to previous
   treatment with fluoxetine, sertraline, venlafaxine, and bupropion
   prescribed by her primary care physician. What further information
   do you need in order to consider treatment recommendations, and
   how will you obtain it? Once available, how will it alter your opinion of your original diagnosis and of treatment options? Describe
   plausible scenarios.

2. During follow-up assessment, you determine that a patient receiving
   an antidepressant for major depression has developed worsening
   insomnia and anxiety. Discuss how you would assess these com-

plaints. How will this inform your reassessment of your diagnosis and current treatment plan?

Additional Reading

Polson N, Scott J: AIQ: How People and Machines Are Smarter Together. New York, St. Martin's Press, 2018 (Accessible discussion of decision making using data and probability, with many examples, including medicine and neuroscience.)
Silver N: The Signal and the Noise: Why So Many Predictions Fail—But Some Don't. New York, Penguin, 2012 (A discussion of predictive modeling with multiple examples. Chapter 8, "Less and Less and Less Wrong," is particularly helpful and includes examples of Bayesian inference in health care.)

Suggested Online Resources for Patients

Depression and Bipolar Support Alliance (DBSA): www.dbsalliance.org (Formerly the National Depressive and Manic-Depressive Association, DBSA has provided balanced information as a national support network for more than three decades. This site provides links to local support groups.)
National Alliance on Mental Illness (NAMI): www.nami.org (Founded by families of patients with chronic mental illness, NAMI offers education and programs for most chronic mental illnesses, including primary thought disorders.)
National Institute of Mental Health (NIMH) Health Topics: www.nimh.nih.gov/health/topics/index.shtml (This page of the NIMH site provides well-curated information on psychiatric disease states and treatments.)

References

American Psychiatric Association: Diagnostic and Statistical Manual of Mental Disorders, 5th Edition. Arlington, VA, American Psychiatric Association, 2013
Amsterdam JD, Fawcett J, Quitkin FM, et al: Fluoxetine and norfluoxetine plasma concentrations in major depression: a multicenter study. Am J Psychiatry 154(7):963–969, 1997 9210747
Bauer M, Tharmanathan P, Volz HP, et al: The effect of venlafaxine compared with other antidepressants and placebo in the treatment of major depression: a meta-analysis. Eur Arch Psychiatry Clin Neurosci 259(3):172–185, 2009 19165525
Cipriani A, Furukawa TA, Salanti G, et al: Comparative efficacy and acceptability of 12 new-generation antidepressants: a multiple-treatments meta-analysis. Lancet 373(9665):746–758, 2009 19185342
Cipriani A, Furukawa TA, Salanti G, et al: Comparative efficacy and acceptability of 21 antidepressant drugs for the acute treatment of adults with major depressive disorder: a systematic review and network meta-analysis. Lancet 391(10128):1357–1366, 2018 29477251
Connolly KR, Thase ME: If at first you don't succeed: a review of the evidence for antidepressant augmentation, combination and switching strategies. Drugs 71(1):43–64, 2011 21175239

de Sousa RT, Zanetti MV, Brunoni AR, et al: Challenging treatment-resistant major depressive disorder: a roadmap for improved therapeutics. Curr Neuropharmacol 13(5):616–635, 2015 26467411

Einarson TR, Arikian SR, Casciano J, et al: Comparison of extended-release venlafaxine, selective serotonin reuptake inhibitors, and tricyclic antidepressants in the treatment of depression: a meta-analysis of randomized controlled trials. Clin Ther 21(2):296–308, 1999 10211533

Ellenberg J: How Not to Be Wrong: The Power of Mathematical Thinking. New York, Penguin, 2014

Keynes JM: Treatise on Probability. London, MacMillan, 1921

Papakostas GI, Fava M, Thase ME: Treatment of SSRI-resistant depression: a meta-analysis comparing within- versus across-class switches. Biol Psychiatry 63(7):699–704, 2008 17919460

Polanczyk G, de Lima MS, Horta BL, et al: The worldwide prevalence of ADHD: a systematic review and metaregression analysis. Am J Psychiatry 164(6):942–948, 2007 17541055

Solmi M, Pigato G, Kane JM, et al: Treatment of tardive dyskinesia with VMAT-2 inhibitors: a systematic review and meta-analysis of randomized controlled trials. Drug Des Devel Ther 12:1215–1238, 2018 29795977

Thase ME, Entsuah AR, Rudolph RL: Remission rates during treatment with venlafaxine or selective serotonin reuptake inhibitors. Br J Psychiatry 178:234–241, 2001 11230034

Thase ME, Corya SA, Osuntokun O, et al: A randomized, double-blind comparison of olanzapine/fluoxetine combination, olanzapine, and fluoxetine in treatment-resistant major depressive disorder. J Clin Psychiatry 68(2):224–236, 2007 17335320

Vandel S, Vandel B, Sandoz M, et al: Clinical response and plasma concentration of amitriptyline and its metabolite nortriptyline. Eur J Clin Pharmacol 14(3):185–190, 1978 365538

Woods SW, Morgenstern H, Saksa JR, et al: Incidence of tardive dyskinesia with atypical versus conventional antipsychotic medications: a prospective cohort study. J Clin Psychiatry 71(4):463–474, 2010 20156410

Ziegler VE, Clayton PJ, Taylor JR, et al: Nortriptyline plasma levels and therapeutic response. Clin Pharmacol Ther 20(4):458–463, 1976 788992

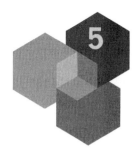

Risks of Jumping
From Molecule
to Mind or Symptom

Abductive Reasoning

In contemporary clinical medicine, it is very easy to get carried away with molecular mechanisms and to use errors in inductive and deductive reasoning to supply a rationale for therapeutic choices. Pharmaceutical companies particularly like to exploit the fact that we have developed some understanding of the receptor sites potentially involved in the efficacy of psychotropic medications (and, in fact, we have come a long way). Clinical observation, however, has always preceded the development of underlying theories to explain results, and through randomized controlled trials (RCTs), abductive reasoning tells us what might be possible to obtain from any pharmacological treatment. When choosing a pharmacological agent for treatment, be guided solely by clinical outcome data (see Chapter 2) and process that data as discussed in Chapters 1 and 4.

The modern scientific method, which was initiated in Muslim countries during the European Dark Ages, developed further during the Enlightenment in the eighteenth century, and refined in the nineteenth and twentieth centuries (see Chapter 1), remains the most effective method to date for developing a rational view of our world. Beginning with an observation, using that observation to propose a hypothesis, experimenting to reject or fail to reject that hypothesis, and returning to observation—with the whole cycle starting again—is the best method we know for inching toward "facts." Pharmacology inherited this tradition, starting with observations of herbs that could be linked to physiological and medicinal changes. Observation must come first, then we can make clumsy and often inaccurate attempts at theory, which then must also be submitted to the scientific method. Modern scientific method uses a serial combination of inductive and then deductive reasoning. In medicine, we often transition from inductive and deductive reasoning to abductive reasoning (again, as discussed in Chapters 1 and 4).

Guided by Observation

We must not lose sight of what we do and do not know. The reason that we use antidepressant medications today is because isoniazid (an early monoamine oxidase inhibitor [MAOI]) noticeably improved the mood of patients treated for tuberculosis, just as imipramine (the first tricyclic antidepressant [TCA]) did for psychotic patients when tested as a better-tolerated substitute for chlorpromazine (López-Muñoz and Alamo 2009; Ramachandraih et al. 2011). We use convulsive therapies for the treatment of severe depression today because they failed to treat schizophrenia but significantly improved a subset of patients later found to have mood disorders (see Chapter 10). Careful, if serendipitous, clinical observations in these cases, followed by tested hypotheses of clinical benefit, led to the knowledge that each treatment improved the moods of people who were also depressed. Only later were monoamine neurotransmitters implicated as potential mechanistic agents for the medications we called antidepressants, and we are still searching for a mechanism for the undoubtable efficacy of electroconvulsive therapy.

When we observe that taking oral doses of amitriptyline is associated with improvement in the syndrome of major depression, and that this observed association can be replicated in RCTs, not only can we use this information to predict positive treatment outcomes for the right patients, we may also seek to understand the mechanisms behind it, in a reductive, simpler way. We look at the building blocks of the association: structures in the brain and the rest of the body that might be involved. This leads to the next level of reduction, such as nerves and blood vessels, and then to a smaller level, molecules such as hormones and neurotransmitters, eventually leading to drug receptor sites that might be involved. This inevitably results in the development of a list of neurotransmitters and receptor sites associated with the action of amitriptyline and similar agents. Efforts are made to distinguish between desirable effects or actions and side effects—that is, actions that are inconsequential to our goal of treatment and may even be annoying or deleterious. The effects on other medications in the body are eventually outlined (see Chapter 6).

Theory Follows Observation

Theories have developed to explain the associations observed in treating mood disorders with TCAs: that norepinephrine and serotonin neurotransmission may be manipulated in some way to produce the clinical improvements we see. Also considered are the side effects, including many mediated through anticholinergic pathways: dry mouth, constipation, tachycardia, blurred vision, and urinary sphincter tightening. Thoughtful pharmacologists have suggested, almost lightheartedly, that perhaps what we refer to as "side effects" are actually the mechanism of action. Regardless of their seriousness, this mind-expanding suggestion should help us maintain our perspective about the depth of our knowledge and the dangers of making assumptions. Although the original theory has evolved to demonstrate its superior claim to action over side effect, early guesses often lead us astray.

Examining how similar clinical outcomes can be obtained from medications with seemingly different mechanisms of action illustrates how perilous it may be to plan treatment based only an agent's (often presumed) mechanism of action. The monoamine theory, which notably remains a theory after 50 years, has left us with more than 30 so-called antidepressants that affect the amount of the neurotransmitters norepinephrine, serotonin, or both in the synaptic cleft. Strikingly, however, quite a scatter remains as to exactly which receptors are responsible for this clinical effect (Table 5–1 lists a sample of antidepressants and some of their receptor binding affinities). Several categories of antidepressants exist: TCAs, which are serotonin-norepinephrine reuptake inhibitor (SNRI) agents; newer second-generation SNRIs such as venlafaxine, duloxetine, and mirtazapine; selective serotonin reuptake inhibitors (SSRIs) such as fluoxetine, sertraline, and citalopram; and MAOIs, which inhibit enzymes that degrade the neurotransmitters, thereby sustaining their action. Add to these somatic treatments such as electroconvulsive therapy, for which no known mechanism exists (and has not been adequately explained by the theories used for medications). If we look superficially at only the proposed mechanism of action, we would miss the final common pathway: downregulation of the postsynaptic terminal. Although we understand this example, when can we be sure we have elucidated or demonstrated the final common pathway in other pharmacological cases? Until fully clarified and clearly linked to symptom outcome, these attempts at elucidation must take a back seat in driving clinical decision making.

TABLE 5–1.   Some antidepressant receptor affinities

Antidepressant	$\alpha_1{}^a$	$\alpha_2{}^a$	$5\text{-HT}_{1A}{}^b$	$5\text{-HT}_{2A}{}^b$	$5\text{-HT}_{2C}{}^b$	mACh	NET	SERT
Bupropion	++					++++		++++
Citalopram	+				++++	+	++	++++
Duloxetine	+	+	++	++++	++++	++	+	+++
Fluoxetine	+			++++	++++	+	++++	
Maprotiline	++++	+		++++	++++	++++		
Mirtazapine	++++	+++++	+++++	++++	+++++	++++		

Note. + = binding affinity; mACh = muscarinic acetylcholine; NET = norepinephrine transporter; SERT = serotonin transporter.
[a]α adrenergic.
[b]Serotonergic.

Emergents and Rational Thought

Emergents, or multiscale processes, make extrapolation from such basic processes impossible with the current cognitive skills we employ. As yet, we are unable to understand how the concept of *mind* develops from neuronal synaptic transmission. Phenomena at one level of organization cannot be fully explained by the simpler processes of lower levels of complexity. The laws of physics lead to the structure of atoms that leads to molecules and the laws of chemistry; to crystals and then polymers; to the laws of biology with larger complex structures, such as cells, the emergence of life, and the laws of physiology; to consciousness and psychology; and then to social and group interaction with anthropology, sociology, and political science. Lower levels of structure inform higher-scale structure, along with the element of chance, and new, more complex forms emerge (Teilhard de Chardin 1955/1975). Explaining the results of the latest local election by quantum theory is not yet possible. We are much more likely to try, and also fail, to understand quantum theory through teleological reasoning, using analogies from the scales we can observe, such as psychology or sociology.

Research into scientific education informs us that as students grow more sophisticated with scientific thinking, they often make significant errors in reasoning across scales, turning to generalized narrative explanations, including teleology, using primarily their understanding of the observable scales (Chi et al. 2012; Scott et al. 2018). Although new information must be considered in the context of existing knowledge (discussed in Chapter 4), *prior probability* biases may inaccurately distort our assessments: people naturally choose explanations that are simple and that match already-known observations. Therefore, our as-yet incomplete understanding of mechanism is likely to lead to errors of logic and to significant errors in judgment about therapeutic recommendations.

With all of our data, we have yet to be able to reliably predict a response bottom-up or from receptor to clinical symptom. The human body and brain appear too complex for us to use only the laws of lower levels of complexity. The emergents that develop at every level of physiology change the nature of the problem so that it cannot be adequately explained by reductionistic thinking. The hope is that someday artificial intelligence and big data will provide tools for such bottom-up extrapolation. This, too, may be unlikely, however, because big data and machine learning are actually association and pattern recognizers, similar to the human brain.

Because we have only limited knowledge of psychotropic mechanism, the limits of reasoning, along with our human cognitive processing style, will not be objective enough compared with the slow, steady progress we can achieve in clinical research using the scientific method and abductive reasoning. Unless the entire multiscale mechanistic explanation for the pharmacological relief of psychiatric syndromes and symptoms is some-day determined, we cannot allow flawed attempts from incomplete mechanistic understanding to supplant clinical results and dictate treatment selection.

Throughout this book, I stress that clinical decisions guided solely by composite results of replicated, double-blind RCTs, which have been analyzed to refine treatment models using Bayesian logic, must take precedence over every other method. That is not to say that we should not attempt to understand theory and to deepen our mechanistic and multistage emergent understanding of the science involved—we should. However, we must also explore the limits to each method of rational thought and how far each approach can actually take us (as discussed in Chapter 1).

Clinicians in training and in practice often debate detailed arguments about clinical efficacy projecting from a proposed mechanism of action and, amazingly, never reference information from RCTs. Part of this influence, again, might be attributed to our friends in the pharmaceutical sales industry. Although clinicians remain grateful to pharmaceutical companies for providing the tools we need to treat our patients, we nevertheless must never forget that these companies can only stay in business by making a profit. Tightly controlled by the FDA, they strive to increase their market shares largely with nuance, including highlighting differences in neurotransmitter effects in the hope that the prescribing clinician might think these data meaningful. Most of these associations are, in fact, spurious, not directly related to clinical outcome, and therefore do not represent rational tools for making a treatment choice. Clinical outcome data from RCTs represent the most useful information about which patients might respond best to which medication. Always use syndrome resolution or improvement—linked to grouped, rather than single, symptom improvement—as the guide for choosing medications for treatment, rather than basing the decision on a proposed mechanism of action with irrational predictions.

Remember this the next time you are presented with a new psychopharmacological agent and told it is clinically different because it has a variable effect on a particular receptor. No one can know if that speculation is true until RCTs are performed and replicated. Be guided only by your own careful review of the clinical outcome data describing the clinical syndromes that the agent might treat in your patients, while awaiting the elucidation and confirmatory experiments of mechanistic explanations that may arrive in the future.

Summary

The practice of medicine most often uses *abductive reasoning*—using incomplete information to form hypotheses and then testing these hypotheses. Observation of clinical benefit, often serendipitous, guides treatment predictions tested in RCTs. Reductionistic attempts to uncover the underlying mechanisms of these clinical outcomes cross scales of complexity. Phenomena at one level of organization cannot be fully explained by the simpler processes of lower levels of complexity, and this often leads to significant errors in reasoning across scales: we choose explanations that are simple and that match known observations, not allowing for emergent properties. Although we look forward to the full delineation of mechanisms underlying our treatments, clinically we cannot allow irrational errors of judgment to misguide us in proposing treatment options for our patients. Rational practitioners must be guided only by the results of RCTs and their meta-analyses, not by flawed down-up extrapolations from proposed mechanisms during this stage of our understanding.

Key Points

- Similar clinical outcomes can often be obtained from medications with seemingly different mechanisms of action.
- Multiscale processes make extrapolation from basic processes impossible with the current cognitive skills we employ.
- Do not allow flawed attempts from incomplete mechanistic understanding to supplant clinical results and dictate treatment selection.
- When choosing a pharmacological agent for treatment, be guided solely by clinical outcome data.

Self-Assessment

1. Emergents

   A. Are also referred to as multiscale processes
   B. Can be explained by lower levels of complexity
   C. Involve lower levels of structure informing higher-scale structure, along with the element of chance
   D. A and C

2. Even as students become more sophisticated in their scientific thinking, they

   A. Often make errors of reasoning across scales
   B. Turn to generalized narrative explanations, including teleology
   C. Use their understanding of already-known, observable scales
   D. All of the above

3. Which of the following are true? (Choose all that apply)

   A. Similar clinical outcomes can only be obtained from treatments with similar mechanisms of action
   B. The receptors responsible for antidepressant efficacy in major depression are fairly standard across antidepressants
   C. Similar clinical outcomes may be obtained from treatments with seemingly different mechanisms of action
   D. It is always clear which receptors are responsible for efficacy and which for side effects

4. Which of the following statements is false? (Choose all that apply)

   A. Isoniazid was an early tricyclic antidepressant.
   B. Imipramine was an early tricyclic antidepressant.
   C. Isoniazid improved mood in patients with tuberculosis.
   D. Imipramine improved mood in patients with psychosis.

5. The human brain is an association and pattern recognizer like (choose all that apply)

   A. All algorithms
   B. Big data
   C. Machine learning
   D. None of the above

Discussion Topics

1. During a pharmaceutical company–sponsored (and FDA-approved) lecture, a psychiatrist tells you that a new antidepressant will be more effective than others for problems with cognition because of its novel effects as an agonist and antagonist, partial and otherwise,

on various serotonergic receptors. What specific data will you need to consider before accepting this claim?

2. Two popular antidepressants are being compared in an industry-sponsored study. One is found to be more efficacious than the other, both in head-to-head and placebo comparisons. Its effects include $5\text{-}HT_{1B}$ receptor partial agonism, whereas the competitor does not have this action. What can you conclude about the mechanism of action based solely on this study? What other data would you like to have?

Additional Reading

Harari YN: 21 Lessons for the 21st Century. New York, Spiegel and Grau, 2018 (Chapter 15, "Ignorance," and Chapter 17, "Post-Truth," are particularly relevant to discussions in this chapter and those of Chapters 1 and 4.)

West G: Scale: The Universal Laws of Growth, Innovation, Sustainability, and the Pace of Life in Organisms, Cities, Economies and Companies. New York, Penguin, 2017 (Enlightening exposition of scaling across several domains, including physiology, by the former head of the Santa Fe Institute, a complexity theory think tank. Chapter 3, especially pages 99–103, contains excellent examples of emergent properties.)

References

Chi MT, Roscoe RD, Slotta JD, et al: Misconceived causal explanations for emergent processes. Cogn Sci 36(1):1–61, 2012 22050726

López-Muñoz F, Alamo C: Monoaminergic neurotransmission: the history of the discovery of antidepressants from 1950s until today. Curr Pharm Des 15(14):1563–1586, 2009 19442174

Ramachandraih CT, Subramanyam N, Bar KJ, et al: Antidepressants: from MAOIs to SSRIs and more. Indian J Psychiatry 53(2):180–182, 2011 21772661

Scott EE, Anderson CW, Mashood KK, et al: Developing an analytical framework to characterize student reasoning about complex processes. CBE Life Sci Educ 17(3):ar49, 2018 30183566

Teilhard de Chardin P: The Phenomenon of Man [Le Phénomene Humain] (1955). Translated by Bernard Wall. New York, Harper Colophon Books, 1975

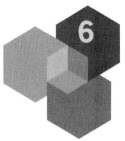

Pharmacokinetics, Pharmacodynamics, and Pharmacogenomics

Although one need not earn a doctorate in pharmacy to practice good clinical psychopharmacology, the more a practitioner remembers from pharmacology class, the more rational he or she can be. Easy familiarity with terms from these fields also helps clinicians as they evaluate published, randomized controlled trials (RCTs). This brief chapter offers a quick review for the rational pharmacologist.

Pharmacokinetics describes how a medication is absorbed, distributed, changed, and excreted from the body over time. *Pharmacodynamics* describes the changes a medication makes on the body through its location, bindings, and chemical interactions (Fan and de Lannoy 2014). *Pharmacogenomics* is the study of how genes affect a person's response to medication.

Pharmacokinetics

As medication enters the body (i.e., by injection, orally, sublingually, transdermally), we are first concerned with how completely and rapidly it is absorbed. *Bioavailability* represents the fraction of the drug that reaches systemic circulation. The speed is measured by the *time to maximal concentration* (t_{max}) of the drug in the blood. Both can be affected by another medication being administered at the same time or by food intake when administered orally. As an example, patients adding a fiber supplement to their regimen may see a reduction in the absorption of a routine medication and an eventual decline in benefit. A medicine may also differ in its bioavailability when it is given through multiple delivery systems or produced by more than one manufacturer, resulting in different serum levels. The FDA, for example, carefully monitors the bioavailability of brand-name medications and intervenes when even the smallest aberrations are detected in and among factories. For generic versions in the United States, however, the bioavailability is allowed to vary up to 20% (20% *higher* or *lower* than the brand bioavailability). Due to the worldwide location of many generic manufacturers, stringent monitoring is not feasible. Therefore, practitioners must consider carefully any generic brands they prescribe and be alert that pharmacies may change brands without informing either the prescriber or the patient, even if a brand has been specified. This may result in clinical changes such as loss of benefit or an increase or decrease in side effects, any of which may indicate a serum level change. Clinicians should educate each patient about these issues so that they can partner in monitoring brand changes (see discussion of Concerta in Chapter 7, "Medications to Treat Cognitive Disorders").

Next, we are concerned with how long it will take for the medication to leave the body—its *elimination*. This is most commonly measured by *half-life*: the time it takes for half of a single dose to leave the blood through excretion or metabolism. The drug may then be localized elsewhere in the body, but in the simplest case we imply it is not (other measurements are used to describe such a situation). The *effective* half-life ($t_{1/2}$) adds the time it takes to also eliminate active metabolites of the drug that sustain the clinical effect. The discussion and references in Chapter 7 (see "Medications to Treat Anxiety Disorders") illustrate how some clinicians make use of these concepts.

Once we know the half-life of a medication, we can use that to extrapolate new information. For most medications, it takes approximately five half-lives ($5 \times t_{1/2}$) to achieve a steady-state serum level concentration ($C_{av,ss}$). This means that given regular administrations of the same dose, the amount in the bloodstream is basically constant after five half-lives (e.g., 5 days [120 hours] for a drug with a $t_{1/2}$ of 24 hours, 60 hours for another with a $t_{1/2}$ of 12 hours). Should the dosage be changed, it also takes five half-lives to reach a new steady-state serum level. Even if the dosage is not changed, a new manufacturer's product likely has a different bioavailability, and this will also alter the serum level. The time it takes to reach maximum serum concentration when the drug is added at steady state ($C_{max,ss}$) is its $t_{max,ss}$. A trough serum level (C_{trough}) is the concentration of the drug in the blood at the end of a dosing period. A peak serum level (C_{max}) represents the highest concentration achieved.

Once $C_{av,ss}$ has been achieved, we then know how long it will take the medication to leave the body if abruptly discontinued, assuming healthy physiological function: five half-lives. This knowledge is essential in determining how much of an overlap will occur when changing medications, how long a patient might see lingering benefits or adverse events, or what a safe rate of discontinuation or taper will be for a medication (again, see "Medications to Treat Anxiety Disorders" in Chapter 7).

Protein binding measures how much of a drug is bound to plasma proteins rather than being free to bind to receptor sites and is usually expressed as a percentage (i.e., fluoxetine is 94%–95% protein bound). Sometimes medication serum levels are measured as *total*, including the fraction bound to these proteins, and sometimes only the *free* level is measured: the part not bound. Clinically, one or the other for each molecule is usually determined to be more helpful in diagnosis and treatment.

Location of metabolism is also important to consider with each patient. A few medications are excreted unchanged (see discussion of lithium and gabapentin in Chapter 7, "Medications to Stabilize Mood"); many more have hepatic metabolism, some have renal metabolism, and yet others use the gastrointestinal system, lungs, or skin. Hepatic or renal insufficiency, for example, may affect the choice of medication for an individual patient. The general health, sex, age, and at times, ethnicity of each patient must be considered with regard to how it will alter the expected pharmacokinetics of the medication chosen (see "Pharmacogenomics" later in this chapter).

Pharmacokinetics can be a lot more detailed, considering additional issues such as compartmental methods, permeability (e.g., across the blood–brain barrier), and volume distribution, as well as much more about metabolism. However, even the few concepts discussed here will offer the clinical psychopharmacologist enough tools to create a rational treatment plan that respects the constraints of the medication chosen to recommend.

Pharmacodynamics

Once a medication is available in the body, we are concerned with the target of that medication: the receptors to which it binds and how well it binds to them. Is the medication an *agonist* for a receptor, meaning that it potentiates the action, or an *antagonist*, meaning that it blocks the action? Some medications are *partial agonists*, meaning they stimulate action weakly, generating a smaller effect than a pure agonist (see discussion of aripiprazole in Chapter 7, "Medications to Treat Psychosis"). The specificity of a receptor describes how many different types of molecules it is likely to accept. Many drugs bind variably to more than one receptor type, a concept known as *selectivity*, and may in fact not bind to all components of a receptor, thus producing a unique effect (see "Medications to Treat Sleep Problems" in Chapter 7). How well a molecule binds to a receptor is defined as *affinity*, which really just means how potent it is. This is described by the equilibrium dissociation constant (K_d): a low K_d identifies strong binding affinity. Marketers may try to convince prescribers that affinity refers to efficacy, when actually it just determines the dosage (Waldman 2002). Potency has no other relevance; explaining to worried patients that the treatments requiring higher dosages are the less potent, "weaker" ones, whereas those with low doses (high potency) are the "stronger" ones, may be helpful.

Therapeutic index is a measure of how close the effective dose of a medication is to its toxic dose. When possible, clinicians prefer a high therapeutic index because the toxic dose is divided by the effective dose. The t_{dur} is the expected duration of pharmacological response.

Be aware of drug–drug interactions that can occur with each prescription, because these may lead to unexpected toxicity or ineffectiveness. Current prescriptions from other providers, including those taken only as needed, must be considered. Drug–drug interactions often involve competition for the serum protein binding noted earlier or the competitive interference or enhancement of one medication with the metabolism of another through the cytochrome P450 (CYP450) enzyme system (Guengerich et al. 2016; Table 6–1). Although most clinicians can keep a few of these important interactions in their heads (see discussion of lamotrigine and valproate in Chapter 7, "Medications to Stabilize Mood") so many are possible that using a database, electronic or paper, should be a routine habit. Many electronic medical records have built-in screens for drug interactions, although you should learn the capabilities of the system included in order to calibrate its accuracy. Some are poor and over- or underestimate risks. Rather than rely solely on these, look up the information in your preferred database prior to prescription and use the chart-based system only as backup. Rational psychopharmacologists never rely simply on the dispensing pharmacist to catch drug–drug interactions, although they welcome their assistance as a second or third failsafe.

Pharmacogenomics

Genetic analysis may hold the promise to help clinicians choose the best treatment for their patients at the outset, resulting in fewer trials in the office or hospital. It is enticing to think we can know in advance which patients will respond to which medications. Although prediction of efficacy is still lagging, current commercially available technology may provide

TABLE 6–1. Incomplete list of CYP450 substrates, inhibitors, and inducers

CYP450	Substrates	Inhibitors	Inducers
3A4	Alprazolam (+3A5), aripiprazole, citalopram, clomipramine, dextromethorphan, diazepam, pimozide, simvastatin, trazodone, verapamil (+3A5), ziprasidone, zolpidem	Erythromycin, fluvoxamine, norfluoxetine, verapamil	Carbamazepine, modafinil, oxcarbazepine, phenobarbital, phenytoin, topiramate
1A2	Caffeine, clomipramine, clozapine, duloxetine, olanzapine, zolpidem	Fluvoxamine	Carbamazepine, cigarette smoking (polycyclic aromatic hydrocarbons), modafinil
2D6	Amphetamine, aripiprazole, atomoxetine, dextromethorphan, duloxetine, risperidone, venlafaxine	Bupropion, fluoxetine, fluvoxamine, HIV antivirals (ritonavir), paroxetine, sertraline, ziprasidone (weak)	Carbamazepine, modafinil
2C19	Citalopram, clomipramine, diazepam, phenytoin	Fluvoxamine, modafinil, oxcarbazepine	Carbamazepine, phenytoin, primidone
2C9	Ibuprofen, losartan, valproic acid, warfarin, zolpidem	Fluvoxamine, paroxetine, sertraline	Carbamazepine, phenytoin, St. John's wort
2B6	Bupropion, ketamine, methadone	Sertraline	Carbamazepine, phenobarbital, phenytoin

some insight into the tolerability of medications for patients. Knowledge of polymorphisms in receptors, transporters, and CYP450 enzymes provides information that may be useful in treatment selection and dosage guidance of some antidepressant and antipsychotic medications (Hicks et al. 2015; Reynolds et al. 2014). Practitioners and systems are currently integrating this information into daily practice, but others have observed that this technology has not developed to the point where it can provide reliable predictions to practitioners or patients and that it comes at a cost (Weinshilboum and Wang 2017). If tolerability cannot be predicted clinically, genetic analysis could provide value for patients in some cases, but because high false-negative and false-positive rates for biomarkers persist, most feel this technology, unfortunately, is not yet reliable enough for routine rational practice (Bousman and Hopwood 2016; Rosenblat et al. 2017). In any case, genetic data should only be considered as part of the comprehensive evaluation and decision making necessary for rational psychopharmacology and should never take precedence.

Summary

Pharmacokinetics concerns how a medication is absorbed, distributed, changed, and excreted from the body over time. *Pharmacodynamics* describes changes a medication makes on the body through its location, bindings, and chemical interactions. *Pharmacogenomics* is the study of how genes affect a person's response to medication and at present may only be useful in predicting tolerability in routine office and hospital practice.

Pharmacokinetics measurements include bioavailability (the amount that reaches circulation), time to full concentration (t_{max}), half-life or time to 50% elimination ($t_{1/2}$) of the original (or parent) molecule, time to 50% elimination adding in all clinically active metabolites (effective half-life), steady-state serum level ($C_{av,ss}$=five $t_{1/2}$); and free, total, and protein-bound levels in the serum. Location of metabolism should be compared with specific health deficits in each patient. Calculation of elimination for each medication prescribed is particularly important when changing medications.

Pharmacodynamics identifies receptors and their specificity, the selectivity of medications for receptors, and actions at the receptor: agonists that potentiate, antagonists that block, and partial agonists that potentiate weakly. Binding affinity (K_d) determines potency—and therefore dosage—but not efficacy. A high therapeutic index means the toxic dose of a medication is much higher than its effective dose. Drug–drug interactions based on protein binding or metabolism through the CYP450 system may influence any combination of medications. These interactions should be determined and compensated for, prior to prescription, with the use of a reliable database.

Key Points

■ Bioavailability, the fraction of the drug that reaches systemic circulation, may be influenced by other medications or supplements, food intake, delivery systems, or production by more than one manufacturer.

■ Effective half-life must be considered when changing medications.

■ Location of metabolism must be compared with the health status of each patient.

■ Possible drug–drug interactions must be predicted by the clinician, using a reliable database prior to prescription.

Self-Assessment

1. A new medication reports a time to maximal concentration (t_{max}) of 3 hours and a half-life ($t_{1/2}$) of 6–10 hours. Due to adverse events, the patient wishes to discontinue it after 3 days. Abrupt cessation being safe, how long will it take the medication to exit her body?

   A. 6–10 hours
   B. 18–30 hours
   C. 30–50 hours
   D. 3 hours

2. When choosing between two medications expected to have similar chances of efficacy, which would patients better tolerate?

   A. The one with a higher therapeutic index
   B. The one with a lower therapeutic index
   C. Therapeutic index is not relevant, so it makes no difference

3. Which of these statements is true? (Choose all that apply)

   A. Binding affinity is a measure of efficacy.
   B. Binding affinity determines potency.
   C. Binding affinity determines dosage.
   D. None of the above

4. Which of the following statements is true? (Choose all that apply)

   A. A medication with no active metabolites will have an effective half-life that is equal to $t_{1/2}$.

   B. A medication with active metabolites will have an effective half-life that is equal to $t_{1/2}$.

   C. A medication with active metabolites will have an effective half-life that is greater than $t_{1/2}$.

   D. A medication with active metabolites will have an effective half-life that is less than $t_{1/2}$.

5. Drug–drug interactions may result from (choose all that apply)

   A. Competition for serum protein binding

   B. Competitive interference through the CYP450 enzyme system

   C. Enhancement of metabolism via the CYP450 enzyme system

   D. Competitive absorption

Discussion Topics

1. A patient proudly brings you a 14-page printout of a pharmacogenomic evaluation she did on her own initiative at a nearby laboratory. She paid $400 for the report, which was not covered by her insurance. It reports efficacy and tolerability scores for each antidepressant she might consider. How might the information be useful, and how will you explain its limitations to her?

2. A patient maintained on an effective and well-tolerated once-daily antipsychotic medication reports that her gastroenterologist has directed her to begin daily fiber supplements. How might you recommend she accomplish this while preserving her clinical response from the antipsychotic?

Additional Reading

Abubakar AR, Chedi BAZ, Mohammed KG, et al: Drug interaction and its implication in clinical practice and personalized medicine. Natl J Physiol Pharm Pharmacol 5:343–349, 2015

Currie GM: Pharmacology, part 1: introduction to pharmacology and pharmacodynamics. J Nucl Med Technol 46(2):81–86, 2018

Currie GM: Pharmacology, part 2: introduction to pharmacokinetics. J Nucl Med Technol 46(3):221–230, 2018 (Intended for nuclear medicine technicians, this and the previous article by Currie offer an excellent discussion of many of the concepts covered in this chapter.).

References

Bousman CA, Hopwood M: Commercial pharmacogenetic-based decision-support tools in psychiatry. Lancet Psychiatry 3(6):585–590, 2016 27133546

Fan J, de Lannoy IA: Pharmacokinetics. Biochem Pharmacol 87(1):93–120, 2014 24055064

Guengerich FP, Waterman MR, Egli M: Recent structural insights into cytochrome P450 function. Trends Pharmacol Sci 37(8):625–640, 2016 27267697

Hicks JK, Bishop JR, Sangkuhl K, et al: Clinical pharmacogenetics implementation consortium (CPIC) guideline for CYP2D6 and CYP2C19 genotypes and dosing of selective serotonin reuptake inhibitors. Clin Pharmacol Ther 98(2):127–134, 2015 25974703

Reynolds GP, McGowan OO, Dalton CF: Pharmacogenomics in psychiatry: the relevance of receptor and transporter polymorphisms. Br J Clin Pharmacol 77(4):654–672, 2014 24354796

Rosenblat JD, Lee Y, McIntyre RS: Does pharmacogenomic testing improve clinical outcomes for major depressive disorder? A systematic review of clinical trials and cost-effectiveness studies. J Clin Psychiatry 78(6):720–729, 2017 28068459

Waldman SA: Does potency predict clinical efficacy? Illustration through an antihistamine model. Ann Allergy Asthma Immunol 89(1):7–11, quiz 11–12, 77, 2002 12141724

Weinshilboum RM, Wang L: Pharmacogenomics: precision medicine and drug response. Mayo Clin Proc 92(11):1711–1722, 2017 29101939

Categories of Medication Used in Clinical Psychopharmacology

Whereas the rest of this book encourages you to think thoroughly, completely, and methodically about data and treatment choice, this chapter contains information on the actual pharmacological tools to be considered. Many sources of this information are available to the clinician, and the case has already been made for evaluating each source with the best scientific method. In this chapter, we add the historical context. Most readers would never read about a historical event without attempting to put it into cultural, historical, and political context. How can we understand the American, French, or Russian revolutions without understanding what preceded them? Similarly, the rational psychopharmacologist should approach the selection of a pharmacological agent for patients only with an understanding of the full range of options for treatment. For this reason, each section in this chapter commences with the earliest available treatments and ends with the most current. The latest or most popular may not always be the best choice, and clinicians must be aware of all the options that came before and after to fully understand the treatment they are offering. Superior efficacy and safety are not always the reasons for changes in prescribing fashions.

Medications to Treat Anxiety Disorders

Anxiety symptoms predominate patient complaints in psychiatry, regardless of the underlying diagnosis. In most cases, anxiety is best treated by treating the primary underlying syndrome; use of additional antianxiety medications is often neither necessary nor desirable (see Chapter 4). This section focuses on the medications used to treat primary anxiety disorder diagnoses, referred to as minor tranquilizers and anxiolytics.

During the nineteenth century, widely available opiates and cannabis, not to mention alcohol, could be used to suppress anxiety prior to the development of legal and more scientifically sanctioned remedies (Horwitz 2009). Popular films and books often allude to taking a shot of brandy "to steady the nerves." The opiate mixture laudanum, familiar to readers of mystery novels, was prescribed, marketed, and sold for various indications, including emotional irritation. Bromides were identified as sedatives and anticonvulsants; by the end of the century they were even more widely used than opiate alkaloids, until toxicity concerns led to the restriction of their use. Barbiturates dominated sedative and anticonvulsant treatment in the first half of the twentieth century, but meprobamate and benzodiazepines, developed in the 1950s and 1960s, respectively, largely replaced them due to risks of overdose and concerns about abuse (López-Muñoz et al. 2005).

Meprobamate, considered the first minor tranquilizer, was heavily marketed as an anxiolytic that was effective without also being sedating. A carbamate related to carisoprodol and methocarbamol, meprobamate actually is sedating and not particularly safer than barbiturates (Rho et al. 1997). By the early to mid-1960s, benzodiazepines had replaced it.

The first synthesized and commercially available benzodiazepines were chlordiazepoxide in 1960 and diazepam in 1963. Causing less respiratory depression than barbiturates, especially when taken orally, they were initially considered to be safer, with less risk of abuse and addiction (Wick 2013). Intravenous administration, however, can still carry a significant risk of central respiratory depression and arrest (Bailey et al. 1986; Forster et al. 1980). The final active metabolite of these two agents, oxazepam, was released in 1965, in addition to nitrazepam. In the 1970s, flurazepam was approved by the FDA and used primarily for sleep; clorazepate was also introduced and has been used for anxiety since its approval. The final benzodiazepines approved in the mid- to late 1970s were clonazepam and lorazepam, both also indicated as anticonvulsants. Lorazepam has been particularly popular in emergency departments because it can be easily delivered intravenously and is quickly and almost completely absorbed from intramuscular injection as well (Griffin et al. 2013). For this reason, many nonpsychiatric physicians are most familiar with it.

The early 1980s brought the release of temazepam, another active metabolite of diazepam, as well as halazepam, alprazolam, and triazolam.

Quazepam, which was largely rejected by providers as an unnecessary "me, too" medication, and midazolam, which found popular use as a sedative for short-term outpatient procedures such as colonoscopies, rounded out the decade. Triazolam, although it offered a very quick onset (0.5–2 hours) and short half-life (2 hours), eventually waned in popularity because the lethal dose is closer to the effective dose than is typical. It has mostly become a tool for dentists seeking sedation of patients during procedures. Alprazolam, which was originally marketed as both an anxiolytic and antidepressant, was broadly accepted, although it fails to treat major depression and may worsen it. It arrived coincident with development of treatment protocols to treat panic disorder, which may have heightened its appeal (Ballenger et al. 1988).

Estazolam and clobazam are the newest benzodiazepines approved by the FDA for marketing in the United States. Estazolam is used exclusively as a sedative-hypnotic. Clobazam, used worldwide for anxiety since 1975 and for epilepsy since 1984, was only approved in Canada in 2005 and in the United States in 2011 for limited use in some forms of epilepsy, as it is in the United Kingdom and additional Commonwealth countries. In India and the United Kingdom, clobazam is also indicated for short-term use against agitation and anxiety in patients with psychosis. Notably, it is specifically approved for use in depressive cases only with concurrent antidepressant treatment, carrying the warning that use of benzodiazepines alone in unstable mood cases may increase the risk of suicide (e.g., Frisium 10 mg tablets [Electronic Medicines Compendium 2018]); this risk should always be considered with each benzodiazepine.

Benzodiazepines may be sorted by half-life, a useful distinction for clinical decision making (Table 7–1). The longer the half-life, the longer it takes to reach a steady-state serum level and the longer the medication persists in the body, even after it is no longer administered. Half-lives also have implications for how patients will tolerate removal of the agent and when they may experience withdrawal after cessation of use, although not necessarily how severe any withdrawal syndrome will be. Half-lives do not describe the length of a desired clinical effect, however.

If we know the half-life of a medication, we can calculate when we expect it to leave the body, allowing for any individual differences in metabolism and excretion, such as patients with liver and kidney function problems (see Chapter 6). As discussed in Chapter 3, assessing hepatic and renal function prior to prescription is essential. Most benzodiazepines are metabolized by the liver, usually to forms that are also psychoactive. Diazepam, for example, has three active metabolites, all of which have been marketed as separate medications: nordiazepam (also called desmethyldi-

TABLE 7–1.   Half-lives and active metabolites of commonly used benzodiazepines

Benzodiazepine	Half-life, hours	Active metabolites	Effective half-life, hours
Alprazolam	6–15	4-Hydroxyalprazolam, α-hydroxyalprazolam (weak)	12–20
Chlordiazepoxide	5–30	Nordiazepam, oxazepam	36–200
Clonazepam	18–60	None	18–60
Clorazepate	40–50	Nordiazepam, oxazepam	36–200
Diazepam	20–48	Nordiazepam, temazepam, oxazepam	24–80
Estazolam	10–24	4-Hydroxyestazolam, 1-oxoestazolam (weak)	12–30
Flurazepam	40–100	Norflurazepam, N_1-hydroxyethylflurazepam	47–250
Lorazepam	12	None	12
Midazolam	1.5–2.5	α_1-Hydroxymidazolam, norflurazepam	1.8–6.4
Oxazepam	5.7–10.9	None	5.7–10.9
Prazepam	29–90	Nordiazepam, 3-hydroxyprazepam, oxazepam	36–200
Temazepam	0.4–0.6	Oxazepam	12
Triazolam	1.5–5.5	None	1.5–5.5

azepam) and temazepam, each further metabolized to oxazepam, which is itself removed by renal excretion. The parent compound has a half-life of 24–48 hours; steady-state levels from routine dosing are accomplished in 5–14 days. The principal metabolite is nordiazepam, which has a 50- to 120-hour half-life, leading to a steady-state serum level in approximately 21 days (Calcaterra and Barrow 2014). Rational planning of the use of all medications includes taking into account the pharmacokinetics and pharmacodynamics of the parent compounds plus those of the active metabolites, resulting in effective half-lives (Boxenbaum and Battle 1995). Because oxazepam is eliminated solely by renal excretion, it can be used more safely in cases of liver compromise (Greenblatt et al. 1975). Temazepam, which also has a shorter effective half-life than nordiazepam ($t_{1/2}$ 5–11 hours in the absence of hepatic compromise), has been utilized as a soporific (Heel et al. 1981).

Matching the length of the effective half-life to the clinical goal is important. As examples, chlordiazepoxide has long been a popular choice for alcohol and benzodiazepine detoxification regimens, largely because its half-life is so long: 5–30 hours for the parent compound and 36–200 hours for the active metabolite desmethyldiazepam, sometimes even longer in geriatric patients (Sachdeva et al. 2015; Vozeh 1981). More than half of the first-day dosage is effectively still present on the second day, and so on; thus, a very slow taper occurs when the medicine is discontinued, greatly reducing the risk of withdrawal. Flurazepam, however, has a similarly long half-life at 47–100 hours, which leads to an undesirable buildup and excessive sedation beyond its intended use as a daily soporific for most patients.

All benzodiazepines have the features of tolerance, rebound, and physiological dependence. Psychological dependence and abuse may or may not occur with use and are not necessarily related to these features. *Tolerance* means that over time, the serum level of the benzodiazepine must be increased to maintain the same clinical effect previously achieved with the initial effective dose and level, apparently due to a decrease in receptor sensitivity (Miller et al. 1988). *Rebound* means that upon rapid or abrupt cessation, the underlying symptoms may return briefly at higher-than-pretreatment severity. This is distinguished from a simple recurrence of the underlying symptoms once treatment is stopped. *Physiological dependence* describes the appearance of a physiological withdrawal syndrome after discontinuation, especially when removal is too rapid (Shader and Greenblatt 1993).

Opiate dependence, by definition, results in a horrific "withdrawal" or discontinuation syndrome following quick cessation of use, but it is not by itself lethal. The saying is that although opiate "withdrawal" will not kill you, you might wish it would; anxiety, sweating, severe muscle cramps, and gastrointestinal rebound predominate. Benzodiazepine withdrawal, in contrast, can be lethal (Lann and Molina 2009) and may even occur with regularly prescribed use, not just from abuse. It is similar to alcohol withdrawal syndrome (Santos et al. 2017), running the risk of tonic-clonic seizures, and may present with severe agitation, anxiety, tremor, irritability, nausea, dry vomiting, diaphoresis (sweating), palpitations, headache, impaired concentration, and muscular discomfort (Pétursson 1994).

Prevention of benzodiazepine withdrawal syndrome must always be on the clinician's mind when choosing, prescribing, and removing benzodiazepines. Patients taking and stopping benzodiazepines must be carefully monitored for unexpected withdrawal symptoms from missed doses, unfilled prescriptions, or prescribing errors from other providers. Patients entering the hospital for surgery or other medical reasons must have their prescription continued or be tapered safely. In the office, assessment of symptoms along with elevated pulse and blood pressure may alert you to the possibility of benzodiazepine withdrawal. If uncertain, always check vital signs in addition to asking the appropriate questions. Unfortunately, patients are all too commonly thrown into benzodiazepine withdrawal by a provider who is not knowledgeable about the varying half-lives of these agents.

In most cases, a reasonable taper schedule for benzodiazepines is 25% every 14 days, but this schedule must be adapted to the clinical situation, taking into account half-lives, dosage, and length of treatment as well as other medications and substances used. For example, alprazolam and lorazepam have shorter half-lives and therefore are quite difficult to taper comfortably when treatment ends. Shorter-acting benzodiazepines that patients have taken for 2–4 months or longer should be tapered more slowly, perhaps over 2–4 months. Alternatively, benzodiazepines with longer actual or effective half-lives, such as clonazepam or diazepam, may be substituted and tapered. Originally choosing, or later switching to, benzodiazepines with longer half-lives is an often-successful strategy for overcoming discontinuation symptoms (e.g., nausea, anxiety, insomnia) that may occur even after a sufficient taper. During and following the taper, attempt to distinguish among rebound, withdrawal, and recurrence of underlying symptoms. All three events may occur near the end of a taper, so slowing the taper further or continuing the medication at a lower dosage may be the better clinical choice (Shader and Greenblatt 1993).

Benzodiazepines are indicated and used in the treatment of seizures, insomnia, muscle spasticity, tremor, and alcohol withdrawal, as well as for anxiety. In the 1970s, this class of medication became the most prescribed in the United States. Later in that decade, awareness of overuse, dependence, and addiction led to calls for more judicious prescribing and stricter monitoring. Unfortunately, this call for careful monitoring (clarity of diagnosis, consideration of alternative treatments [including psychotherapy], regularly scheduled visits, and therapeutic endpoints) has become misconstrued by many to imply that benzodiazepine use is made safer simply by restricting it to short-term use. Long-term use may be indicated in some cases, however (Stevens and Pollack 2005; Veronese et al. 2007; Worthington et al. 1998), and both long- and short-term use must be properly assessed and monitored.

Benzodiazepines are generally thought of as well tolerated, but side effects do occur. Sedation can be a problem, especially if dosing is too high or early in treatment before the patient develops tolerance to this side effect (Lucki et al. 1986). This may have implications for patients' driving safety and work performance. Geriatric patients receiving any benzodiazepine have an increased risk of falls and a 24% increased incidence of hip fractures, the greatest risk being within the first 2–4 weeks of use (Wagner et al. 2004). Although treatment of anxiety with benzodiazepines can improve cognitive function (Fabre and Putman 1988), short-term use of benzodiazepines may also cause transient cognitive impairment, as seen with anticholinergic and antihistaminic agents (Tannenbaum et al. 2012). Further research is attempting to determine whether long-term memory impairment persists after discontinuation of use, allowing for withdrawal. To date, conclusive evidence of this is lacking, because many early studies suffered from methodological problems. Clearer studies have not found a clinically significant link (Gray et al. 2016; Stewart 2005). Also remember that benzodiazepines are cross tolerant with barbiturates and alcohol and that, although they can thus be used in treating the withdrawal syndromes of these two agents, concomitant use may result in lethal overdose.

The suggestion that β-blockers such as propranolol could be used for treatment of anxiety was first published in 1966 (Granville-Grossman and Turner 1966). Subsequent attempts to demonstrate not only greater safety but also enhanced efficacy of β-blockers over benzodiazepines have been pursued (Turner 1989), and propranolol has become commonly thought of as efficacious, particularly among nonspecialists. Unfortunately, sufficient supportive data are not available (Steenen et al. 2016). Although propranolol does seem effective in reducing tremor and other peripheral symptoms of anxiety, compelling randomized controlled trials (RCTs) showing a central anxiolytic effect are lacking. This leads to the possibility that suppressing the physical symptoms of anxiety may help patients appear calmer to themselves and others, therefore reducing a fear cycle provoked by these symptoms.

β-Blockers may offer an advantage in treating PTSD, through a differential effect on memory reconsolidation as compared with other anxiety treatments (Brunet et al. 2008; Lonergan et al. 2013; Schwabe et al. 2013). Further studies to confirm and measure the extent of this effect, and its applicability to the most severe traumatic memories, are needed, however (Brunet et al. 2018; Burbiel 2015; Steenen et al. 2016). Risks of β-blockers include worsening or promotion of depressed mood (Huffman and Stern 2007; Patten 1990); they are usually contraindicated in patients with asthma and other chronic obstructive pulmonary diseases, certain heart failures, diabetes mellitus, symptomatic bradycardia, and atrioventricular block (Pozzi 2000; Zafrir and Amir 2012). Lethal acute heart failure may result from rapid discontinuation in the absence of an adequate multiweek taper (Prichard and Walden 1982). Use of β-blockers to treat anxiety disorders should be carefully considered, given the current level of evidence for sufficient efficacy.

Although serotonin-norepinephrine reuptake inhibitors (SNRIs), including tricyclic antidepressants (TCAs), and selective serotonin reuptake inhibitors (SSRIs) are generally referred to as *antidepressants*, they are quite effective in the treatment of anxiety disorders, even in the absence of mood symptoms. Each of these is discussed more thoroughly in the next section; here they are mentioned only in the context of anxiety treatments.

Imipramine was one of the first medications found to treat panic disorder (Klein 1967; Pohl et al. 1982). Additional SNRIs, such as its secondary amine form desipramine and amitriptyline, plus monoamine oxidase inhibitors (MAOIs) and SSRIs, particularly sertraline and paroxetine, have demonstrated similar efficacy, as well as for generalized anxiety disorder (GAD) and social anxiety (Canton et al. 2012). Unlike earlier anxiolytics, the effects of these agents take at least 1–2 weeks, and often 4–6 weeks, to occur. They must be taken daily, although usually only once daily, and cannot be used only as needed. Given their demonstrated efficacy, lack of abuse potential, and relative safety, TCAs, SNRIs, and SSRIs are considered by many to be first-line treatments for anxiety disorders in children, adolescents, and adults (Katzman et al. 2014; Wehry et al. 2015) and useful long term (Batelaan et al. 2017).

The gabaminergic agent (affecting the neurotransmitter GABA) gabapentin has been reported to have efficacy in treating social anxiety disorder (Pande et al. 1999). No RCTs of gabapentin in the treatment of GAD have been published, and it has not been found particularly effective in other anxiety disorders (Berlin et al. 2015). Pharmacologically, gabapentin has some distinguishing features; it is excreted unchanged by the kidney, with a half-life of about 5 hours given adequate renal function. It enters the body through carrier-mediated absorption: a specific molecule ferries it from the gastrointestinal tract into the bloodstream. When this carrier is fully saturated, no further gabapentin can be absorbed. The maximum dose that can enter the body within a 5-hour period is approximately 1,400–1,600 mg, which is a safe dose; thus, problems from overdose are not possible in the absence of renal dysfunction.

Unlike SNRIs and SSRIs, but more like benzodiazepines, gabapentin can be taken only as needed and must be taken three or four times a day for sustained use because clinical benefits wear off after 5 hours. Several attempts have been made to develop long-acting versions of gabapentin, but so far these formulations have either failed in concept (e.g., gabapentin gastric-retentive, marketed as Gralise) or have only recently been able to provide useful correlation of diurnal serum levels with the short-acting form (e.g., gabapentin enacarbil extended-release formulation, marketed as Horizant). The latter form appears to have greater bioavailability, so dosing is one-third that of the standard short-acting gabapentin (Swearingen et al. 2018).

Side effects such as nausea, sedation, and dizziness may occur from gabapentin early in use, so low doses such as 100 mg should be used with the standard short-acting form. Weekly, doses may be increased by 100 mg until the more standard 300–1,200 mg dose is reached and tolerance to side effects is achieved. If gabapentin is to be used as needed for social performance anxiety, doses of 300–400 mg are often necessary and reasonably well tolerated, although test doses are recommended before use for performances, presentations, or scholastic tests. If used in this way, patients should take the dose 2 hours prior to the event, because peak levels are achieved in 120 minutes.

One interesting footnote in the treatment of anxiety is the 5-HT_{1A} agonist buspirone. Buspirone is marketed as a nonaddicting anxiolytic; the common saying is that it has everything you would want in a medication except efficacy. It does not affect GABA and lacks the dangers of opiates, barbiturates, carbamates, and benzodiazepines. Also, unlike these agents, any positive effect on anxiety takes 2–4 weeks, similar to SNRIs, SSRIs, and TCAs (as noted earlier) and the treatment of major depression (discussed later). Buspirone cannot, therefore, be used for rapid or brief treatment of anxiety. In fact, the effect is so weak that buspirone is indicated only for the treatment of GAD, although it enjoyed brief popularity as a potentiating agent for SSRIs and SNRIs that failed as monotherapies.

Medications to Treat Major Depression

In evaluating the selection of antidepressants, we must consider the actual syndrome we are treating and not confuse it with the symptom of depressed mood. Would we usually treat depression in bipolar disorder with an antidepressant? When we choose antidepressants to treat "depression," we often mean the syndrome major depression. Clarifying this with patients should help them understand why antidepressants might not be the best choice for every symptom of depressed mood. If the neurovegetative symptoms that antidepressants treat (per RCTs) are not present, we do not expect a beneficial response in mood. The only exception is a diagnosis of dysthymic disorder, which responds 50% of the time (Kocsis et al. 1997).

Other than amphetamines, the earliest use of antidepressant medications began around 1953 and included MAOIs and TCAs. As mentioned in Chapter 5, isoniazid, a nonspecific MAOI, was the first medication identified as treating symptoms of clinical depression, and the TCA imipramine followed quickly, after failing as a more tolerable alternative to chlorpromazine for psychosis. Other early MAOIs developed exclusively for psychiatric use included isocarboxazid, phenelzine, and tranylcypromine. These agents are named for their interference with the function of the monoamine oxidase enzyme, located in the synaptic cleft, that degrades the monoamine neurotransmitters epinephrine, norepinephrine, and 5-hydroxytryptophan (a serotonin precursor). Although isoniazid use in the treatment of depression faded quickly due to hepatotoxicity, these other MAOIs were approved by the FDA for marketing. Problems using them quickly developed, however, because use with sympathomimetic agents or concomitant dietary intake of the amino acid tyramine leads to dangerous elevations in blood pressure. This practically limited their use unless patients could reliably adhere to a strict, tyramine-free diet (Table 7–2). At the same time, success with TCAs in treating the same symptoms led to minimal use of MAOIs, although some researchers and practitioners believed MAOIs superior to TCAs for treating treatment-resistant depression (rather circular logic, because *treatment-resistant* meant not responding to TCAs at that time). Efforts were made to develop specific and reversible MAOIs that could be safer: in the mid-2000s, the MAOI selegiline was developed in transdermal delivery form and approved by the FDA for the treatment of major depression. Absorbed into the blood transdermally, selegiline bypasses first-pass metabolism by the liver. This leads to a reduced risk of hypertensive crisis when tyramine is present in the gut, provided low to moderate dosages (6 mg every 24 hours or less) are used (Lee and Chen 2007). Despite aggressive marketing, however, selegiline never really caught on with providers, who by then often used the better-tolerated and still-safer SSRIs and newer SNRIs.

TCAs, named for their structure, dominated psychopharmacology in the late 1960s, 1970s, and 1980s. The tertiary amines imipramine, amitriptyline, and doxepin, followed by the next-generation secondary amines nortriptyline and desipramine, allowed treatment of major depression with less reliance on convulsive therapies, against which they had to repeatedly demonstrate comparative efficacy (see Chapter 10). Protriptyline and trimipramine were also used, although less frequently, failing to really distinguish themselves with globally accepted niche indications. Amoxapine, which received U.S. marketing approval in 1992, is an active metabolite of the antipsychotic loxapine and similarly failed to find a

TABLE 7–2. Common foods to avoid in tyramine-free diet

Avoid aged, cured, dried, fermented, salted, smoked, pickled, and spoiled foods. Also avoid monosodium glutamate, nitrates, nitrites, meat tenderizers, yeast, and yeast extracts.

Meats	Pepperoni, salami, liverwurst, liver, bacon, hot dogs, luncheon meat, mincemeat
Dairy	Sour cream, yogurt, cheeses (cheddar, Swiss, Roquefort, Stilton, mozzarella, blue, brick, brie)
Seafood	Shrimp paste, caviar
Nuts	All
Vegetables	Snow peas, fava and broad beans, sauerkraut, pickles, olives, avocados, stinky tofu, tempeh
Sauces	Miso, soy, teriyaki
Grains	Sourdough bread
Alcoholic beverages	All

Note. This list may still not be complete; help patients identify specific foods in their diets using common databases.

niche. Clomipramine, developed in the early 1960s and approved in Europe in 1970, was never approved for marketing as an antidepressant in the United States, perhaps due to a crowded field. It became more popular as the earliest pharmacological treatment for OCD and has been approved for such in the United States.

Although miraculous for many patients, TCAs' heavily anticholinergic and antihistaminic side effects (e.g., sedation, 30–40 lb weight gain, dry mouth, constipation, urinary retention, blurred vision) and their ability to elongate the QRS complex and cause cardiac death in overdose were of constant concern. Because TCAs were placed in the hands of patients who often evidenced suicidal risk, limited amounts were prescribed at a time. Even when effectively reducing the risk of suicide, these agents' poor tolerability led to the practice of treating symptoms for about a year, tapering and stopping their use, and then monitoring for recurrence—which would necessitate resumption of the same medication.

Trazodone was briefly popular in the mid-1980s as a novel compound antidepressant, described as a serotonin receptor antagonist and reuptake inhibitor (Fagiolini et al. 2012). It causes heavy sedation at doses of 50–150 mg, which is problematic because the fully effective antidepressant dosage is often 300–450 mg. Trazodone was explored as a potentiator of other antidepressants in difficult-to-treat cases and, as discussed later, as a tool to reduce sexual side effects from SSRIs. It finally found its broadest use as a sedative. It also carries a risk of priapism (spontaneous and sustained penile erection), more rarely reported with some other psychotropic medications (Thompson et al. 1990). Although the incidence of this side effect has been difficult to determine, it has been reported as high as 12% in some populations (Warner et al. 2001).

As a result, the appearance of the SSRI fluoxetine in 1987 was a welcome step forward. Fluoxetine offered, for the first time, an effective and well-tolerated antidepressant. Unlike the MAOIs and TCAs that required expert titration over weeks or months, the 20-mg fluoxetine capsule or pill was the starting *and* usually the final dosage, so practitioners with much less experience could manage it. In addition, fluoxetine raised little to no concern about death from overdose.

Because of these simple but important changes, fluoxetine—followed in 1992 by sertraline and paroxetine—greatly expanded public acceptance not only of antidepressant treatment but also of depression itself. Prozac, the U.S. brand name for fluoxetine, became a cultural meme, often the tagline for any reference to needing mental health care. The popular press book *Listening to Prozac* (Kramer 1993) and its counterpoint *Talking Back to Prozac* (Breggin and Breggin 1994) illustrated how treatment that was once mentioned only in hushed terms was now discussed candidly. Depression became less stigmatized as potential patients sought help. Nonpsychiatrists became the major prescribers of antidepressants (Mark et al. 2009).

Fluoxetine and the other SSRIs have similar efficacy to TCAs—neither better nor worse. What revolutionized the treatment of major depression was not efficacy but the dramatic improvement in tolerability. No longer did patients experience a 30- to 40-lb weight gain or increased sedation. In fact, fluoxetine was at first thought by some to induce weight *loss*. Studies later confirmed that patients who were switched from TCAs to fluoxetine were losing the weight they had gained from the TCAs. Similarly, although clinicians could count on the sedation from TCAs aiding insomnia in patients with depression early in treatment, this no longer occurred. Fluoxetine was then accused of causing insomnia. Further work clarified that fluoxetine was not inducing insomnia in the vast majority of patients but merely was not sedating them as the TCAs had done. In 1994, a paper proposed that because patients with depression, some early in treatment, might still be experiencing insomnia, trazodone could be added to sedate them (Nierenberg et al. 1994). This became an overnight fad that continues to this day, unfortunately sometimes also in patients with bipolar depression (we must always fully understand the rationale for our choices and not just follow the crowd). Over the decades, many attempts to show additional benefits or harms from fluoxetine and other SSRIs have led to the result that SSRIs are of average efficacy in treating major depression, with relatively low side effect profiles.

The other significant change ushered in by these first three SSRIs was in the duration of treatment. Again, because of the serious side effects of the TCAs, patients were often treated for only 12–18 months at a time and were then monitored for recurrence, which then provoked reinstitution of treatment. Once patients receiving fluoxetine, sertraline, or paroxetine improved to the point of remission and tolerated the medication very well, they came to resist these "drug holidays," asking to remain on the medication rather than risking relapse into debilitating and painful major depression. The profession responded, and studies showing sustained efficacy for long-term use were completed. Chronic, sustained treatment became the fashion, and recurrences declined. When clinicians explore the reasons for the significant increase in the prescription of antidepressants over the past several decades, long-term use appears to be a significant factor (Moore et al. 2009).

Other SSRIs became available. Citalopram, initially unavailable in the United States because it killed beagle dogs in early toxicity tests, became a very popular SSRI in the rest of the world once it was determined that a different metabolism in humans made it safer (U.S. Food and Drug Administration 2012). It was introduced into the United States in 1998, followed by its biologically active racemic fraction, escitalopram, in 2002. The function and results of these two preparations are the same, but the later, purer version requires about half the dose strength. Fluvoxamine was approved in the United States in 1994. Although it was used elsewhere for the treatment of major depression, the manufacturing company chose to initially market it in the United States specifically for OCD, but practitioners were allowed to (and often did) choose it to treat major depression (see "Medications to Treat Impulse-Control Problems" later in this chapter).

Although SSRI side effects are few, several do require further discussion: reduction in sexual desire, anorgasmia, and discontinuation syndrome. The use of TCAs, MAOIs, and SNRIs can also lead to sexual side effects. The responsible mechanism of action has yet to be confirmed, but the SSRIs most specific for enhancing serotonin transmission, paroxetine and citalopram, have been implicated as carrying the greatest risk for sexual side effects, and SNRIs and bupropion have measurably lower risks in the totality of studies. Although erectile dysfunction is reported from antidepressants, the incidence is lower than that for anorgasmia and low desire. Note that the incidence of these latter two sexual side effects is about 30%–60% in controlled studies, but only if the participants are asked directly about them. If sexual desire and performance questions are not included in the assessment, self-report incidence is significantly lower. When evaluating the potential side effects of new antidepressants, determine whether the study participants were asked directly about sexual side effects. Pharmaceutical representatives have been known to exploit this difference to imply their product has fewer sexual side effects than competitors (Higgins et al. 2010; Jing and Straw-Wilson 2016). Several pharmacological strategies have been investigated for reversing or limiting these sexual side effects, with little demonstrated effect shown in RCTs (e.g., trazodone, cyproheptadine, yohimbine, amantadine); a switch to another antidepressant, such as bupropion, appears to be more helpful (Clayton et al. 2001; Michelson et al. 2000). Some clinicians have proposed drug holidays to relieve this side effect, but given that most SSRIs achieve steady-state serum levels in 5 days (and much longer with fluoxetine), such holidays are really not helpful for most patients.

Discontinuation syndrome was first recognized in the early 1980s as "withdrawal" from TCAs that occurred once a drug was no longer being taken, especially abruptly (Dilsaver and Greden 1984), and was subsequently attributed to each category of antidepressant that involved the enhancement of serotonergic transmission (Agelink et al. 1997; Curtin et al. 2002; Peabody 1987). We generally reserve the term *withdrawal* to refer to medically dangerous syndromes caused by the absence of an agent (e.g., alcohol, barbiturates, and benzodiazepines), so the term *discontinuation syndrome* is more accurate here (Schatzberg et al. 1997). By 2005, SSRIs, MAOIs, TCAs, and SNRIs all carried changes in medication labeling reflecting this phenomenon, but the syndrome is most closely identified with the SSRIs, which are most commonly used and lack many other annoying side effects. Discontinuation syndrome involves flu-like symptoms, such as nausea, dizziness, headaches, fatigue, and possibly vertigo and myalgias; paresthesia, including "electric shocks"; and anxiety and agitation (Berber 1998; Black et al. 2000; Warner et al. 2006). Loss of the clinical benefit provided by the antidepressant may also occur, of course, and the patient's mood may drop precipitously. These symptoms can be very frightening, so the possibility of discontinuation syndrome from self or prescribed cessation of serotonergic medications, especially when rapid, or from missed doses of those with shorter half-lives (e.g., venlafaxine), must be discussed at the time of initial treatment planning. Patients should also be advised in advance that the syndrome is quickly reversible by resuming the medication and is not lethal. Some patients will not find this risk acceptable, and that will inform their treatment choice.

The risk of discontinuation syndrome is minimized either by choosing medications with long half-lives (e.g., fluoxetine) that "taper" themselves over weeks or by prescribing a reasonable taper schedule. Taking half-life into account, reduce the dose by the minimum increment possible every 14 days, even halving the final dose or prescribing it every other day for the final 14 days. Some patients will be more sensitive to discontinuation symptoms than others, and the symptoms may be more noticeable as the lowest doses are reached. In these cases, after prescribing the lowest dose every other day for 14 days, you may find it effective to stretch the taper by giving the same dose every 3 days for 14 days, then every 4 days, and so on, until the symptoms are absent or minimal. Another frequently effective strategy is to change from an agent with a shorter half-life to an alternative with a longer one, especially fluoxetine (which has the longest). If the shorter half-life agent is stopped when the fluoxetine is begun, however, discontinuation syndrome may still occur, because it takes fluoxetine about 6 weeks to reach a steady-state serum level. Thus, this strategy requires adding fluoxetine to the medication being tapered. Give both medications for 6 weeks until fluoxetine is fully established, then abruptly stop both medications. The fluoxetine will linger in the body for about another 6 weeks and will block the discontinuation syndrome from the first agent. The fluoxetine must be stopped at the same time as the first agent to allow it to begin its taper, otherwise it will take months to eliminate it with an unnecessarily extended taper. You should be fairly certain that the diagnosis of major depression is correct, because this taper plan involves overlapping two antidepressants for 6 weeks, which may provoke mood cycling in patients with bipolar disorder. The possibility of inducing serotonin syndrome (see Chapter 11) must also be considered. The key to minimizing the risk of discontinuation syndrome is the serotonergic agent leaving the body slowly (Schatzberg et al. 2006). Of course, if the underlying major depression has not been adequately treated or returns, these decisions must be made in the context of protecting the patient from the risks of the illness as well.

Another way to avoid discontinuation syndrome is by choosing an antidepressant that does not affect serotonin. Bupropion, described as a norepinephrine-dopamine reuptake inhibitor, is also a releasing agent for norepinephrine and dopamine and, through active metabolites, a nicotinic acetylcholine receptor antagonist. Again, these receptor descriptions are listed for classification reasons and not as a proven mechanism of action for the clinical outcome. Thus, bupropion does not affect serotonin, giving it an almost unique status in contemporary psychopharmacology. This, plus its effect on dopamine, has been theorized to lead to another demonstrated clinical feature mentioned earlier—a potential effect on reversing the sexual side effects of SSRIs. When added to SSRI treatment, bupropion offers a more than 50% chance of improved sexual desire and orgasmic function. When used alone, it has a very low incidence of sexual side effects and has been found to enhance sexual desire and performance (Jing and Straw-Wilson 2016; Modell et al. 1997; Montgomery 2008).

Bupropion was released in the United States in 1989 as a short-acting antidepressant taken three times a day. In 1996, it became available in a twice-daily sustained-release form and in 2003 as a once-daily extended-release pill. Due to its effect on reducing nicotine use, it was marketed separately as Wellbutrin for treating major depression and as Zyban for smoking cessation. Aplenzin, a hydrobromide-based version (compared with the standard hydrochloride) that allows once-daily strengths of 174 mg (equivalent to 150 mg of the hydrochloride version), 348 mg (300 mg of hydrochloride version), and 522 mg (450 mg of hydrochloride version), debuted in the United States in 2008. Forfivo XL, which appeared in the United States in 2012, offers 450 mg of the hydrochloride-based version in one extended-release pill. For this reason, practitioners must be aware that bupropion, bupropion SR, bupropion XL, Wellbutrin, Wellbutrin SR, Wellbutrin XL, Zyban, Aplenzin, and Forfivo XL all have the exact same active ingredient and should never be combined; toxic levels predispose to seizures. This illustrates why clinicians should never prescribe or refill other practitioners' prescriptions unless absolutely sure they know exactly what they are prescribing. Patients also are not likely to know this information and may have medications at home that they think are safe to add to a prescription, for example, taking an old prescription of Zyban when they feel the urge to smoke while also receiving bupropion. As discussed in Chapters 3 and 12, practitioners must clarify with patients, at every visit, every medication they have available at home or by refill and explain any duplications or interactions.

Two additional clinical points can be illustrated by the history of the development of bupropion for human use: making erroneous assumptions based on 1) warnings from the FDA or 2) the experimenter's choice of dosing for pivotal studies (those presented to the FDA seeking marketing approval). First, in the mid-1980s, when bupropion was in Phase II and III studies prior to its release in the United States, a Phase III study testing efficacy and safety in patients with bulimia showed an unexpectedly high risk of seizure: 6 of 40 study participants. Approval was put on hold, and thousands more patients were studied for safety. This level of seizure activity was never replicated, yet the FDA only allowed release for treatment of major depression with a strong warning about (and contraindication with) seizures in its medication guide. We know bupropion lowers the sei-zure threshold in humans, so this is a reasonable precaution. Unfortu-nately, many fail to recognize that this risk of seizures is also true of every other antidepressant available, none of which carries this same degree of warning (Steinert and Fröscher 2018). Practitioners must learn that bu-propion carries an additional risk in patients with seizure disorders and in overdose but must not assume it is the only antidepressant that carries this risk, which, sadly, has occurred. Always recall that the absence of data or, in this case, the absence of *reference to data*, is not a negative or positive result; each medication must be remembered for its own risks. Do not over-simplify or fall for clinical gossip (see Chapter 2). Again, relying solely upon the FDA medication guide is inadequate.

Second, bupropion was initially available in 100-mg and 150-mg strengths, either strength given three times a day. The FDA recommended safe dosages as 100 mg or 150 mg three times a day, based on the pivotal studies submitted, and a maximum total daily dosage of 450 mg. When the sustained-release version was developed, it was tested in strengths of 100 mg and 200 mg to be given twice a day at least 8 hours apart. Patients should be reminded that this means 8 hours not only between the morning and afternoon or evening doses but also between the evening and morning doses. Therefore, based on these pivotal studies, the FDA recommended a maximum safe dosage of the sustained-release version as 400 mg/day. When the extended-release version, 150 mg and 300 mg, was tested, dos-ages up to 450 mg/day were again tried and found safe, and thus the FDA again recommended 450 mg/day as the highest safe dosage (Table 7–3). All these versions have same active ingredient; their differences are based solely on pill or capsule strength and experimental formulation. Do not be confused or misled by experimental design or bureaucracy. Instead, noting details will expose the situation rationally.

Patients, and some providers, believe that the FDA reviews all known data and makes comprehensive suggestions about each drug it approves or denies. Actually, the FDA responds to studies that are *submitted* when seeking initial approval and to data *submitted* for postmarketing review when a particular committee meets to make a decision. The FDA is not a clearinghouse for all ongoing information about a medication, and its comments are not always as comprehensive or current as assumed, al-though it is making progress with postmarketing surveillance.

After the popular emergence of SSRIs, new SNRIs, similar to the older TCAs, began to appear. Venlafaxine became available in the United States in late 1993 but had difficulty finding widespread use because of its ex-tremely short half-life and uncomfortable discontinuation symptoms. As

TABLE 7–3. FDA-approved maximum dosages for bupropion formulations

Bupropion	150 mg	Three times a day
Bupropion SR (sustained release)	200 mg	Twice a day, ≥8 hours apart
Bupropion XL (extended release)	450 mg	Once a day

a result, dosing was three times a day as opposed to the once a day used with SSRIs and older TCAs. Also, many patients reported feeling the discontinuation side effects (particularly nausea and dizziness) three times a day. A once-daily long-acting version was released in 1997 that was far better tolerated as long as patients were warned about the prominent discontinuation side effects if they stopped taking their medication abruptly or forgot doses. Venlafaxine's active metabolite desvenlafaxine (released in the United States in 2008) further increased tolerability by reducing the 10% chance of first-week nausea. Along with promising remission data, these changes led to broader acceptance and the search for additional new SNRIs. Duloxetine was approved in the United States in 2004. Its clinical characteristics are similar to venlafaxine hydrochloride, although duloxetine affects norepinephrine relative to serotonin at a fixed ratio across the dosage range. Venlafaxine affects serotonin more strongly at lower doses; the percentage affecting norepinephrine increases as doses increase above the standard 150-mg dose (Shelton 2018).

As clever marketers have pointed out, duloxetine can have a beneficial nonnarcotic effect on treating pain, and for this reason many nonpsychopharmacologists favor its use when selecting antidepressants. What is less well known is that the same benefit has been demonstrated for every SNRI, including the TCAs; the benefit exists in treating *neuropathic* and other central pain syndromes, including fibromyalgia (Obata 2017). Therefore, changing from one SNRI to another merely to treat pain, even neuropathic pain, is not rational.

More recent SNRIs include milnacipran and levomilnacipran, which preferentially inhibit norepinephrine over serotonin. The former is approved in the United States and Australia for fibromyalgia (Palmer et al. 2010) but is approved for major depression in Europe and Japan (Nakagawa et al. 2009). Levomilnacipran, its more potent L-enantiomer, was approved for adults with major depression in the United States in 2013. As with citalopram and escitalopram, the two medications contain the same active ingredient (Bruno et al. 2016).

The tetracyclic agent maprotiline is sometimes listed with the TCAs, although it is currently considered a selective norepinephrine reuptake inhibitor, along with atomoxetine, reboxetine, and viloxazine (used in Europe from 1976 to early 2000s but no longer produced). Maprotiline is a weaker inhibitor of serotonin reuptake than of norepinephrine and is still available, although it has largely been forgotten by most practitioners. Reboxetine has never been approved for marketing in the United States, although it is available in some countries in Europe and elsewhere. Conflicting reports show no efficacy or adequate efficacy for it compared with placebo (Cipriani et al. 2009; Medicines and Healthcare Products Regulatory Agency 2011). Atomoxetine has failed to show sufficient efficacy in treating major depression but has been approved by the FDA for treating ADHD (Kratochvil et al. 2005).

Other antidepressants are classified as *atypical* because they do not fit neatly into the TCA, SSRI, SNRI, MAOI, or other categories of description. Mirtazapine became available in the United States 1996 as a unique noradrenergic and specific serotonergic antidepressant. It has many effects at the synapse, which, remember, we are using more for classification than for predicting clinical response. Mirtazapine creates an increase in 5-HT_1 neurotransmission by blocking 5-HT_2 and 5-HT_3 heteroreceptors, plus it enhances norepinephrine release due to blockade of presynaptic autoreceptors through antagonism of α_2-adrenergic receptors (de Boer 1996; Watanabe et al. 2011). Mirtazapine also has one of the more unique side effect profiles in psychopharmacology: more side effects occur at lower (15–30 mg) than higher doses (45–60 mg), particularly increased appetite (with probable weight gain) and increased sedation. Oncologists sometimes prescribe low dosages to help chemotherapy patients with appetite and sleep. Therefore, in psychiatry, start treatment at 45 mg because starting lower may lead to excessive sedation for some patients, so much so that they may refuse to raise the dose despite an explanation. Emotion often trumps logic if it is counterintuitive. Similarly, when discontinuing mirtazapine, a taper of the dose will likely lead to more side effects than found in discontinuation syndrome. Either cessation without taper or a rapid 3-day taper is usually preferable. Remember, a cross taper of a longer-acting SSRI may also help with serotonergic discontinuation syndrome.

Nefazodone, introduced to the U.S. market in 1994, is still available in generic form in the United States but is not available in Canada. It has been largely abandoned since 2003 due to a rare risk of hepatotoxicity. Vilazodone can be listed as an SSRI but is also a 5-HT_{1A} receptor partial agonist. Clinically, little distinguishes vilazodone from other options; it has been available in the United States since 2011. Vortioxetine, considered a serotonin receptor modulator and an inhibitor of the serotonin transporter, was approved in the United States and Europe in 2013 and in Canada in 2014. Interestingly, its U.S. brand name Brintellix was changed to Trintellix in 2016 to avoid confusion with the platelet aggregation inhibitor brand named Brilinta. Outside of North America, it is still sold as Brintellix. Efforts are under way to demonstrate that vortioxetine may improve cognitive processing speed, independent of its effect on mood, when used to treat major depression (McIntyre et al. 2014). In 2018, this effect was added to its labeling by the FDA. Because we expect all symptoms of a syndrome to respond to primary treatment, and cognitive impairment is a hallmark of major depression, more studies clearly demonstrating the superiority of vortioxetine over other antidepressants in improving processing speed are sought (Katona et al. 2012; Mahableshwarkar et al. 2015).

Perhaps the most recent breakthrough in the pharmacological treatment of major depression is ketamine—not necessarily as a treatment itself but certainly as a research tool. Used for half a century for anesthesia, particularly in children and animals, it is known to have hallucinogenic properties and can be a drug of abuse, although ketamine does not produce as severe an emergence delirium as its analogue and predecessor phencyclidine (Li and Vlisides 2016). Not until 2006 was it observed to rapidly reverse the symptoms of major depression (Zarate et al. 2006). Due to low bioavailability from oral and rectal dosing, ketamine is administered intravenously. Remarkably, even single doses have been observed to reverse depressed mood and suicidal ideation within 24 hours in patients with major depression, the benefits lasting up to a week (Murrough et al. 2013, 2015). A recent Cochrane meta-analysis was less enthusiastic, noting the still-limited number of studies, with those available having little replication and often inadequate blinding (McCloud et al. 2015). Ketamine appears to noncompetitively antagonize the NMDA receptor, one type of glutamatergic receptor, in two ways (Orser et al. 1997). Interestingly, ketamine is composed of the enantiomers S(+) and R(–). The S(+) isomer esketamine appears to be better tolerated and more effective in anesthesia, whereas the R(–) form is more tolerable and potent for the treatment of major depression (Li and Vlisides 2016; Zhang et al. 2014). It is a novel antidepressant compound, structurally and neurochemically, and therefore a potentially valuable research tool to better understand the pathophysiology of the disorder and to discover treatments that are similar but better tolerated and easier to use.

Unfortunately, enthusiasm over ketamine for the treatment of major depression has already tempted too many practitioners into questionable practice. Clinics have popped up all over the United States selling treatments for $350–$1,000 each, often without adequate evaluation or supervision (Thielking 2018). Even if this burst of treatment is motivated by compassion and duty rather than greed, it seriously outstrips the science available. The American Psychiatric Association, in an attempt to rein in this practice, has released a set of standards for ketamine use that stresses an evidence-based approach in the face of limited data (Sanacora et al. 2017). The United States approved esketamine nasal spray for limited adjunctive use with an oral antidepressant in 2019, despite concerns about the risk that it provoked very disturbing dissociative symptoms (Correia-Melo et al. 2017). The FDA mandated that it be given in the office by a practitioner, who must then monitor the patient for 2 hours after administration. The patient may not take the mediation home, given additional concerns about abuse (U.S. Food and Drug Administration 2019).

Rapastinel, an NMDA receptor glycine site partial agonist, has demonstrated efficacy for major depression in phase II studies. The antidepressant effects at this early stage of investigation appear to be long lasting, as well as particularly helpful for cognition. Although ketamine and other NMDA receptor agents have shown a high risk of psychotomimetic side effects, rapastinel has not (although research continues). Rapastinel received "breakthrough therapy" designation by the FDA in 2016, which accords it expedited review (Donello et al. 2019; Moskal et al. 2014, 2017; Preskorn et al. 2015; Ragguett et al. 2019; U.S. Food and Drug Administration 2018; Vasilescu et al. 2017). In 2019, however, data from three acute Phase III trials showed lack of efficacy, and recruitment by the manufacturer for studies in the treatment of depression have been abandoned (ClinicalTrials.gov 2019; Psychiatry and Behavioral Health Learning Network 2019).

In this section, antidepressants have been discussed as though they are only efficacious in treating major depression (see Table 7–4 for characteristics of those most commonly used). This feature gave this group of mixed structures and neurochemical effects a name. In psychopharmacology, some names are structural (e.g., TCA), some are related to observed neurochemical effects (e.g., SNRI), and some to observed clinical action (e.g., antidepressant). Thus, some medicines carry two labels, such as both SSRI and antidepressant. When naming by clinical action or result, the habit has been to award the name to the first demonstrated clinical effect. This is why some *antidepressants* also treat anxiety disorders and OCD. When considerable confusion resulted after anticonvulsants were also found to be effective as mood stabilizers and antimigraine agents, they were renamed *neuromodulators* so practitioners would quit arguing with and confusing

TABLE 7–4.   Characteristics of commonly used antidepressants

Antidepressant	Starting dose, mg	Average dose, mg	Daily maximum dose,[a] mg	Common side effects
Bupropion	100–150	300	400–450	Dry mouth, constipation
Citalopram	20	40–60	60	Sexual, discontinuation syndrome
Desvenlafaxine	50	50	100	Sexual, discontinuation syndrome, gastrointestinal
Duloxetine	20	60–80	120	Sexual, nausea, discontinuation syndrome
Escitalopram	5	20	20	Sexual, discontinuation syndrome
Fluoxetine	20	20–40	80	Sexual, gastrointestinal
Fluvoxamine	50	150	300	Sexual, discontinuation syndrome
Paroxetine	10–20	40–60	80	Sexual, discontinuation syndrome, anticholinergic
Sertraline	25–50	150	300	Sexual, gastrointestinal, discontinuation syndrome
Venlafaxine XL	37.5	150	225–375[b]	Sexual, discontinuation syndrome, gastrointestinal, hypertension
Vortioxetine	10	10–20	20	Gastrointestinal, anticholinergic, discontinuation syndrome, sexual, abnormal dreams

[a]These values may exceed published maximum doses when supported by the literature and clinical necessity, while maintaining safety. Be particularly alert for toxicities.

[b]Due to pivotal study choices, 225 mg is the maximum for extended-release (XL) and 375 mg is the maximum for immediate-release forms, although it is the same parent compound.

each other. Again, explaining this to patients helps them understand why they should take an antidepressant when they are not depressed.

Medications to Treat Psychosis

Whereas medications used to treat anxiety are often referred to as *minor tranquilizers*, those prescribed to treat psychosis are commonly referred to as *major tranquilizers* as well as *neuroleptics* and *antipsychotics*. If we think of the term *tranquilizer* to imply an antianxiety effect, this can be achieved with both major and minor classes, but medicines that specifically treat psychosis are distinguished by this separate therapeutic advantage (see King and Voruganti 2002).

The antihypertensive agent reserpine was discovered in the 1950s to calm and reverse psychotic symptoms in affected patients. Due to its hypotensive effects (its original indication) and its ability to deplete monoamines and lead to depressive symptoms, reserpine could not be used in many cases; by the 1960s, it was relegated to a role as a research tool in psychopharmacology (Preskorn 2007).

By 1952, chlorpromazine, developed from promethazine and originally used as an anesthetic in France, was found to also reverse the positive symptoms of psychosis. *Positive symptoms* are features we wish were not present, such as hallucinations and delusions. In contrast, *negative symptoms* are missing features, such as blunted affect, poverty of speech and thought content, apathy, anhedonia, poor socialization, and loss of motivation (Foussias and Remington 2010). Chlorpromazine is a phenothiazine derivative, as are many subsequent antipsychotic medications. Its action in blocking dopaminergic D_2 receptors led to the dopamine theory of psychosis (Carpenter and Davis 2012).

The success with chlorpromazine, despite its significant sedation, postural hypotension, and Parkinson-like side effects, led to the rapid development and release of several new antipsychotics by 1975 (Shen 1999). Among the most successful were haloperidol, trifluoperazine, thioridazine, thiothixene, and fluphenazine. Haloperidol, a butyrophenone, was particularly well known and used across many specialties (Granger and Albu 2005). It has less sedation than chlorpromazine but more acute movement side effects (discussed later). Thioridazine was popular among psychiatrists as well; like chlorpromazine, it is sedating and carries a side effect of retinopathy at dosages greater than 800 mg/day (Richa and Yazbek 2010).

These earlier medications are known as *first-generation antipsychotics* (FGAs). This generally means they carry the highest risk of tardive dyskinesia (TD; Cornett et al. 2017) and are primarily associated with D_2 blockade. Clinically, they have their best outcome on the positive symptoms of psychosis and are significantly less effective on the negative symptoms. They are further subdivided by their dosing and side effect profiles into high- and low-potency FGAs.

Low-potency means higher doses are necessary to produce clinical effect (up to 800 mg for thiothixene and chlorpromazine). Low-potency agents carry similar side effect profiles: sedation, orthostatic hypotension, and greater anticholinergic side effects (i.e., dry mouth, constipation, urinary retention). *Higher-potency* agents reverse psychotic symptoms at lower doses (5–10 mg for haloperidol, 1–5 mg for trifluoperazine). They also have characteristic side effect profiles: less sedation but more akathisia (restless agitation), acute dystonic reactions, and extrapyramidal syndrome (EPS). EPS, also called pseudoparkinsonian side effects, includes cogwheel rigidity, bradykinesia, and resting "pill-rolling" tremor.

Both potencies of FGA or "typical" antipsychotics often lead to excessive weight gain, increased nicotine use (see "Chapter 9, "Nicotine"), and elevated prolactin levels, which can lead to gynecomastia and galactorrhea as well as decreased fertility after intercourse (Marken et al. 1992). In practice, this infertility is reversed when the medication is reduced or discontinued; patients may not realize that some method of birth control should be continued if conception is not in their plans. Some side effects of FGAs may be modified by adding additional medications. For example, EPS may be ameliorated by adding anticholinergic agents such as diphenhydramine, trihexyphenidyl, and benztropine or the glutamate receptor antagonist amantadine (DiMascio et al. 1976). Use of these agents may worsen TD, however, although some limited evidence indicates this exacerbation may reverse with their discontinuation (Desmarais et al. 2014). Screening for movement disorders with a neurological examination and standard scales, such as the Abnormal Involuntary Movement Scale, can help detect and counter TD, tremor, and other EPS symptoms (Citrome 2017; Munetz and Benjamin 1988).

The "atypical" or second-generation antipsychotic (SGA) medications, introduced with clozapine, are distinguished from the older antipsychotics by having a lower risk of TD (<1% annually compared with 5% annually), greater efficacy with the negative symptoms of psychosis, and, with some, fewer EPS symptoms (Correll et al. 2004; Waln and Jankovic 2013). Clozapine was developed in 1958 in Switzerland but was not approved in the United States until 1990 because of concern it could produce neutropenia and eventual life-threatening agranulocytosis (Atkin et al. 1996; Crilly 2007). As in most of Europe, it was released with the requirement that weekly complete blood counts be obtained and presented to a registry and pharmacy prior to weekly release of the medication to a patient (Honigfeld et al. 1998). The U.S. registry was revised in 2016 and became the Clozapine Risk Evaluation and Mitigation Strategy.

Current practitioner requirements for clozapine include registration plus documented education and testing about the risk of neutropenia. Also required is blood monitoring of a patient's absolute neutrophil count weekly for the first 6 months, every 2 weeks for the next 6 months, and then monthly for the duration of treatment, provided it remains within parameters (U.S. Food and Drug Administration 2020). Once again, this may illustrate how publicizing one risk of one medication may lead the unaware clinician to false security about other problems and medications. In fact, the risk of severe neutropenia is similar in all antipsychotics (Crilly 2007; Ingimarsson et al. 2016), and all patients receiving them should be monitored initially and then episodically. The FDA did not trust physicians to monitor clozapine without strict requirements (Crilly 2007). Unfortunately, these mandates also helped deemphasize the need to monitor similar medications and to look for additional adverse events, such as diabetic ketoacidosis and gastrointestinal hypomotility (Cohen et al. 2012). Rational psychopharmacologists must comply with—but not rely solely upon—governmental polices to fully understand the risks of treatments they are providing. Otherwise, informed consent and patient safety may be compromised.

Clozapine was found to be a particularly effective antipsychotic, especially with the negative and mood-related symptoms of psychosis. It also showed a 30% chance of reversing psychosis that had previously been unresponsive to treatment, compared with a 4% chance with chlorpromazine in this population (Kane et al. 1988). This improved effect of SGAs on negative symptoms, well demonstrated clinically in RCTs, is theorized to be a result of effects on serotonin receptors, a feature that carries implications for their use in mood disorders that include thought disorder symptoms, such as bipolar disorder (Fornaro et al. 2016).

In fact, many pharmaceutical companies have attempted successfully to increase their market share by marketing the SGAs for mood disorders, especially affective-based psychoses. Some have even gone so far as to seek FDA approval for promoting SGAs as monotreatment for bipolar disorder, overlooking standard mood stabilizers (López-Muñoz et al. 2018). Some supporting studies are compromised by design; others are accepted (Goodwin et al. 2016). Even if SGAs are found to have comparable efficacy with mood stabilizers, they still carry the risk of permanent TD, EPS, and prolactin elevation (Peuskens et al. 2014), something traditional mood stabilizers do not (see "Medications to Stabilize Mood"). Any clinicians planning to use SGAs in this way must discuss these additional risks with patients and seek their agreement prior to prescription.

The serotonergic activity of atypical antipsychotics appears strongest at the lowest dosages and is suppressed at higher dosages by dopaminergic activity (Remington and Kapur 1999). As I mentioned in Chapters 2 and 4, SGAs have been found useful in potentiating the effects of antidepressant treatment in treatment-resistant cases, usually at lower dosages (Barbee et al. 2004; Lane et al. 1998; Philip et al. 2008). This may also explain why, early in their use, reports of treatment-induced mania were published that initially confused practitioners because antipsychotics usually have been considered treatments for manic psychosis (Baldaçara et al. 2007; Nolan and Schulte 2003). Serotonin stimulation at low dosages would be expected to destabilize a patient with bipolar disorder, possibly into mania, although this might not always be the explanation (Benyamina and Samalin 2012; Ichikawa et al. 2001; Kavoor et al. 2014; Rachid et al. 2004).

Clozapine also has more side effects related to antihistaminic and anticholinergic activity, and it lowers the seizure threshold even more than antidepressants and other antipsychotics (which all increase seizure risk). The weight gain from it is significant, the mean being 30 lb, as is excessive salivation, which may lead to constant drooling or choking. Postural hypotension and sedation also are often problematic. Its benefit is in new efficacy, especially with negative symptoms, plus a very low rate of EPS and TD. Titration of clozapine is very slow, starting at 25 mg three times a day and progressing to no more than 300 mg three times a day, if well tolerated, safe, and necessary, all with ongoing monitoring through the registry. The concomitant use of anticonvulsants is often suggested (Nucifora et al. 2017).

Although clozapine was an important breakthrough, many patients declined or could not tolerate it. In 1993, the United States approved the marketing of the second available SGA, risperidone. Like clozapine and many medications in this group, risperidone weakly blocks D_2 and offers potent postsynaptic 5-HT_2 receptor blockade. The neurochemical effects of this clinically defined group of antipsychotics differ. Unfortunately, EPS problems (especially muscle rigidity) are common with risperidone, particularly at the higher target dosages initially suggested by the FDA: 4–8 mg/day for adult schizophrenia (U.S. Food and Drug Administration 2009). Rather quickly, lower dosages of 2–4 mg/day were adopted that reduced the incidence of EPS (Kopala et al. 1997). Time to first antipsychotic response appears to be short, 5–6 days, so this medication might be an option when rapid effect is of prime importance (Mousavi et al. 2013). Risperidone's active metabolite, paliperidone, was released in long-acting oral form in 2007 so it could be given only once a day. Both produce the highest degree of hyperprolactinemia of any of the SGAs (Leucht et al.

2013), as well as more movement disorders, a possible reason patient drop-out for the drug is 47% for risperidone, although many reviewed studies used the higher and more poorly tolerated initial dosage recommendations (Komossa et al. 2011).

Olanzapine, which entered the U.S. market in 1996, carries a similar neurochemical profile to clozapine, and although its side effects are also similar, they are milder. Whereas clozapine is a low-potency medication, olanzapine, at 10–20 mg nightly, is high potency but offers sedation and less EPS than risperidone (Meyer and Simpson 1997). Like clozapine, it is known for causing weight gain (Tschoner et al. 2009).

Quetiapine was introduced in the United States in 1997. Although another atypical antipsychotic, it has a side effect profile similar to the low-potency FGAs, particularly thioridazine, with its degree of sedation. It was originally directed for twice-daily dosing, but it became rapidly apparent that patients could not tolerate the daytime sedation. Bedtime dosing, also adequate, became the rule. A brief titration, even with bedtime dosing, is still necessary, because quetiapine is about twice as sedating the first week as later. Therefore, half the target dose may be given for the first 7 days before moving to the full dose (≤ 800 mg), 200–400 mg being most common. Sadly, too many nonpsychopharmacologists prescribe lower doses of 25–100 mg solely for sleep, an irrational practice given far-safer options that do not carry a risk of TD or weight gain (see "Medications to Treat Sleep Problems" section). Some clinicians, as noted previously, like to provide sedation at night for their patients even though it has little to do with the primary outcome of treatment, and quetiapine may certainly provide this when indicated.

In 2008, an extended-release version of quetiapine was released that confused less-careful prescribers. Compared with the rapid onset of sedation of the immediate-release preparation, the extended-release form delays sedation by about 4 hours. Patients taking it at bedtime, therefore, experience no particular sedation (which is therapeutically acceptable), but the sedation that is triggered 4 hours into their sleep persists into the middle of the next day, preventing many from attending work or school. The extended-release version should be administered about 4 hours prior to bedtime, around dinner time for most people. No preferential clinical benefit is had by using this form, and the immediate-release version is easier for most patients to manage.

Ziprasidone was approved in Sweden in 1998, although concerns about electrocardiological QT prolongation delayed its U.S. approval until 2001. Its absorption is enhanced by food intake at the time of dosing. Ziprasidone is more difficult to tolerate at lower than higher doses. Thus, early titration may be difficult because many patients will refuse to move to higher doses, expecting worse side effects. Starting with 40–60 mg twice a day with quick titration up to 80 mg twice a day might be more successful than slower titration regimens (Mattei et al. 2011). Little else distinguishes the oral form from its fellow atypical antipsychotics, except maybe lower weight gain (Tschoner et al. 2009) and less sedation.

Ziprasidone, however, was the first SGA to be developed into a short-acting intramuscular version. This produces more rapid antipsychotic effects than intramuscular preparations of older antipsychotics (Sheehan 2003). Initial use of the intramuscular form at 20 mg may be repeated after 4 hours, for a daily maximum of 40 mg (roughly equivalent to 160 mg of oral), which may then be followed by twice-daily oral doses of 80 mg. This allows quick initiation of treatment in emergency situations (Sheehan 2003) or avoidance of the bothersome side effects of lower doses.

Sometimes referred to as a third-generation antipsychotic, the atypical antipsychotic aripiprazole became available in the United States in 2002 and in the United Kingdom in 2004. For classification purposes, it is not a traditional D_2 blocker but rather a functionally selective D_{2L} partial agonist (Shapiro et al. 2003). Because of this feature, many were hopeful that, in addition to reversing psychosis, aripiprazole might not lead to TD. Unfortunately, postmarketing surveillance and studies revealed it carries a risk similar to that of other SGAs, another illustration of how clinical medicine is guided by RCT results and not by theory (Carbon et al. 2018; Peña et al. 2011). A high-potency antipsychotic, aripiprazole's longer half-life ($t_{1/2}$ 75 hours for the parent drug and 94 for its active hepatic metabolite dehydroaripiprazole [Winans 2003]) means that final steady-state serum levels are not achieved for 16–20 days. This may delay full therapeutic effect as well as leave a lingering taper of about 3 weeks after abrupt cessation, both of which must be taken into account when switching medications.

Asenapine, first available for U.S. clinicians in 2009, has less risk of weight gain and prolactin elevation than many SGAs. Its sedation is close to but less than that of olanzapine (Leucht et al. 2013). Meta-analysis of studies comparing asenapine with placebo and olanzapine show it to be efficacious, although mostly inferior to the active comparator, albeit with a safer metabolic profile (Orr et al. 2017). Asenapine is the only antipsychotic medication available in sublingual form. This was developed to exploit its enhanced bioavailability through buccal absorption (35%) compared with oral (2%). Although it dissolves rapidly, it requires more cooperation than medications well absorbed with oral preparations. Enhanced adherence was not found in the referenced study.

Lurasidone entered the U.S. market in 2010 and Europe in 2014 and has been found effective in acute and maintenance treatment of primary psychoses, such as schizophrenia (Tandon et al. 2016). Its half-life of 20–40 hours allows once-daily (evening) dosing between 40 mg and 160 mg, and like quetiapine, its absorption is greatly enhanced with food intake (Loebel and Citrome 2015). Like aripiprazole, lurasidone appears to have a low risk of weight gain (Meyer et al. 2017) and is as well tolerated as most drugs in this class.

Sertindole, amisulpride, and zotepine require footnotes in a discussion of SGAs. Sertindole, which was initially approved in Europe in 1996, had its approval revoked in 1998, followed by restricted reintroduction in 2002. It has never been approved in the United States. Although efficacy has been established (Leucht et al. 2013), concerns over QT prolongation and a high number of associated cardiac deaths (similar to QT prolongation concerns that delayed the approval of quetiapine) led to this outcome (Muscatello et al. 2014). Sertindole should not be used in older patients or those with demonstrated or potential QT interval problems or other cardiac illness. Electrocardiograms are required prior to administration and during treatment in places where it is still available.

Amisulpride was released in the 1990s and is used in Europe, Israel, Mexico, and English-speaking countries except for the United States and Canada, apparently skipping these two countries for business reasons (Psychiatric Times 2004). Efficacy has been demonstrated, but it significantly raises prolactin levels (Curran and Perry 2001; Zhang et al. 2013). FDA approval is currently being sought for its use in postoperative nausea and vomiting (Drugs.com 2019). Also not approved for psychosis in the United States, zotepine has not demonstrated sufficient efficacy due to a limited number of brief studies (Subramanian et al. 2010), and it is no longer available in Germany or the United Kingdom. Its use is mostly limited to Japan.

More than 40% of patients receiving FGAs or SGAs gain weight, with the low-potency FGAs clozapine and olanzapine apparently leading to the greatest gains (Worrel et al. 2000). As noted, aripiprazole, lurasidone, and asenapine show less risk of causing this in RCTs. The risk of metabolic syndrome in patients with primary psychoses treated with antipsychotic medications has been well documented. The American Diabetes Association, American Psychiatric Association, American Association of Clinical Endocrinologists, and North American Association for the Study of Obesity published joint monitoring guidelines in 2004, and others have proposed various monitoring plans (American Diabetes Association et al. 2004; Riordan et al. 2011). Most agree that weight, body mass index (BMI), and waist circumference should be monitored in all patients receiving antipsychotic medication, as well as fasting and 2-hour postprandial blood sugars, hemoglobin A1C, and lipid profiles (discussed in Chapter 12).

Because major tranquilizers are sometimes sedating, be sure to distinguish among sedating patients, calming patients, and reversing patients' psychosis. Many RCTs and review articles mention use of these agents for agitation, but not specifically reversal of psychosis. Keep in mind which symptoms are targeted, agitation or psychosis, when planning treatment and measuring response. Hospital staff given "use as needed" (prn) orders for antipsychotic medications may not use them judiciously, incorrectly equating a quiet, mollified patient with one recovering from psychosis.

Similarly, the concept of rapid neuroleptization was popular during the late 1970s and early 1980s—the idea that rapidly raising serum levels of antipsychotic medications actually produced quicker clinical improvement than the traditional dosing schedules. Within a few years, it became clear that this was a failed initiative with FGAs, because psychosis reversed at the same rate independent of how fast adequate serum levels were achieved. Sedation of the patient made it appear they had improved sooner (Belmaker et al. 1980; Coffman et al. 1987). The short-acting intramuscular forms of the SGAs ziprasidone and, to a lesser degree, olanzapine stand out as the most effective and well-tolerated agents, however, truly offering almost immediate response (Brook et al. 2000; Zimbroff et al. 2005). Four SGAs are available as oral dissolving tablets: clozapine, risperidone, olanzapine, and ziprasidone. Remember that though some patients may prefer them to swallowing pills, dissolving tablets do not act any more rapidly than oral (swallowed) tablets; they are not absorbed sublingually and must enter the gastrointestinal system for absorption (Montgomery et al. 2012; Seager 1998).

Complete antipsychotic response to an oral FGA or SGA will take 4–6 weeks, with the greatest rate of improvement occurring within the first 2 weeks for most medications. Improvement has been demonstrated to begin between the first few days and the first week of treatment, although many clinicians would still find this early result incomplete (Table 7–5). It has been argued, however, that treatment failure from oral dosing might be ascertained at 2 weeks rather than waiting the full 4–6 weeks (Agid et al. 2006). The needs of the patient should guide this strategy, given that premature switching, especially more than once, may actually delay a robust outcome.

In contrast to rapid neuroleptization, so-called depot injections of antipsychotic medications strive for sustained rather than rapid response. The first popular form was an intramuscular injection of fluphenazine decanoate that debuted in 1968. It was primarily used to improve compliance in patients with schizophrenia who would not take their medication

TABLE 7–5. **Time to significant antipsychotic response for commonly used antipsychotics**

Antipsychotic	Time to response, *days*
Aripiprazole	14–21
Olanzapine	10–14
Quetiapine	10–14
Lurasidone	10–14
Risperidone	5–6
Ziprasidone intramuscular	<1
Ziprasidone oral	10–14

daily. It was given every 3–6 weeks; many clinicians felt that these regular visits helped to solidify their therapeutic alliance with patients, further enhancing compliance (Crocq 2015). In the 1980s, haloperidol decanoate followed and was also found to be helpful when given every 2–4 weeks (Kane et al. 2002). Its cost, however, was often prohibitive compared with fluphenazine decanoate, which continued to be broadly used until the arrival of the SGAs.

Long-acting intramuscular SGAs were introduced with risperidone in 2003 for biweekly use and required coadministration with the oral form during the first 3 weeks. Long-acting injectable olanzapine was released in 2008 for use every 2–4 weeks and does not require oral supplementation (Kane et al. 2010). Paliperidone palmitate debuted in 2009 and can be given every 4 weeks without oral backup. A 3-month version was approved in the United States in 2015, and its therapeutic profile appears to be as good as the monthly version (Savitz et al. 2016). Long-acting injectable aripiprazole arrived in 2013; it requires 3 weeks of oral supplementation and may be given every 6 weeks (remember its long half-life). Studies have shown it has superior efficacy and tolerability to paliperidone palmitate (Miyamoto and Fleischhacker 2017). Long-acting injectables can provide a better chance at sustained treatment with potentially fewer side effects due to relatively constant serum levels. They also appear to lead to fewer relapses, according to naturalistic studies, although the differences are not as easily demonstrated in RCTs (Brissos et al. 2014: Kishimoto et al. 2014).

Medications to Stabilize Mood

Insufficient consensus has been found on the properties a medication must have to be labeled a "mood stabilizer." Some pharmaceutical companies, largely for purposes of marketing, have called antipsychotic medications "mood stabilizers" because of their antimanic properties (mania being a form of psychosis). This section considers a *mood stabilizer* to be a single medication that prevents or reduces spontaneous pathological elevations *and* depressions of mood or the more common mixed state. This does not mean that major depression, previously called unipolar depression, is included, and medications that treat it, antidepressants, would also not be included.

Although we accept small perturbations of mood in healthy individuals, we have valid criteria for defining abnormal levels of high and low mood. At one time, we thought that unstable mood disorders, such as bipolar disorder, could not be diagnosed unless a clear manic state (elevation) had been demonstrated. We now know that recurrent episodes of bipolar depression, and those with mixed features, occur much more commonly than clear elevations and that this old criterion led to misdiagnosing many patients. It is also now clearer that symptoms such as increased sleep and increased appetite, possibly along with mixed features such as rapid thinking or other psychotic symptoms, often describe bipolar depression rather than major depression. Because the use of an antidepressant medication in bipolar depression may provoke rapid cycling or mania, the preferential use of mood stabilizers, when major depression is not a clear diagnosis, should be considered (Akiskal and Pinto 1999; Judd et al. 2002; Mason et al. 2016).

The story of how lithium was found to be effective in the treatment of mania due to high concentrations of the element occurring in the drinking water of communities with low rates of crime and mental illness appears apocryphal (Parker et al. 2018). Although lithium was involved in many natural curative springs in the nineteenth and early twentieth centuries, its early use for mental illness in the United States and Denmark was forgotten until resurrected in Australia in 1949. The well-known toxicity from lithium led to hesitancy regarding its use, especially in the United States, but a small but growing number of researchers persisted in obtaining data, with impressive results (Shorter 2009). Lithium was eventually approved by the FDA for marketing of the bipolar indication in 1970 and prevention of relapse in 1974, later than many other countries; some feel it is still underused (Post 2018). Publications such as the *Handbook of Lithium Therapy* (Johnson 1980) were a major tool in educating prescribers in the safe treatment of patients with lithium and helped facilitate its introduction into mainstream psychiatric office and hospital practice.

The salt form of lithium, a naturally occurring element, comes in citrate and carbonate forms. Although identical in bioavailability, the liquid citrate form has been reported to possibly offer better gastrointestinal tolerance than the carbonate, but the carbonate pill or capsule form is more commonly prescribed (Guelen et al. 1992; Vasile and Shelton 1982). Originally given three times a day, the twice-daily form (Lithobid or sustained release) is now the standard, usually prescribed with food to limit nausea. Some clinicians believe that once-daily dosing is preferable to reduce toxicity, especially renal (Singh et al. 2011). Reviews of the literature do not confirm this practice but show no evidence to discourage it, which may even improve compliance (Abraham et al. 1992; Carter et al. 2013). Diarrhea is a common side effect, as is polyuria, which sometimes reaches the level of diabetes insipidus. Hand tremor is also a common and particularly annoying side effect for many patients (Baek et al. 2014). Weight gain, despite exercise and food intake, may also be a problematic health risk of long-term treatment (Baptista et al. 1995; Gitlin 2016).

Therapeutic serum levels for mood stabilization and prophylaxis are listed at 0.5–1.2 mEq/L. These serum levels must be drawn 12 hours after a dose, although 10–14 hours will accommodate the limitations of real life for most patients, who should be counseled to delay laboratory visits until this timing can be accomplished. A serum level of 0.8–1.2 mEq/L represents the best combination of strongest clinical effect and avoidance of lithium toxicity for many patients. Because polyuria is a common side effect, patients should replace fluids regularly using electrolyte solutions to avoid volume and electrolyte depletion that will add to the risk of toxicity. Also, the human kidney was not developed to manage lithium and, due to the element's size, will treat it like sodium: retaining it in hyponatremic states and releasing it in hypernatremia. Therefore, explain to patients that their intake of table salt (sodium chloride) should not significantly change once the proper dose and level of lithium have been established. Cooking with table salt *plus* adding it at the table equates with 4 g of daily sodium intake. Using salt either during cooking *or* adding it at the table equals 2 g daily, and not using salt in either case is a zero-sodium diet (obviously rough estimates). Warn patients that if they change these categories, their lithium will need to be monitored more frequently. A reduction in dietary sodium may raise their lithium level and increase toxicity; an increase in dietary sodium intake may lower their lithium level to a subtherapeutic one. Remind patients of this before any scheduled hospitalizations, because well-meaning hospital staff, ignorant of this issue, may attempt to improve a patient's health by changing his or her diet. Lithium is also excreted in sweat, so any extreme alteration of exercise might also lead to changes in lithium level, requiring closer monitoring than usual.

Symptoms of toxicity that are not life threatening include severe tremor and nausea and may occur with serum levels in the expected therapeutic range (Foulser et al. 2017). Vomiting for any reason while taking lithium is dangerous, because it can provoke a cascade of electrolyte disturbances that might quickly lead to dangerous toxicity. As levels reach 1.3–1.5 mEq/L and higher, most patients' toxicity worsens and may begin to include confusion and ataxia. Levels of 1.8 mEq/L and higher are life threatening and a medical emergency requiring hospitalization and measures up to and including hemodialysis (Gitlin 2016). Astute clinicians will avoid taking patients anywhere near toxicity by measuring their renal function prior to prescription and monitoring it and their 12-hour serum levels regularly: at least every 3 months and upon dosage and brand changes. Because lithium may lower levels of circulating thyroxine, a thyroid-stimulating hormone (TSH) test should also precede treatment and be monitored regularly. A transient rise in TSH during the first year of treatment, followed by normalization, is expected. TSH levels not normalizing after 8–12 months, or continuing to rise rapidly, require endocrine consultation. Patients are also at risk for hyperparathyroidism, so serum calcium, phosphorus, and parathyroid hormone levels should also be monitored at baseline and along with at least quarterly TSH, estimated glomerular filtration rate (eGFR), and serum levels of lithium, creatinine, and sodium (McKnight et al. 2012).

Lithium is exclusively eliminated by the kidney, so any decrease in kidney function will allow buildup and potential toxicity. Lithium is widely characterized as causing renal impairment beyond the side effect of polyuria. Data supporting and rejecting this assertion are almost balanced, especially when treatment schedules developed after 1980 are considered, although recently, large databases have again suggested a link; further study with large prospective databases is still necessary (Gupta and Khastgir 2017; Kessing et al. 2015; Post 2018). However, the incidence of chronic kidney disease (CKD) in the United States is 14%, most commonly caused by hypertension and diabetes mellitus (National Institute of Diabetes and Digestive Diseases 2016). Estimates of the potential incidence of lithium-induced CKD, at worst, are low (Gong et al. 2016; McKnight et al. 2012). Be aware that many patients who need to be treated for unstable mood may have or be at risk for developing CKD, apart from lithium exposure, and make sure you neither give lithium to a patient who already has a lowered eGFR nor treat a patient with lithium while this develops. A declining eGFR or sustained serum creatinine level above normal requires renal evaluation from an internist or nephrologist. A patient in this dilemma may need to be switched gradually from lithium to alternative treatments, because merely using lower serum levels may still lead to toxicity in the face of progressive renal insufficiency (especially considering other ongoing causes of CKD) or eliminate the mood-stabilizing effects of the drug. Thoughtful consideration must be given to treatment changes by all concerned, because alternative treatments will need to be as effective (Davis et al. 2018; Hajek et al. 2011).

Once lithium was accepted by the profession as a valid and safe treatment for mood instability, it was the only agent in its class until the anti-kindling effects of anticonvulsant medications were theorized to provide a similar effect in bipolar disorder (Ballenger and Post 1978b, 1980; Post et al. 1982). *Kindling* is the observation that the seizure threshold in the brain becomes lower and lower with each successive seizure, a process also linked to alcohol withdrawal syndrome (Ballenger and Post 1978a; Goodwin and Ghaemi 1999). Carbamazepine, a popular anticonvulsant at the time (late 1970s and early 1980s), was first proposed as an effective mood stabilizer in Japan, and subsequent RCTs over decades have confirmed its efficacy (Okuma and Kishimoto 1998; Post et al. 2007). This opened the door to a significant list of new mood stabilizers, many eventually labeled "neuromodulators" because they may affect slow-acting receptors in groups of neurons rather than fast-acting single ones.

Carbamazepine, although important as a breakthrough treatment, actually has significant limitations regarding dosing and side effects. Enzymatic induction increases its own rate of metabolism, making it difficult to maintain therapeutic trough levels of 8–12 µg/mL (Chen and Lin 2012; McNamara et al. 1979; Pynnönen et al. 1980). Note that for most anticonvulsants, the therapeutic serum levels for treating unstable mood are usually higher than those employed for controlling seizures. Also, a small risk of aplastic anemia was associated with carbamazepine (López-Muñoz et al. 2018; Weisler 2006). This risk is present for many anticonvulsants, and white blood cell counts should always be monitored during treatment. Originally given four times a day due to its short half-life, a sustained-release twice-daily capsule of carbamazepine became available in 1996 and was approved for bipolar treatment marketing in 2004. Sedation, dizziness, and malaise are common side effects, so it is often best to start with bedtime dosing for the first 2 weeks, check serum drug and sodium levels along with complete blood counts every 2 weeks, and then follow with dose escalation as indicated. These same laboratory tests need to be ordered at least every 3 months, or sooner when brand or clinical changes dictate.

Valproate was found between 1966 and 1970 to have antimanic properties (Emrich et al. 1980; Lambert et al. 1966). Various forms were approved in France, Germany, and the United Kingdom between 1968 and 1973 before entering the U.S. market in 1983 (López-Muñoz et al. 2018). In an RCT (Bowden et al. 1994), the better-tolerated divalproex sodium version demonstrated that it, as well as lithium, was superior to placebo in the treatment of mania; FDA approval for marketing this indication followed in 1995. Divalproex sodium is a twice-daily enteric-coated preparation; a once-daily extended-release version (Depakote ER) was released in 2000.

Serum levels should always be used to guide treatment with divalproex sodium, the initial steady-state serum level being reached after 5 days (Zaccara et al. 1988). Target therapeutic levels are at least 50–100 μg/mL at trough, and most studies eventually supported levels of 85–125 μg/mL (Allen et al. 2006; Stoner et al. 2001). It is reasonable to begin dosing with 500 mg nightly and to obtain a serum level along with liver function tests (serum glutamic-oxaloacetic transaminase, serum glutamic-pyruvic transaminase, alkaline phosphatase) and pancreatic measurements (amylase) 1 week later. Doses to achieve therapeutic range can then be extrapolated for the short term. As with carbamazepine, the levels will likely drop over weeks to months, possibly through enzymatic induction; monitoring every 3 weeks or so is indicated to maintain this therapeutic range. After the first 6–12 months, levels can be checked quarterly unless symptoms or brands change. Nausea is usually avoided with this gradual titration.

Hepatotoxicity is rare but still a concern with divalproex sodium and appears to occur more commonly in younger patients (Cotariu and Zaidman 1988). The FDA has also issued a warning concerning pancreatitis, although the risk is also rare (Gerstner et al. 2007). In fact, sustained or extreme amylase elevations are most likely to be due to other causes and should prompt referral for proper diagnosis. Divalproex sodium also may be teratogenic, so patients planning pregnancy in the near future should consider alternatives; fertile female patients not planning pregnancy and engaging in intercourse will want to maintain effective contraception should they accept this risk (Gotlib et al. 2017).

Due to its depletion of carnitine, valproic acid may also lead to high serum ammonia levels that are often asymptomatic, but sedation may occur (Vázquez et al. 2014). Once identified, correction has been reported with oral replacement of L-carnitine, 250–990 mg three times a day, which also may guard against hepatic toxicity (Belousova 2017; Cattaneo et al. 2017; Mock and Schwetschenau 2012). After enthusiastic debate, researchers have found consensus that valproate also may lead to polycystic ovarian syndrome, a risk that should be discussed with female patients (Genton et al. 2001; Gotlib et al. 2017; Isojärvi et al. 2002; Joffe et al. 2006). As with many anticonvulsants, neutropenia, thrombocytopenia, and hyponatremia may rarely develop, so patients should also be monitored for these risks as well as for weight gain (Bowden and Singh 2005).

In the 1980s, when lithium was the only available mood stabilizer, the FGAs were often used to quell manic symptoms during the first week or so while waiting for a response to the lithium. These major tranquilizers had significant side effects (see "Medications to Treat Psychosis"), so many clinicians began utilizing the benzodiazepine anticonvulsant clonazepam in their place (Chouinard et al. 1983). This afforded patients rapid tranquilization with no risk of TD or other movement disorders. Clonazepam also began to be used in maintenance treatment, particularly as a supplement and in cases of schizoaffective disorder (Chouinard 1987; Mashiko et al. 2004).

I began this section by distinguishing mood stabilizers from antimanic agents such as antipsychotics. Although clonazepam does show fewer depressive recurrences in bipolar disorder than FGAs (Sachs 1990) and efficacy in reducing the recurrence of major (or unipolar) depression, studies demonstrate it is less effective in preventing bipolar depressive symptoms for many patients (although it may still play a role in treatment-resistant cases). Dosing begins at 0.5 mg three times a day, and total daily dosages have been reported useful in the range of 2.5–6.0 mg divided three times a day (Morishita 2009; Morishita and Aoki 2002). As a benzodiazepine (see "Medications to Treat Anxiety Disorders"), all of the risks associated with this class are relevant, including physiological dependence and cross tolerance. A slow taper is always necessary when discontinuing clonazepam.

Lamotrigine entered the market in Ireland in 1990 and in the United States in 1994 as a new and hopefully safer anticonvulsant (López-Muñoz et al. 2018). Studies in the United States that were started about that time to explore its use for bipolar disorder showed positive results and eventually confirmed its efficacy (Weisler et al. 2008). Lamotrigine offers improvement not only of mania but also of depressive episodes, although it does appear more useful adjunctively than when used as monotherapy (Bowden and Singh 2012; Geddes et al. 2009; Goodwin et al. 2004). A very slow titration is necessary because rapid elevation of serum level appears to provoke dangerous skin rashes such as the rare Stevens-Johnson syndrome (0.04% incidence on lamotrigine; <5% lethal); initiating treatment and reaching a therapeutic level takes weeks to months (Bloom and Amber 2017; Joe et al. 2009). Largely for this reason, lamotrigine is not a viable solution for treating acute mania as a single agent. Caution also is urged regarding rapid increases in serum levels that may be caused by switching from brand name to generic or the reverse, or among brands of generic formulations (Parker 2016, 2018).

Studies in Germany and the United States have determined that a safe rate of titration in adults begins with 25 mg/day for 14 days, followed by an increase of 50 mg/day every 14 days until a therapeutic level is reached. If a patient is also receiving valproate, which elevates the level of lamotrigine by blocking its metabolism, the rate is slower: 25 mg every other day for 14 days, daily for another 14 days, then increased by 25 mg/day every 14 days up to the final therapeutic level (Guberman et al. 1999; Leary et al. 2018; Schmidt and Krämer 1994). Lamotrigine entered markets as a twice-daily medication based on epileptologists' concern that serum levels would not be sustained with once-daily dosing despite its pharmacokinetics (elimination half-life 25–30 hours). After a few years the concern was relaxed, and once-daily dosing of the immediate-release version became standard, although a sustained-release form eventually became available.

To avoid risky rapid elevations of serum levels, advise patients to dose once daily and to never move two doses closer together; if necessary, always move them further apart. For example, if a patient forgets to take his medication one morning, advise him to not take the missed dose later that same day but to return to his regular dosing schedule the next morning. Also, if a patient has missed taking her lamotrigine for 5 or more consecutive days, for any reason, retitration from the beginning is essential to reduce the risk of serious rash. Among the mood stabilizers, lamotrigine is best known for medically significant rashes, but this risk is not exclusive to lamotrigine and may occur with any aromatic anticonvulsant, including carbamazepine and oxcarbazepine (Blaszczyk et al. 2015). Any rash that develops in patients receiving these agents should be evaluated with concern, but most will resolve spontaneously or with discontinuation of the medication. Patients with fever, deterioration of mucous membranes, blisters, or rashes that are painful or spreading rapidly need emergency services within 24 hours (Guberman et al. 1999). Although most cases of serious rash develop during the first 2 months of treatment, there are case reports of Stevens-Johnson syndrome developing after long periods of stable treatment; maintain alertness throughout treatment with aromatic anticonvulsants (Jha et al. 2017; Mockenhaupt et al. 2005).

Gabapentin became available in the United States in 1993 for the adjunctive treatment of epilepsy. Many open studies and case reports have found it to be a promising mood stabilizer, yet sufficient RCTs have not been performed to confirm this. Given gabapentin's safety and tolerability (see discussion in "Medications to Treat Anxiety Disorders"), it has been suggested more than once that so many favorable reports may indicate a possible role as an adjunctive treatment in refractory cases or for patients with comorbid anxiety (Botts and Raskind 1999; Carta et al. 2003; Vieta et al. 2006). Others have been less optimistic (Carey et al. 2008). In the interest of good science, the handful of RCTs testing gabapentin for bipolar disorder have been of low quality in design or size, and meta-analyses have also been criticized (Berlin et al. 2015; Calabrese et al. 2002; Mayo-

Wilson et al. 2017; Pichler et al. 2015). The manufacturer settled a lawsuit in the United States in 2004 for marketing the drug without sufficient data (Fullerton et al. 2010). In 2017, researchers registered a new meta-analysis to address this issue (Houghton et al. 2017). Hopefully, sufficient RCTs of good quality will be identified, or eventually performed, and will help determine the question of efficacy and proper usage.

Topiramate, released in 1996, showed initial promise treating unstable moods in various states during open-label trials (Calabrese et al. 2001; Suppes 2002). Unfortunately, it represents another case with a dearth of high-quality RCTs that might confirm these early results (Pigott et al. 2016). Very slow titration with topiramate is necessary to limit impaired concentration as an early side effect (Sommer et al. 2013). Topiramate may suppress appetite, so it is indicated for obesity as well as for migraine headaches and epilepsy. Some have proposed that it might be used to help patients who gained weight with other psychotropic treatments (Mahmood et al. 2013). Topiramate also inhibits carbonic anhydrase, which leads to carbonated beverages tasting flat, a feature that may annoy some patients. This action also may produce a generally mild to moderate metabolic acidosis and contributes to kidney stone formation at an incidence of 2.1% (Dell'Orto et al. 2014; Gupta et al. 2017; Mirza et al. 2009). Paresthesia and visual distortions are other reported side effects, although a recent review of visual field defects found no statistical difference with placebo (Ford et al. 2017; Silberstein 2017).

Oxcarbazepine is structurally related to carbamazepine (a 10-keta analogue). It was approved in the United States in 2000 for epilepsy, following use in Europe and the United Kingdom. Manufacturers have not sought an indication to market it for unstable mood, but a limited number of studies have been performed, and some efficacy has been reported (Hirschfeld and Kasper 2004; López-Muñoz et al. 2018; Vasudev et al. 2008, 2011). Unlike carbamazepine, oxcarbazepine does not induce its own metabolism, so serum levels are more stable and the side effect profile is generally milder (Hellewell 2002). Monitoring for blood dyscrasia is still recommended, however, because case reports of its occurrence have been published (Hsiao et al. 2010; Milia et al. 2008). Also, although many anticonvulsants may lower serum sodium levels, oxcarbazepine is exceptionally likely to do so, with a 29.9% incidence being reported. Once established, this effect is usually persistent (Dong et al. 2005; Kumar and Gopalakrishnan 2016). Hyponatremia (sodium level <136 mmol/L at most laboratories) may be asymptomatic until the most critical stages, so regularly monitor the sodium levels of every patient receiving oxcarbazepine. Although mild hyponatremia may be addressed with fluid restriction or dosage reduction, moderate or severe hyponatremia (sodium level <125 mmol/L) is of acute medical concern and requires referral to an emergency center that day to be evaluated by a specialist who will also know how to avoid osmotic demyelination syndrome should a bolus of hypertonic saline be necessary, as with normal volume hyponatremia (Ball and Iqbal 2016; Hoorn and Zietse 2017).

Some anticonvulsants have been found useful for stabilizing moods, but many more have not, including zonisamide, phenytoin, pregabalin, tiagabine, levetiracetam, and retigabine. Once again, assuming a class effect would be erroneous. Sufficient evidence for donepezil and verapamil is lacking (Fountoulakis et al. 2017; Grunze et al. 2018; López-Muñoz et al. 2018). As discussed earlier (see "Medications to Treat Psychosis"), caution should be exercised when considering use of typical and atypical antipsychotics as monotherapy for unstable mood, especially at low dosages. Clozapine, despite its many side effects, does appears to have sufficient data to support its use as monotherapy, and some limited evidence has been found for quetiapine, olanzapine, and risperidone, although all four carry a risk of TD (Li et al. 2015; Lindström et al. 2017).

Medications to Treat Cognitive Disorders

A demand exists for medications that improve cognition, particularly concentration and memory. Cognitive symptoms such as impairment of these occur in many of our diagnostic categories and are not limited to ADHD or dementia. Although we strive to help patients with these symptoms, we best serve them by treating syndromes rather than individual symptoms, as I have discussed. Improvement of the underlying syndrome is expected to improve each component symptom, including cognition when applicable. This section, therefore, is devoted to medications that are used to treat cognitive symptoms when they represent the primary syndrome, such as dementia or ADHD.

As mentioned previously (see Chapters 3 and 4), diagnoses of ADHD are made clinically, not with neuropsychological testing, using the criteria in DSM-5 (American Psychiatric Association 2013). Some forms of psychological testing can determine whether a patient has problems concentrating, but they cannot confirm a diagnosis. Unless you seek additional information about cognitive deficits, use of psychological testing solely to diagnose ADHD is not indicated and represents unnecessary expense and trouble for the patient. ADHD is also not accurately diagnosed based merely on the presence of impaired concentration or on response to treatment: stimulants will enhance concentration in normal persons as well as those with ADHD and other diagnoses (Linssen et al. 2014). A clinical interview, including a complete history and formal mental status examination, should lead to a correct diagnosis, applying the full DSM-5 criteria for the disorder. Once a diagnosis has been made, treatment may proceed.

ADHD was originally called, among other things, "hyperactive/hyperkinetic syndrome" and then "minimal brain dysfunction" (Mahone and Denckla 2017). Original descriptions focused more on behavior than on actual cognition. Because the terminology has changed over the past near-century, I use *ADHD* here to refer to the symptoms listed as this syndrome in DSM-5, no matter what term was in practice when a specific medication was introduced. Also, most ADHD medications involve a variation on amphetamines and vary mostly in enantiomer, duration of action, and method of delivery, so this section, more than others, refers to the brand names of the preparations in an effort to better distinguish them.

The first use of medication that specifically focused on behavioral disturbances in children was Benzedrine (D-amphetamine+L-amphetamine) (Bradley 1937), reported about the same time that amphetamine was being considered for the short-term treatment of depressed mood (Anderson 1938). As is often the case, this was a serendipitous observation, because the author had intended to treat headaches in his pediatric patients with DL-amphetamine. Additional data on the effects of DL-amphetamine and D-amphetamine followed (Bradley 1950), focused still on the behavioral observations of the children being subdued (50%–60%) and noting that only 5% showed "an acceleration of school progress only."

Bradley's investigations were largely ignored until the early 1960s, but they are now considered seminal in our understanding and treatment of ADHD (Strohl 2011). The intervening years were focused mostly on medications to tranquilize, such as phenobarbital, meprobamate, hydroxyzine, and the major tranquilizer chlorpromazine. Methylphenidate, at the time, was only noted to be helpful in overcoming the sedative side effects of these medications that further inhibited academic performance (Ayd 1957). Its use to treat primary symptoms was reported in 1963, and in addition to its effects on behavior, attention was given to its enhancement of learning (Conners and Eisenberg 1963). Methylphenidate became a more popular treatment for ADHD than dextroamphetamine (Dextrostat, Dexedrine) and multiplied into a dizzying array of preparations and delivery systems, all jockeying for market share (Stevenson and Wolraich 1989).

Methylphenidate has a half-life of 4 hours, time to peak of 1.9 hours, and clinically is experienced with an abrupt onset and abrupt halt to benefit, sometimes with rebound events such as moodiness and anergy (Kolar et al. 2008). Adderall attempts to take the edge off the square wave "on-off" response to methylphenidate; it is a mixture of amphetamines, including dextroamphetamine saccharate, amphetamine aspartate monohydrate, dextroamphetamine sulfate, and amphetamine sulfate, yielding a 3:1 ratio of D- to L-amphetamine (Drugs.com 2018a). Each component has a different time to peak and half-life, so a smoother increase and decrease in the serum level (and thus benefits and side effects) is achieved, still over a 4-hour period. The extended-release form, which arrived in 2001, may extend the period of treatment to 10–12 hours. The generic preparations of Adderall are generally labeled "amphetamine salts" by pharmacies. An alternative strategy to managing rebound in children, adolescents, and adults may be changing preparations with an eye toward longer-acting, more sustained preparations at the lowest effective doses.

In addition to problems with rebound, many children and adolescents did not like having to take a second dose at school, further encouraging efforts to deliver stimulants in long-acting form (Cascade et al. 2008). Ritalin SR and LA, Concerta (methylphenidate osmotic release oral system [OROS]) and Metadate CD represent early attempts to extend the effect of a single morning dose of methylphenidate throughout the day, usually for 8–12 hours. Ritalin SR (t_{max} 4.7 hours), although absorbed more slowly, does not quite reach the same peak serum levels as immediate release (Birmaher et al. 1989; Patrick et al. 1989). Concerta's OROS system delivers methylphenidate in three steps: 1) a coating for immediate effect, 2) osmotic delivery of 30% of the dose in the first internal compartment, and 3) release of the remaining 70%. It is found to be as effective as the immediate-release and more effective than the sustained-release formulations (Biederman et al. 2006; Keating et al. 2001; Swanson et al. 2003). This means that the dose equivalencies for the OROS form with immediate or other sustained-release preparations often skew higher, up to 54–108 mg daily for some adults. A problem developed when the FDA approved generic versions of Concerta that did not use the OROS technology, because other forms release methylphenidate in different manners with varying results (Lally et al. 2016). When choosing the generic form, take care to determine which technology is used and specify a manufacturer to the pharmacist. The market is constantly changing, so practitioners must research the available options at the time of prescription. Biphasic release is used in Metadate CD (1st, 30%; 2nd, 70%) and Ritalin LA (1st, 50%; 2nd, 50%) (Haertling et al. 2015).

An effort to provide only the efficacious D-enantiomer, although of no additional clinical benefit, resulted in the dexmethylphenidate hydrochloride form (Focalin and Focalin XR) (Markowitz et al. 2006). Daytrana delivers methylphenidate in patch form (Findling and Dinh 2014); applied to the hip once daily, it has only a small following. Methylin is methylphenidate available in both short-acting oral solution and chewable tablets. Quillivant XR, another liquid form, debuted in 2010 along with QuilliChew ER, another chewable form, in 2016. Pemoline was introduced to the United States in 1975 as a stimulant for the treatment of ADHD symptoms but was discontinued in 2003 after FDA warnings about a small but significant risk of fatal liver failure (U.S. Food and Drug Administration 2002).

Dextroamphetamine (Zenzedi) has not disappeared, however, and long-acting versions are also available (beginning with Dexedrine Spansules, also available in generic). A short-acting liquid form (Procentra) was released in 2008, and a long-acting liquid (Dyanavel XR) was approved in 2016 that demonstrated 13 hours of benefit in RCTs (Childress et al. 2018, 2019). Dextroamphetamine's parent compound, lisdexamfetamine, was released in the United States as a prodrug (Vyvanse) in 2007. A prodrug is one that is not pharmacologically active until it is metabolized into an active metabolite—in this case, dextroamphetamine. The theory is that this extra step delays onset of action in useful ways, lasting up to 12 hours after a dose (Cowles 2009; Najib 2009). An intranasal version has been developed (Ermer et al. 2011) but is not available, although chewable tablets are. Another short-acting preparation available in the United States since 2015 is Evekeo, made of equal portions of D- and L-amphetamine with the hope of causing less CNS excitation and less appetite suppression (Childress et al. 2015; Drugs.com 2018b). Adzenys XR-ODT (extended-release orally disintegrating tablet), released in 2016, is a 3:1 ratio of D- to L-amphetamine with 50% immediate-release and 50% extended-release microparticles (U.S. Food and Drug Administration 2017). It is a long-acting preparation that may last 10–12 hours; the fact that it also an oral dissolving tablet is really only valuable in avoiding pill swallowing. Recall also that the time to peak and length of action of some stimulants may be delayed by food intake (Auiler et al. 2002).

Originally, practitioners were guided to begin with a short-acting preparation, find the lowest effective dose, and then determine how long each dose was effective (and therefore how many doses per day were necessary). With the advent of long-acting preparations, most patients would be switched to one of these once the individual dose of the short-acting form was determined. Reference expected dose equivalencies when changing to a long-acting product. However, many clinicians now begin with titration of the long-acting forms, a method supported by some practice guidelines (Huss et al. 2017).

The medications covered so far in this section are all stimulants; although their therapeutic effects appear to begin immediately, evaluate their efficacy and tolerability 14–30 days after initiation or dosage change and at least every 90 days thereafter for maintenance treatment. Stimulants may be drugs of abuse (Heal et al. 2013), so prescriptions should not be refilled early or replaced for any reason, something important to discuss with the patient at the time of the first prescription. It also may be necessary to discuss daily versus episodic dosing (as needed or only on school days or workdays, skipping weekends and vacations). College students may prefer short-acting versions that they can dose to match their study times, whereas those with regular jobs often prefer long-acting preparations they can dose once in the morning. Parents, concerned about risk and tolerability, may agree to treatment for academic reasons while giving less importance to family time (Ibrahim and Donyai 2015; Shyu et al. 2016). Planned drug holidays may be helpful in addressing tolerability issues, such as suppressed appetite, but when added to the imperfection of human compliance, these may result in the compromise of a full response. Time spent with family and friends is important, and improving function in these social environments should be discussed as a part of treatment planning. The patient or family may still choose intermittent treatment, and discussion of its possible limitations is merited. Some clinicians have utilized planned holidays to help older adolescents and adults better self-assess the value of their medication; this also would seem apparent from inadvertently missed doses or other lapses in compliance (Ibrahim and Donyai 2018; Ibrahim et al. 2016).

Other categories of medication have been tried for treating ADHD symptoms. Clonidine (Catapres, now also Kapvay), an older α-adrenergic antihypertensive, has for several decades been tried as a treatment for ADHD as well as various behavioral disorders in children. Its use is highly individualized (Ming et al. 2011). It is not always well tolerated, often lowering blood pressure and inducing sedation. Currently, the evidence for its efficacy is considered weak (Gorman et al. 2015). Guanfacine, another α-adrenergic antihypertensive (Seedat 1985), began marketing as an ADHD treatment in 2009. A sustained-release form (Intuniv) became available in 2013 in the United States and Canada (Huss et al. 2016). Although its efficacy is established (Joseph et al. 2017), guanfacine sometimes also is difficult to tolerate due to hypotension and sedation.

For many years, clinicians viewed antidepressants, particularly imipramine and desipramine, as treatments for ADHD and prescribed them widely for this. Part of the reason may be that the syndrome of major depression does involve impaired concentration. Also, hardly any psychotropic medications were approved to treat children and adolescents other than antidepressants, stimulants, and major tranquilizers. Today, use of major depression treatments other than bupropion is not considered indicated for ADHD (Otasowie et al. 2014).

Bupropion (see "Medications to Treat Major Depression") is not only a successful treatment for major depression but also, potentially, for ADHD symptoms independent of mood (Verbeeck et al. 2017). Atomoxetine (Strattera) is a selective norepinephrine reuptake inhibitor approved by the FDA in 2002 to treat ADHD, having failed to demonstrate efficacy for major depression (Kratochvil et al. 2005). Atomoxetine and bupropion are options when you are concerned that stimulants might worsen the depressive or anxiety symptoms of another disorder (Clemow et al. 2017). They can be given once a day, show sustained benefit throughout the day without rebound, are not controlled substances, and have no abuse potential (Upadhyaya et al. 2013; Wilens et al. 2005a). Clinicians must remember, however, that the time for a complete response with each of these two agents is longer than generally expected with stimulants, 2–6 weeks, and that each must be taken daily (Reimherr et al. 2005).

Modafinil, a nonstimulant that appears to affect many catecholamines, was first used in France in the early 1990s for the treatment of narcolepsy and is now approved in the United States for that disorder as well as shift-work sleep disorder and sleep apnea. Interest in using it to treat ADHD is high, but few RCTs have addressed this question. Review and meta-analysis show it might have efficacy with fewer cardiovascular side effects, although appetite suppression and insomnia are common effects (Minzenberg and Carter 2008; Wang et al. 2017). The rare appearance of Stevens-Johnson syndrome in studies for ADHD led the FDA to decline approval for this indication (Wood et al. 2013).

With the exception of atomoxetine and bupropion, most medications to treat ADHD symptoms may suppress appetite. In younger patients, weight monitoring is important. Stimulants may also interfere with sleep (Hvolby 2015) and raise blood pressure, particularly in adults (Biederman et al. 2006; Findling et al. 2001; Westover and Halm 2012; Wilens et al. 2005b). All adult patients considered for stimulant treatment must have their blood pressure reliably checked by the provider prior to treatment and at each and every office visit (as discussed in Chapter 3), and many recommendations have been made for the same in children and adolescents (Samuels et al. 2006; Stowe et al. 2002).

Stimulants for ADHD were originally developed for and studied in children, so studies of efficacy are not always tailored to adult usage. For example, to limit the cost of expensive Phase II and Phase III studies (see Chapter 2), many older RCTs began gathering data 2 hours after a dose, assuming that it takes that amount of time for a child to have breakfast, take their medication, and arrive to start the school day. For adults, the timing requirement might be different, but few data are available to guide prescribers beyond pharmacokinetics. In some recent studies, however, testing 30 minutes after dosing was included (Childress et al. 2019).

ADHD and impairment in executive function are sometimes confused. ADHD represents the symptom spectrum outlined in DSM-5 criteria, whereas impairment in executive function is not a separate diagnosis but refers to impairment in the set of cognitive abilities necessary to complete a plan or goal (Banich 2009; Willcutt et al. 2005). It may be subsumed under ADHD and other diagnoses, such as mood and neurological disorders, including autism spectrum and Parkinson's disease, but it does not characterize an entire syndrome. Treatment of impaired executive function involves aggressive efforts to treat the underlying condition, such with as dopamine for Parkinson's disease, anticholinesterase inhibitors for dementia, methylphenidate or atomoxetine for ADHD, and venlafaxine for major depression (Ni et al. 2013; Rabinovici et al. 2015; Tian et al. 2016). As a further illustration, modafinil has been reported to improve executive dysfunction in patients with narcolepsy but not in healthy, non-sleep-deprived students (Fernández et al. 2015; Schwartz et al. 2004).

As the incidence of dementia increases, clinicians and patients are desperately seeking treatments that restore memory. Thus far, no such medications are available, but treatments that appear to delay cognitive decline in cases of Alzheimer's disease, vascular dementia, Lewy body dementia, and frontotemporal dementias are available. Reversible anticholinesterase inhibitors and the NMDA receptor antagonist memantine—but not statins or anti-inflammatory medications—appear to delay, not halt, progression in clinically diagnosed cases of dementia (O'Brien et al. 2017). They do not appear to help patients regain lost function, although some industry-sponsored studies may come close to such claims (Laver et al. 2016). Prior to treatment, any reversible causes of cognitive decline should be addressed (see Chapter 3), particularly anticholinergic treatments for other indications that may be compromising cognition.

Tacrine was the first anticholinesterase inhibitor approved for the treatment of dementia, in 1993, but due to hepatotoxicity it is no longer available in the United States, United Kingdom, or Europe (National Institutes of Health 2018; O'Brien et al. 2017). Donepezil followed, with an indication for use in Alzheimer's disease. Its long half-life (70 hours) allows it to be given once a day, a choice most families caring for a patient at home almost always make. As with most anticholinesterase inhibitors, nausea is the most common side effect.

Rivastigmine, available since 1997 in capsule and patch form but no longer in liquid form, shows good clinical results in delaying cognitive decline in Alzheimer's and Parkinson's diseases. The twice-daily dosing with severe nausea, however, was a limiting factor until a once-daily, better-tolerated transdermal form was developed in 2007. Beyond Alzheimer's disease, it also is approved for Lewy body and Parkinson's dementias. Galantamine debuted in Sweden in 2000, followed shortly by use in the rest of Europe and the United States, United Kingdom, Canada, and Japan. Its half-life requires twice-daily oral dosing, and it is similar to rivastigmine and donepezil in benefits and side effects, but it may be the best tolerated by many (Colovic et al. 2013; Fisher et al. 2017). When used for the treatment of dementia, galantamine's original brand name was Reminyl, which was changed in 2005 to Razadyne to avoid confusion with Amaryl, prescribed to treat diabetes mellitus. Also in that year an extended-release form was approved.

Memantine, the NMDA receptor antagonist, was developed in Germany and approved there for dementia in 1989. It entered Japan in 2000, the United Kingdom and Europe in 2002, and the United States in 2003. Because the initial study design added memantine to donepezil that had already been initiated, early dosing directions followed this same plan. Since then, some studies testing memantine as monotherapy have found a very small effect in a small sample, but only one study was not sponsored by industry (Matsunaga et al. 2015). Memantine used as monotherapy or in combination with anticholinesterase inhibitors has been recommended, however, particularly in moderate to severe Alzheimer's disease (Kishi et al. 2017; O'Brien et al. 2017). An extended-release form became available in 2014, and an extended-release memantine/donepezil preparation was released in 2015.

The question of whether to pharmacologically treat prodromal mild cognitive impairment often comes up. Initially promising, treatment with anticholinesterase inhibitors has yet to demonstrate a delay in progression to dementia, although treatment of mild cases of dementia will likely be satisfactory (Knopman and Petersen 2014; Sanford 2017). Practitioners, patients, and families must understand that although data showed that one large group of patients receiving anticholinesterase inhibitors had slower progression of dementia than a large group not receiving them, we cannot know whether an anticholinesterase inhibitor is actually effective in an individual patient. Therefore, unless tolerability or compliance is an issue (e.g., with multiple daily doses), switching medications merely to seek greater benefit after several years of treatment is actually contraindicated. Clinical decline may accelerate temporarily and is never reversed as one anticholinesterase inhibitor is stopped and another begun. If warranted for tolerability reasons, a switch from one to another should be rapid to avoid a period of subtherapeutic serum levels (Maelicke 2001; Massoud et al. 2011). Eventual decline, however, is always expected.

Some have discussed the length of time a patient should receive anti-cholinesterase inhibitors. Mild and moderate stages of dementia show the best results, and doses may have to be raised or memantine added, if not already used, for severe dementia. Many clinicians think that as the terminal stage of Alzheimer's disease is reached, prolonging the situation further is cruel as well as ineffective and suggest discontinuing treatment (Deardorff et al. 2015).

Medications to Treat Sleep Problems

When rational psychopharmacologists treat sleep, they hope that treating the underlying condition will correct insomnia as part of complete syndrome improvement. Primary sleep disorders exist, but the vast majority of sleep problems mental health professionals encounter are secondary to a linked syndrome. As noted previously, some medications used to treat these syndromes carry sedation as a side effect. This has led some clinicians to count on providing sedation as part of their treatment regimen, such as with trazodone (discussed in the "Medications to Treat Major Depression" section). Providing some short-term sleep assistance to patients who have severe insomnia due to another disorder is not completely contraindicated, but be sure that adding a medication addressing only sleep will not compromise the clinical success of the primary treatment or add debilitating, unnecessary side effects.

Medications that are used primarily for insomnia are called *hypnotics, sedative-hypnotics,* or *soporifics.* Their history overlaps with that of the antianxiety agents discussed earlier. Inadequate efforts were made to aid sleep with alcohol and opiates before the introduction of chloral hydrate in 1869 (Gauillard et al. 2002). The first medication targeted mostly as a hypnotic, chloral hydrate is rapidly absorbed from the gastrointestinal tract; resulting gastrointestinal irritation is minimized by administering it with food. Elimination is primarily renal. At the usual bedtime dosage of 0.5–2 g, sedation develops within 20–60 minutes. Its half-life is very brief, whereas that of its active metabolites are 8–12 and 67 hours. Doses of 5–10 g have been reported as lethal. Chloral hydrate was used into the middle of the twentieth century, but in the twenty-first century it has been almost completely abandoned due to safety concerns of overdose, abuse, carcinogenicity, and genotoxicity (Gauillard et al. 2002).

Potassium bromide was used for sedation, as well as seizures and anxiety, in the late nineteenth century (Balme 1976). Unusually, a large single dose is not effective because it works through accretion by replacing chloride. Sedation occurs as intoxication begins. Dangerous toxicity might follow closely behind, so its use in insomnia disappeared in the late 1960s (Ban 1969, 2006, 2013).

The barbiturate barbital, marketed as Veronal, was discovered to be an effective sedative-hypnotic around the turn of the nineteenth to twentieth century (Norn et al. 2015). The most widely used barbiturate, however, has been phenobarbital, first used as a sedative in 1912 and ultimately most often as an anticonvulsant (López-Muñoz et al. 2005). Like benzodiazepines, barbiturates have a variety of half-lives and speeds of action, and many have been used for brief and intermediate anesthesia, including prior to electroconvulsive therapy. Some also have been the tool for capital punishment, which illustrates the lethal risk of overdose or combination with cross-tolerant agents (see discussion of benzodiazepines in "Medications to Treat Anxiety Disorders"). Intentional and accidental lethal overdose led to barbiturates being left behind as soporifics for daily use.

As noted previously (see "Medications to Treat Anxiety Disorders"), many of the benzodiazepines have found more use as soporifics than as treatments for anxiety. Although diazepam, clonazepam, lorazepam, and alprazolam are prescribed by many practitioners for sleep, they are more commonly used for other indications. Flurazepam, temazepam, triazolam, and estazolam have become specifically identified as treatments for insomnia due to their half-lives and because none of them is a preferred treatment for other disorders. Flurazepam, initially popular in the 1970s, has such a long effective half-life (half-life of the parent compound plus that of each active metabolite) that it can be debilitating during the day in terms of cognition and social function (Adam and Oswald 1984). For this reason, better options have replaced it. Temazepam, an active diazepam metabolite released in the 1980s, has a more appropriate half-life and, prior to arrival of the newer gabaminergic agents, was quite popular at both 15-mg and 30-mg doses. Triazolam was popular in the 1980s and 1990s due to its rapid achievement of peak serum level and therefore sedation. As mentioned earlier, however, the therapeutic dose is unusually close to the lethal dose.

Some practitioners may prescribe one benzodiazepine for daytime use, such as for anxiety, and a different one at bedtime for sleep. The action and result are the same, but this possibly justifiable practice must still be examined because it may be safer to use only one benzodiazepine at a time, dosed to cover both situations. If the justification for this polypharmacy is half-lives, a plan that changes dosing times and uses uneven dosing (i.e., less during the day, more at night) can often be established with one agent. Remember also that benzodiazepines may worsen mood and are cross tolerant with barbiturates, alcohol, and each other. They may be abused recreationally, and a severe and potentially dangerous withdrawal syndrome may occur with inadequate taper after sustained use. The risk/benefit ratio of using benzodiazepines purely for soporific purposes must be thoughtfully considered and thoroughly discussed with patients during treatment planning.

Given the risks of the soporifics reviewed so far, many practitioners were pleased to see the development of new, somewhat safer agents late in the twentieth century. Zolpidem, introduced to the United Kingdom in 1988 and to the United States in 1992, binds to $GABA_A$ receptors—as do the benzodiazepines, but to different subunits. Peak serum levels are achieved in less than 2 hours, and terminal half-life (the time it takes for the serum level to be halved after reaching equilibrium) is 1.5–3.2 hours. Its excretion into breast milk is extremely low (Pons et al. 1989). Zolpidem does not offer significant reduction in anxiety, anticonvulsant properties, or muscle relaxation (Salvà and Costa 1995).

Zolpidem was originally believed to carry no rebound or withdrawal effects and to show no gender differences in metabolism. Starting dosages were recommended as 10 mg nightly for all but geriatric patients. However, later research demonstrated delayed metabolism in female patients that resulted in higher morning concentrations and thus measurements of unsafe driving and impaired work performance in females the morning after use. This problem appears to be exacerbated by modified-release preparations. Lower initial dosages of 5 mg nightly are now recommended for females, and individual titration may then cautiously proceed (Farkas et al. 2013; U.S. Food and Drug Administration 2013).

Media reports have been made of people experiencing somnambulism from zolpidem: walking, sometimes driving, or eating while not being awake or fully alert. It appears that this is neither unique to zolpidem nor common (Singh et al. 2015). Such idiosyncratic reactions to soporifics may occur with any agent and will necessitate reevaluation neurologically and pharmacologically.

Clinicians have seen people taking high doses of zolpidem (160 mg/day or higher) alone or with other substances for attempted recreational purposes. Those engaging in this behavior often have a history of abusing other substances. Such high doses lead to cognitive impairment, seizures, psychosis, and withdrawal symptoms, often necessitating cross-tolerant detoxification, such as with a long-acting benzodiazepine (Chiaro et al. 2018; Eslami-Shahrbabaki et al. 2014). It has not yet been established whether the abuse occurs while merely seeking recreational intoxication, while attempting to sleep during intractable insomnia, or is the result of a distinct property of zolpidem, although investigation continues (Licata et al. 2011; Roehrs and Roth 2016; Schwienteck et al. 2017). As with all soporifics, careful patient selection and ongoing monitoring are essential.

Several agents with similar pharmacodynamics yet different pharmacokinetics followed zolpidem: zaleplon, a very-short-acting soporific, and the longer-acting eszopiclone. Released in the United States in 1999, zaleplon has a very short time to peak serum level of 0.9–1.5 hours and a half-life of 1 hour with no active metabolites. This makes it more useful for helping patients achieve initial sleep than in sustaining it (Beer et al. 1994; Heydorn 2000). Due to its short half-life, residual impairment the next day is uncommon (Dinges et al. 2018; Dooley and Plosker 2000). Zaleplon may be a preferred choice for patients who are outliers in terms of next-day impairment from zolpidem and eszopiclone. Patients should be advised in advance that sleep latency is extremely brief with zaleplon and that they should be prepared to go to bed and sleep quickly after dosing. Because it lasts only about 2 hours, approved dosing during the night might be appropriate when more than 2 hours remain for sleeping, such as in cases of late insomnia (early morning awakening). Dosage is similar to that of zolpidem, 5 or 10 mg nightly, and zaleplon may offer a lower risk of falls and fall-related injuries (Tom et al. 2016).

Eszopiclone, approved by FDA in 2004, also achieves peak absorption rapidly (t_{max} 1 hour) but has a longer half-life of 6 hours, which is also longer than zolpidem. Therefore, it can be helpful in both initiating and sustaining sleep, provided that the longer half-life does not impair patients the following day. Recommended dosing is 2–3 mg, again right at bedtime (1–2 mg for geriatric patients) (Brielmaier 2006).

Ramelteon, unlike the previous three medications, does not bind to GABA receptors and is classified separately as a melatonin (MT) agonist, attaching to MT_1 and MT_2 receptors in the suprachiasmatic nucleus. Ramelteon was approved for marketing by the FDA in 2005. It is not thought to have any properties of abuse or dependence and may be helpful with reducing sleep latency and sustaining sleep. What is unusual about ramelteon is that it does not induce sedation. Its positive effects on sleep may take a week or longer to occur, even with nightly dosing. Patients should understand, therefore, that it is not a quick fix to any insomnia symptoms (Neubauer 2008). Usual dosing is 8 mg nightly.

Another new compound, suvorexant, approaches the treatment of insomnia with a novel mechanism of action—it blocks the action of orexins A and B, hypothalamic neuropeptides responsible for wakefulness. In other words, it acts not by inducing sedation but by blocking signals that keep patients awake. Understanding the potential mechanism of action before any medication is developed to use it and before RCTs confirm efficacy is exciting, as happened with suvorexant (Herring et al. 2016). As I have stressed in all other psychopharmacological cases, scientists have extrapolated from clinical results to infer mechanisms of action. Happily, however, with suvorexant we have both a mechanism of action and clinical data supporting its efficacy.

Approved in the United States in 2014, suvorexant has a time to peak of 120–180 minutes that can be delayed 90 minutes by food intake near dosing. Absorption is greater in women and in obese patients (BMI >30 kg/m^2), which may inform lower doses in these populations, particularly patients belonging to both groups. With a terminal half-life of 9–13.5 hours, it has no active metabolites, so next-day impairment is generally not noted. The dosage in the absence of renal and hepatic impairment is 10–20 mg nightly; higher doses have been associated with mild and reversible adverse neurological events, such as hallucinations, sleep paralysis, somnambulism, and cataplexy. Suvorexant is contraindicated when narcolepsy is a comorbid condition. Withdrawal and dependence have not been demonstrated (Norman and Anderson 2016; Rhyne and Anderson 2015; Sutton 2015). Further experience, observations, and studies will be necessary in order to determine its abuse potential. Other orexin-based treatments may eventually be developed.

Only one other medication targeted for sleep is in common use: Silenor, a reformulation of the old sedating TCA doxepin. Rather than a step forward, Silenor is an example of a company trying to find a new market for a decades-old drug originally used for a completely different indication. In this case, the manufacturer is taking advantage of the sedative side effects of TCAs (discussed in "Medications to Treat Major Depression"). This best illustrates how knowing and understanding the chemical name of the medication, not just the brand name, is essential in understanding the value of a medication, its history, and how it may or may not be safe to prescribe. A clinician would never want to prescribe Silenor alongside doxepin or in cases of bipolar disorder or certain cardiac diseases, such as heart block.

Medications to Treat Impulse-Control Problems

Rather than focus on child and adolescent behaviors, in this section I address compulsive behaviors such as OCD and substance abuse problems. Prior to the 1980s, OCD was treated only with psychotherapy, because no other treatment had been found to be effective. The TCA clomipramine was then confirmed uniquely effective for treating OCD symptoms, even in the absence of major depression (Kellner 2010; Thorén et al. 1980). The response to treatment for OCD took longer than that for major depression, and higher doses were also necessary. Approval for marketing to treat OCD, but not major depression, was granted in the United States in 1989, although clomipramine had been available for the treatment of depression in Europe for almost two decades by then. As a result, U.S. practitioners began using it at about the same time SSRIs were found to have efficacy in OCD. Whereas early comparator studies often found clomipramine to be more effective than SSRIs against OCD, later studies showed that efficacy rates for both are similar (Bandelow et al. 2008; Pigott and Seay 1999). TCAs (as noted in the "Medications to Treat Major Depression" section) do have more anticholinergic, antihistaminic, and cardiovascular side effects than SSRIs, and for this reason, clomipramine may not be a first choice.

Based on RCTs, five—and only five—SSRIs have been demonstrated effective in OCD: fluoxetine, fluvoxamine, escitalopram, sertraline, and paroxetine (Bandelow et al. 2008). The dosages required for the greatest effect in adults are up to 300 mg/day for fluvoxamine and sertraline, 80 mg/day for fluoxetine and paroxetine, and 40 mg/day for escitalopram. Given the high dosages, clinicians should be mindful of and alert for any signs of serotonin syndrome (see Chapter 11). It may also take up to 16 weeks to see the full effect, so only a very slow titration will lead to the greatest effects at the lowest possible doses. A patient may respond to one treatment better than another, so switching agents to compare outcomes is reasonable. Slow titration is still required, however, as is consideration of discontinuation syndrome, unless a gradual cross taper is prescribed. It may take several years, then, to try all five treatment options fully. If a patient is satisfied with the first or second agent, further trials are not necessary.

Although standard treatment for alcohol dependence involves detoxification followed by 12-step support groups, efforts have been made to find pharmacological treatments to minimize alcohol consumption. The first attempt was an aversive one: disulfiram. Ethanol is oxidized to acetaldehyde by alcohol dehydrogenase, then acetaldehyde is oxidized to acetic acid by aldehyde dehydrogenase (ALDH). Disulfiram, first marketed in Denmark and approved by the FDA in 1951, is taken voluntarily to discourage use of alcohol by inhibiting ALDH. This leads to a buildup of acetaldehyde and many unpleasant physical symptoms: flushing, throbbing in the head and neck, headache, respiratory difficulties, nausea, copious vomiting, sweating, thirst, chest pain, palpitation, dyspnea, hyperventilation, tachycardia, hypotension, syncope, marked uneasiness, weakness, vertigo, blurred vision, and confusion. Severe reactions may include respiratory depression, cardiovascular collapse, arrhythmias, myocardial infarction, acute congestive heart failure, unconsciousness, convulsions, and death. Disulfiram is contraindicated in patients with cardiovascular disease or known sensitivities, including to rubber. The effects often last 30–60 minutes but may last up to several hours depending on how long alcohol is in the blood (Daily Med 2017).

Disulfiram does not reduce the desire to use ethanol and should only be used—with a patient's full understanding of the risks and consequences—as a tool to provide extra incentive to refrain from impulsive drinking. It should never be taken when alcohol is already in the body. It may also provoke a reaction when ethanol is ingested in food, such as a sauce or dessert (e.g., cherries jubilee, bananas Foster), or a medication (e.g., cough syrups) or from skin contact, including alcohol used to clean a wound or from aftershave, perfume, and cologne. Reactions may occur up to 14 days after disulfiram has been discontinued.

In 1994, the FDA approved marketing the opiate antagonist naltrexone to reduce the use of alcohol in patients with alcohol dependence. Meta-analysis has shown it has a small effect on the reduction of severe drinking (17%) and decrease in drinking days (4%) when used in oral form (Rösner et al. 2010b). Statistical significance for the intramuscular form or the opiate antagonist nalmefene (available in Europe) was not found (Rösner et al. 2010b). Its potential for liver toxicity in an already vulnerable population has been explored, and most studies report little additional concern except in cases of advanced liver disease (Antonelli et al. 2018; Leggio and Lee 2017; Marrazzi et al. 1997). The limited benefits joined with the cost, however, may still make naltrexone of limited value for many patients struggling with alcoholism.

The only other treatment approved for reducing alcohol use is acamprosate, which has shown modest improvement with a fairly strong safety profile (Plosker 2015; Rösner et al. 2010a). It was approved for marketing in Europe in 1989 and in the United States in 2004. A 15% reduction in relapse after detoxification has been observed with its use, as well as a 9% reduction in any drinking over 3–12 months of use. It may be more effective the closer it is used to detoxification (Kalk and Lingford-Hughes 2014). Diarrhea is the most common side effect, and with its thrice-daily dosing, compliance might be an issue. Acamprosate is largely eliminated through renal excretion, so it is contraindicated in patients with renal insufficiency (Saivin et al. 1998).

Topiramate also has been suggested for the treatment of alcohol abuse (Baltieri et al. 2008; Guglielmo et al. 2015), although it has many potential side effects (see "Medications to Stabilize Mood"). One recent meta-analysis failed to find efficacy for topiramate as well as for nalmefene, acamprosate, or naltrexone (Palpacuer et al. 2018); another found it moderately helpful, especially compared with the latter two (Blodgett et al. 2014). Further study on these four agents appears warranted.

Summary

Medications are labeled by their chemical structure, clinical benefit, receptor affinity, and presumed or confirmed mechanism of action. Therefore, many pharmaceuticals have several labels. An understanding of medicinal treatment options includes their historical context; ultimately, use is based solely upon composite results of RCTs and valid meta-analyses. Maintaining familiarity with replicated peer-reviewed data is crucial. Also, a firm knowledge of pharmacokinetics and pharmacodynamics (see Chapter 6) is essential in rational psychopharmacology, allowing practitioners to predict timing of responses, minimize risk of toxicities, and distinguish among rebound, withdrawal, and recurrence of underlying symptoms.

Key Points

■ Knowing the history of medications is important when considering their use.

■ Treat diagnosed syndromes rather than treating each symptom separately.

■ Choose medications with effective half-lives that match the clinical goals.

■ Prevent withdrawal and discontinuation syndrome by considering the effective half-lives of medications when changing and stopping them.

■ Depressed mood is a symptom not always associated with major depression.

■ Always confirm the generic names of medications before continuing another provider's prescriptions.

■ Warnings about a single risk do not imply that it occurs only with that medication or is the only risk of that medication.

■ Keep the targeted symptoms in mind when assessing outcome.

■ Various brands of the same generic medication may not utilize the same technology.

■ Do not change anticholinesterase inhibitor agents merely to seek greater efficacy.

Self-Assessment

1. Which of the following offers clinical advantages over standard alternatives?

    A. Sublingual preparations
    B. Oral dissolving tablets
    C. Chewable tables
    D. None of the above

2. Seizure threshold is lowered by (choose all that apply)

    A. Bupropion
    B. Clozapine
    C. Antipsychotics
    D. Antidepressants

3. Blood dyscrasias, such as neutropenia and agranulocytosis, are more common with (choose all that apply)

    A. Anticonvulsants
    B. Antidepressants
    C. Antipsychotics
    D. Soporifics

4. Medically threatening rashes occur mostly with

    A. Lamotrigine
    B. Carbamazepine
    C. Oxcarbazepine
    D. All of the above

5. Reversible anticholinesterase inhibitors

    A. Reverse memory impairment
    B. Are clearly effective with mild cognitive impairment
    C. Should not be changed, except for compliance or tolerability
    D. Are not effective in mild dementia

Discussion Topics

1. An 18-year-old college freshman presents with academic problems at the local university. She did well at her small-town high school but now is struggling to make the A grades in college she expected. She borrowed an Adderall from a friend and thought she concentrated better on it. She has diagnosed herself with ADHD and wants you to prescribe treatment. How will you proceed?

2. A male patient with major depression and no comorbidities did not respond to selective serotonin reuptake inhibitors until bupropion was added at 300 mg. Discuss the options for proceeding, considering length of treatment, number of agents used, and management for discontinuation syndrome, side effects, and recurrence.

Additional Reading

Drug Facts and Comparisons. Philadelphia, PA, Lippincott Williams and Wilkins, 2017 (Available in print, and subscription available for online consultation. Excellent, unbiased resource for dosage, form availability, pill and capsule strengths, and pictures.)

King C, Voruganti LNP: What's in a name? The evolution of the nomenclature of antipsychotic drugs. J Psychiatry Neurosci 27(3):168–175, 2002 12066446 (A delightful exploration and discussion of the history and dilemma of naming psychoactive medication categories, particularly those treating psychosis, that expounds upon the discussion of the issue in this chapter.)

Schatzberg AF, Nemeroff CB: The American Psychiatric Association Publishing Textbook of Psychopharmacology, 5th Edition, Revised. Washington, DC, American Psychiatric Publishing, 2017

References

Abraham G, Delva N, Waldron J, et al: Lithium treatment: a comparison of once- and twice-daily dosing. Acta Psychiatr Scand 85(1):65–69, 1992 1546552

Adam K, Oswald I: Effects of lormetazepam and of flurazepam on sleep. Br J Clin Pharmacol 17(5):531–538, 1984 6733001

Agelink MW, Zitzelsberger A, Klieser E: Withdrawal syndrome after discontinuation of venlafaxine. Am J Psychiatry 154(10):1473–1474, 1997 9326838

Agid O, Seeman P, Kapur S: The "delayed onset" of antipsychotic action—an idea whose time has come and gone. J Psychiatry Neurosci 31(2):93–100, 2006 16575424

Akiskal HS, Pinto O: The evolving bipolar spectrum. Prototypes I, II, III, and IV. Psychiatr Clin North Am 22(3):517–534, 1999 10550853

Allen MH, Hirschfeld RM, Wozniak PJ, et al: Linear relationship of valproate serum concentration to response and optimal serum levels for acute mania. Am J Psychiatry 163(2):272–275, 2006 16449481

American Diabetes Association, American Psychiatric Association, American Association of Clinical Endocrinologists, et al: Consensus development conference on antipsychotic drugs and obesity and diabetes. Diabetes Care 27(2):596–601, 2004 14747245

American Psychiatric Association: Diagnostic and Statistical Manual of Mental Disorders, 5th Edition. Arlington, VA, American Psychiatric Association, 2013

Anderson EW: Further observations on Benzedrine. Br Med J 2(4044):60–64, 1938

Antonelli M, Ferrulli A, Sestito L, et al: Alcohol addiction: the safety of available approved treatment options. Expert Opin Drug Saf 17(2):169–177, 2018 29120249

Atkin K, Kendall F, Gould D, et al: Neutropenia and agranulocytosis in patients receiving clozapine in the UK and Ireland. Br J Psychiatry 169(4):483–488, 1996 8894200

Auiler JF, Liu K, Lynch JM, et al: Effect of food on early drug exposure from extended-release stimulants: results from the Concerta, Adderall XR Food Evaluation (CAFE) Study. Curr Med Res Opin 18(5):311–316, 2002 12240794

Ayd FJ Jr: Emotional problems in children; the uses of drugs in therapeutic management. Calif Med 87(2):75–81, 1957 13446749

Baek JH, Kinrys G, Nierenberg AA: Lithium tremor revisited: pathophysiology and treatment. Acta Psychiatr Scand 129(1):17–23, 2014 23834617

Bailey PL, Andriano KP, Goldman M, et al: Variability of the respiratory response to diazepam. Anesthesiology 64(4):460–465, 1986 3083722

Baldaçara L, de Castro Ferrari MC, Monteiro BF, et al: Hypomania induced by atypical antipsychotics among schizophrenic patients: report of three cases. Pharmacopsychiatry 40(4):169–170, 2007 17694481

Ball SG, Iqbal Z: Diagnosis and treatment of hyponatraemia. Best Pract Res Clin Endocrinol Metab 30(2):161–173, 2016 27156756

Ballenger JC, Post RM: Kindling as a model for alcohol withdrawal syndromes. Br J Psychiatry 133:1–14, 1978a 352467

Ballenger JC, Post RM: Therapeutic effects of carbamazepine in affective illness: a preliminary report. Commun Psychopharmacol 2(2):159–175, 1978b 352607

Ballenger JC, Post RM: Carbamazepine in manic-depressive illness: a new treatment. Am J Psychiatry 137(7):782–790, 1980 7386656

Ballenger JC, Burrows GD, DuPont RL Jr, et al: Alprazolam in panic disorder and agoraphobia: results from a multicenter trial. I. Efficacy in short-term treatment. Arch Gen Psychiatry 45(5):413–422, 1988 3282478

Balme RH: Early medicinal use of bromides (Sir Charles Locock). J R Coll Physicians Lond 10(2):205–208, 1976 1107530

Baltieri DA, Daró FR, Ribeiro PL, et al: Comparing topiramate with naltrexone in the treatment of alcohol dependence. Addiction 103(12):2035–2044, 2008 18855810

Ban TA: Psychopharmacology. Baltimore, MD, Williams and Wilkins, 1969

Ban TA: The role of serendipity in drug discovery. Dialogues Clin Neurosci 8(3):335–344, 2006 17117615

Ban TA: Bromides. International Network for the History of Neuropsychophar-macology, October 24, 2013. Available at: http://inhn.org/drugs/bromides.html. Accessed September 29, 2019.

Bandelow B, Zohar J, Hollander E, et al: World Federation of Societies of Biological Psychiatry (WFSBP) guidelines for the pharmacological treatment of anxiety, obsessive-compulsive and post-traumatic stress disorders—first revision. World J Biol Psychiatry 9(4):248–312, 2008 18949648

Banich MT: Executive function: the search for an integrated account. Curr Dir Psychol Sci 18(2):89–94, 2009

Baptista T, Teneud L, Contreras Q, et al: Lithium and body weight gain. Pharmacopsychiatry 28(2):35–44, 1995 7624385

Barbee JG, Conrad EJ, Jamhour NJ: The effectiveness of olanzapine, risperidone, quetiapine, and ziprasidone as augmentation agents in treatment-resistant major depressive disorder. J Clin Psychiatry 65(7):975–981, 2004 15291687

Batelaan NM, Bosman RC, Muntingh A, et al: Risk of relapse after antidepressant discontinuation in anxiety disorders, obsessive-compulsive disorder, and post-traumatic stress disorder: systematic review and meta-analysis of relapse prevention trials. BMJ 358:j3927, 2017 28903922

Beer B, Ieni JR, Wu WH, et al: A placebo-controlled evaluation of single, escalating doses of CL 284,846, a non-benzodiazepine hypnotic. J Clin Pharmacol 34(4):335–344, 1994 8006201

Belmaker RH, Lerner Y, Ebstein RP: Rapid neuroleptization reconsidered. Am J Psychiatry 137(1):129–130, 1980 6101520

Belousova ED: The decreased level of plasma carnitine in patients with epilepsy [in Russian]. Zh Nevrol Psikhiatr Im S S Korsakova 117(6):106–110, 2017 28745680

Benyamina A, Samalin L: Atypical antipsychotic-induced mania/hypomania: a review of recent case reports and clinical studies. Int J Psychiatry Clin Pract 16(1):2–7, 2012 22122647

Berber MJ: FINISH: remembering the discontinuation syndrome. Flu-like symptoms, insomnia, nausea, imbalance, sensory disturbances, and hyperarousal (anxiety/agitation). J Clin Psychiatry 59(5):255, 1998 9632038

Berlin RK, Butler PM, Perloff MD: Gabapentin therapy in psychiatric disorders: a systematic review. Prim Care Companion CNS Disord 17(5):10, 2015 26835178

Biederman J, Mick E, Surman C, et al: A randomized, placebo-controlled trial of OROS methylphenidate in adults with attention-deficit/hyperactivity disorder. Biol Psychiatry 59(9):829–835, 2006 16373066

Birmaher B, Greenhill LL, Cooper TB, et al: Sustained release methylphenidate: pharmacokinetic studies in ADHD males. J Am Acad Child Adolesc Psychiatry 28(5):768–772, 1989 2793805

Black K, Shea C, Dursun S, Kutcher S: Selective serotonin reuptake inhibitor discontinuation syndrome: proposed diagnostic criteria. J Psychiatry Neurosci 25(3):255–261, 2000 10863885

Blaszczyk B, Lason W, Czuczwar SJ: Antiepileptic drugs and adverse skin reactions: an update. Pharmacol Rep 67(3):426–434, 2015 25933949

Blodgett JC, Del Re AC, Maisel NC, et al: A meta-analysis of topiramate's effects for individuals with alcohol use disorders. Alcohol Clin Exp Res 38(6):1481–1488, 2014 24796492

Bloom R, Amber KT: Identifying the incidence of rash, Stevens-Johnson syndrome and toxic epidermal necrolysis in patients taking lamotrigine: a systematic review of 122 randomized controlled trials. An Bras Dermatol 92(1):139–141, 2017 28225977

Botts SR, Raskind J: Gabapentin and lamotrigine in bipolar disorder. Am J Health Syst Pharm 56(19):1939–1944, 1999 10554911

Bowden CL, Singh V: Valproate in bipolar disorder: 2000 onwards. Acta Psychiatr Scand Suppl (426):13–20, 2005 15833096

Bowden CL, Singh V: Lamotrigine (Lamictal IR) for the treatment of bipolar disorder. Expert Opin Pharmacother 13(17):2565–2571, 2012 23140205

Bowden CL, Brugger AM, Swann AC, et al: Efficacy of divalproex vs lithium and placebo in the treatment of mania. JAMA 271(12):918–924, 1994 8120960

Boxenbaum H, Battle M: Effective half-life in clinical pharmacology. J Clin Pharmacol 35(8):763–766, 1995 8522631

Bradley C: The behavior of children receiving Benzedrine. Am J Psychiatry 94(3):577–585, 1937

Bradley C: Benzedrine and Dexedrine in the treatment of children's behavior disorders. Pediatrics 5(1):24–37, 1950 15404645

Breggin PR, Breggin GR: Talking Back to Prozac. New York, St. Martin's Press, 1994

Brielmaier BD: Eszopiclone (Lunesta): a new nonbenzodiazepine hypnotic agent. Proc Bayl Univ Med Cent 19(1):54–59, 2006 16424933

Brissos S, Veguilla MR, Taylor D, et al: The role of long-acting injectable antipsychotics in schizophrenia: a critical appraisal. Ther Adv Psychopharmacol 4(5):198–219, 2014 25360245

Brook S, Lucey JV, Gunn KP: Intramuscular ziprasidone compared with intramuscular haloperidol in the treatment of acute psychosis. J Clin Psychiatry 61(12):933–941, 2000 11206599

Brunet A, Orr SP, Tremblay J, et al: Effect of post-retrieval propranolol on psychophysiologic responding during subsequent script-driven traumatic imagery in post-traumatic stress disorder. J Psychiatr Res 42(6):503–506, 2008 17588604

Brunet A, Saumier D, Liu A, et al: Reduction of PTSD symptoms with pre-reactivation propranolol therapy: a randomized controlled trial. Am J Psychiatry 175(5):427–433, 2018 29325446

Bruno A, Morabito P, Spina E, et al: The role of levomilnacipran in the management of major depressive disorder: a comprehensive review. Curr Neuropharmacol 14(2):191–199, 2016 26572745

Burbiel JC: Primary prevention of posttraumatic stress disorder: drugs and implications. Mil Med Res 2:24, 2015 26504586

Calabrese JR, Keck PE Jr, McElroy SL, et al: A pilot study of topiramate as monotherapy in the treatment of acute mania. J Clin Psychopharmacol 21(3):340–342, 2001 11386499

Calabrese JR, Shelton MD, Rapport DJ, et al: Bipolar disorders and the effectiveness of novel anticonvulsants. J Clin Psychiatry 63(suppl 3):5–9, 2002 11908919

Calcaterra NE, Barrow JC: Classics in chemical neuroscience: diazepam (Valium). ACS Chem Neurosci 5(4):253–260, 2014 24552479

Canton J, Scott KM, Glue P: Optimal treatment of social phobia: systematic review and meta-analysis. Neuropsychiatr Dis Treat 8:203–215, 2012 22665997

Carbon M, Kane JM, Leucht S, et al: Tardive dyskinesia risk with first- and second-generation antipsychotics in comparative randomized controlled trials: a meta-analysis. World Psychiatry 17(3):330–340, 2018 30192088

Carey TS, Williams JW Jr, Oldham JM, et al: Gabapentin in the treatment of mental illness: the echo chamber of the case series. J Psychiatr Pract 14(suppl 1):15–27, 2008 19034206

Carpenter WT Jr, Davis JM: Another view of the history of antipsychotic drug discovery and development. Mol Psychiatry 17(12):1168–1173, 2012 22889923

Carta MG, Hardoy MC, Hardoy MJ, et al: The clinical use of gabapentin in bipolar spectrum disorders. J Affect Disord 75(1):83–91, 2003 12781355

Carter L, Zolezzi M, Lewczyk A: An updated review of the optimal lithium dosage regimen for renal protection. Can J Psychiatry 58(10):595–600, 2013 24165107

Cascade E, Kalali AH, Weisler RH: Short-acting versus long-acting medications for the treatment of ADHD. Psychiatry (Edgmont Pa) 5(8):24–27, 2008 19727272

Cattaneo CI, Ressico F, Valsesia R, et al: Sudden valproate-induced hyperammonemia managed with L-carnitine in a medically healthy bipolar patient: essential review of the literature and case report. Medicine (Baltimore) 96(39):e8117, 2017 28953637

Chen CH, Lin SK: Carbamazepine treatment of bipolar disorder: a retrospective evaluation of naturalistic long-term outcomes. BMC Psychiatry 12:47, 2012 22620289

Chiaro G, Castelnovo A, Bianco G, et al: Severe chronic abuse of zolpidem in refractory insomnia. J Clin Sleep Med 14(7):1257–1259, 2018 29991431

Childress AC, Brams M, Cutler AJ, et al: The efficacy and safety of Evekeo, racemic amphetamine sulfate, for treatment of attention-deficit/hyperactivity disorder symptoms: a multicenter, dose-optimized, double-blind, randomized, placebo-controlled crossover laboratory classroom study. J Child Adolesc Psychopharmacol 25(5):402–414, 2015 25692608

Childress AC, Wigal SB, Brams MN, et al: Efficacy and safety of amphetamine extended-release oral suspension in children with attention-deficit/hyperactivity disorder. J Child Adolesc Psychopharmacol 28(5):306–313, 2018 29211967

Childress AC, Kando JC, King TR, et al: Early onset efficacy and safety pilot study of amphetamine extended-release oral suspension in the treatment of children with attention-deficit/hyperactivity disorder. J Child Adolesc Psychopharmacol 29(1):2–8, 2019 30575407

Chouinard G: Clonazepam in acute and maintenance treatment of bipolar affective disorder. J Clin Psychiatry 48(suppl):29–37, 1987 3312180

Chouinard G, Young SN, Annable L: Antimanic effect of clonazepam. Biol Psychiatry 18(4):451–466, 1983 6407539

Cipriani A, Furukawa TA, Salanti G, et al: Comparative efficacy and acceptability of 12 new-generation antidepressants: a multiple-treatments meta-analysis. Lancet 373(9665):746–758, 2009 19185342

Citrome L: Clinical management of tardive dyskinesia: five steps to success. J Neurol Sci 383:199–204, 2017 29246613

Clayton AH, McGarvey EL, Abouesh AI, et al: Substitution of an SSRI with bupropion sustained release following SSRI-induced sexual dysfunction. J Clin Psychiatry 62(3):185–190, 2001 11305705

Clemow DB, Bushe C, Mancini M, et al: A review of the efficacy of atomoxetine in the treatment of attention-deficit hyperactivity disorder in children and adult patients with common comorbidities. Neuropsychiatr Dis Treat 13:357–371, 2017 28223809

ClinicalTrials.gov: Study of Rapastinel as monotherapy in patients with MDD. Updated July 19, 2019. Available at: https://clinicaltrials.gov/ct2/show/NCT03560518. Accessed February 27, 2020.

Coffman JA, Nasrallah HA, Lyskowski J, et al: Clinical effectiveness of oral and parenteral rapid neuroleptization. J Clin Psychiatry 48(1):20–24, 1987 3542982

Cohen D, Bogers JP, van Dijk D, et al: Beyond white blood cell monitoring: screening in the initial phase of clozapine therapy. J Clin Psychiatry 73(10):1307–1312, 2012 23140648

Colovic MB, Krstic DZ, Lazarevic-Pašti TD, et al: Acetylcholinesterase inhibitors: pharmacology and toxicology. Curr Neuropharmacol 11(3):315–335, 2013 24179466

Conners CK, Eisenberg L: The effects of methylphenidate on symptomatology and learning in disturbed children. Am J Psychiatry 120(5):458–464, 1963 14051237

Cornett EM, Novitch M, Kaye AD, et al: Medication-induced tardive dyskinesia: a review and update. Ochsner J 17(2):162–174, 2017 28638290

Correia-Melo FS, Argolo FC, Araújo-de-Freitas L, et al: Rapid infusion of esketamine for unipolar and bipolar depression: a retrospective chart review. Neuropsychiatr Dis Treat 13:1627–1632, 2017 28790825

Correll CU, Leucht S, Kane JM: Lower risk for tardive dyskinesia associated with second-generation antipsychotics: a systematic review of 1-year studies. Am J Psychiatry 161(3):414–425, 2004 14992963

Cotariu D, Zaidman JL: Valproic acid and the liver. Clin Chem 34(5):890–897, 1988 3131043

Cowles BJ: Lisdexamfetamine for treatment of attention-deficit/hyperactivity disorder. Ann Pharmacother 43(4):669–676, 2009 19318601

Crilly J: The history of clozapine and its emergence in the US market: a review and analysis. Hist Psychiatry 18(1):39–60, 2007 17580753

Crocq MA: A history of antipsychotic long-acting injections in the treatment of schizophrenia [in French]. Encephale 41(1):84–92, 2015 25598520

Curran MP, Perry CM: Amisulpride: a review of its use in the management of schizophrenia. Drugs 61(14):2123–2150, 2001 11735643

Curtin F, Berney P, Kaufmann C: Moclobemide discontinuation syndrome predominantly presenting with influenza-like symptoms. J Psychopharmacol 16(3):271–272, 2002 12236637

Daily Med: Antabuse–disulfiram tablet. May 11, 2017. Available at: https://dailymed.nlm.nih.gov/dailymed/drugInfo.cfm?setid=f0ca0e1f-9641–48d5–9367-e5d1069e8680. Accessed September 29, 2019.

Davis J, Desmond M, Berk M: Lithium and nephrotoxicity: a literature review of approaches to clinical management and risk stratification. BMC Nephrol 19:305, 2018 12236637

de Boer T: The pharmacologic profile of mirtazapine. J Clin Psychiatry 57(suppl 4):19–25, 1996 8636062

Deardorff WJ, Feen E, Grossberg GT: The use of cholinesterase inhibitors across all stages of Alzheimer's disease. Drugs Aging 32(7):537–547, 2015 26033268

Dell'Orto VG, Belotti EA, Goeggel-Simonetti B, et al: Metabolic disturbances and renal stone promotion on treatment with topiramate: a systematic review. Br J Clin Pharmacol 77(6):958–964, 2014 24219102

Desmarais JE, Beauclair L, Annable L, et al: Effects of discontinuing anticholinergic treatment on movement disorders, cognition and psychopathology in patients with schizophrenia. Ther Adv Psychopharmacol 4(6):257–267, 2014 25489477

Dilsaver SC, Greden JF: Antidepressant withdrawal phenomena. Biol Psychiatry 19(2):237–256, 1984 6324897

DiMascio A, Bernardo DL, Greenblatt DJ, et al: A controlled trial of amantadine in drug-induced extrapyramidal disorders. Arch Gen Psychiatry 33(5):599–602, 1976 5066

Dinges DF, Basner M, Ecker AJ, et al: Effects of zolpidem and zaleplon on cognitive performance after emergent Tmax: a randomized placebo-controlled trial. Sleep 42(3):258, 2018 30576525

Donello JE, Banerjee P, Li YX, et al: Positive N-methyl-D-aspartate receptor modulation by rapastinel promotes rapid and sustained antidepressant-like effects. Int J Neuropsychopharmacol 22(3):247–259, 2019 30544218

Dong X, Leppik IE, White J, et al: Hyponatremia from oxcarbazepine and carbamazepine. Neurology 65(12):1976–1978, 2005 16380624

Dooley M, Plosker GL: Zaleplon: a review of its use in the treatment of insomnia. Drugs 60(2):413–445, 2000 10983740

Drugs.com: Adderall. October 1, 2018a. Available at: https://www.drugs.com/pro/adderall.html. Accessed September 29, 2019.

Drugs.com: Evekeo. October 1, 2018b. Available at: https://www.drugs.com/pro/evekeo.html. Accessed September 29, 2019.

Drugs.com: Barhemsys approval status. July 8, 2019. Available at: https://www.drugs.com/history/barhemsys.html. Accessed September 29, 2019.

Electronic Medicines Compendium: Frisium, 10 mg tablets. July 6, 2018. Available at: https://www.medicines.org.uk/emc/medicine/8298. Accessed September 29, 2019.

Emrich HM, von Zerssen D, Kissling W, et al: Effect of sodium valproate on mania. The GABA-hypothesis of affective disorders. Arch Psychiatr Nervenkr (1970) 229(1):1–16, 1980 6778456

Ermer JC, Dennis K, Haffey MB, et al: Intranasal versus oral administration of lisdexamfetamine dimesylate: a randomized, open-label, two-period, crossover, single-dose, single-centre pharmacokinetic study in healthy adult men. Clin Drug Investig 31(6):357–370, 2011 21539403

Eslami-Shahrbabaki M, Barfeh B, Nasirian M: Persistent psychosis after abuse of high dose of zolpidem. Addict Health 6(3–4):159–162, 2014 25984284

Fabre LF, Putman HP 3rd: Depressive symptoms and intellectual functioning in anxiety patients treated with clorazepate. J Clin Psychiatry 49(5):189–192, 1988 2896666

Fagiolini A, Comandini A, Catena Dell'Osso M, et al: Rediscovering trazodone for the treatment of major depressive disorder. CNS Drugs 26(12):1033–1049, 2012 23192413

Farkas RH, Unger EF, Temple R: Zolpidem and driving impairment—identifying persons at risk. N Engl J Med 369(8):689–691, 2013 23923991

Fernández A, Mascayano F, Lips W, et al: Effects of modafinil on attention performance, short-term memory and executive function in university students: a randomized trial. Medwave 15(5):e6166, 2015 26135067

Findling RL, Dinh S: Transdermal therapy for attention-deficit hyperactivity disorder with the methylphenidate patch (MTS). CNS Drugs 28(3):217–228, 2014 24532028

Findling RL, Short EJ, Manos MJ: Short-term cardiovascular effects of methylphenidate and Adderall. J Am Acad Child Adolesc Psychiatry 40(5):525–529, 2001 11349696

Fisher A, Carney G, Bassett K, et al: Tolerability of cholinesterase inhibitors: a population-based study of persistence, adherence, and switching. Drugs Aging 34(3):221–231, 2017 28138912

Ford L, Goldberg JL, Selan F, et al: Comprehensive review of visual defects reported with topiramate. Clin Ophthalmol 11:983–992, 2017 28579749

Fornaro M, Stubbs B, De Berardis D, et al: Atypical antipsychotics in the treatment of acute bipolar depression with mixed features: a systematic review and exploratory meta-analysis of placebo-controlled clinical trials. Int J Mol Sci 17(2):241, 2016 26891297

Forster A, Gardaz JP, Suter PM, et al: Respiratory depression by midazolam and diazepam. Anesthesiology 53(6):494–497, 1980 7457966

Foulser P, Abbasi Y, Mathilakath A, et al: Do not treat the numbers: lithium toxicity. BMJ Case Rep 2:2017, 2017 28576914

Fountoulakis KN, Grunze H, Vieta E, et al: The International College of Neuro-Psychopharmacology (CINP) treatment guidelines for bipolar disorder in adults (CINP-BD-2017), part 3: the clinical guidelines. Int J Neuropsychopharmacol 20(2):180–195, 2017 27941079

Foussias G, Remington G: Negative symptoms in schizophrenia: avolition and Occam's razor. Schizophr Bull 36(2):359–369, 2010 18644851

Fullerton CA, Busch AB, Frank RG: The rise and fall of gabapentin for bipolar disorder: a case study on off-label pharmaceutical diffusion. Med Care 48(4):372–379, 2010 20195173

Gauillard J, Cheref S, Vacherontrystram MN, et al: Chloral hydrate: a hypnotic best forgotten [in French]? Encephale 28(3 Pt 1):200–204, 2002 12091779

Geddes JR, Calabrese JR, Goodwin GM: Lamotrigine for treatment of bipolar depression: independent meta-analysis and meta-regression of individual patient data from five randomised trials. Br J Psychiatry 194(1):4–9, 2009 19118318

Genton P, Bauer J, Duncan S, et al: On the association between valproate and polycystic ovary syndrome. Epilepsia 42(3):295–304, 2001 11442143

Gerstner T, Büsing D, Bell N, et al: Valproic acid-induced pancreatitis: 16 new cases and a review of the literature. J Gastroenterol 42(1):39–48, 2007 17322992

Gitlin M: Lithium side effects and toxicity: prevalence and management strategies. Int J Bipolar Disord 4(1):27, 2016 27900734

Gong R, Wang P, Dworkin L: What we need to know about the effect of lithium on the kidney. Am J Physiol Renal Physiol 311(6):F1168–F1171, 2016 27122541

Goodwin FK, Ghaemi SN: Bipolar disorder. Dialogues Clin Neurosci 1(1):41–51, 1999 22033232

Goodwin GM, Bowden CL, Calabrese JR, et al: A pooled analysis of 2 placebo-controlled 18-month trials of lamotrigine and lithium maintenance in bipolar I disorder. J Clin Psychiatry 65(3):432–441, 2004 15096085

Goodwin GM, Haddad PM, Ferrier IN, et al: Evidence-based guidelines for treating bipolar disorder: revised third edition recommendations from the British Association for Psychopharmacology. J Psychopharmacol 30(6):495–553, 2016 26979387

Gorman DA, Gardner DM, Murphy AL, et al: Canadian guidelines on pharmacotherapy for disruptive and aggressive behaviour in children and adolescents with attention-deficit hyperactivity disorder, oppositional defiant disorder, or conduct disorder. Can J Psychiatry 60(2):62–76, 2015 25886657

Gotlib D, Ramaswamy R, Kurlander JE, et al: Valproic acid in women and girls of childbearing age. Curr Psychiatry Rep 19(9):58, 2017 28726062

Granger B, Albu S: The haloperidol story. Ann Clin Psychiatry 17(3):137–140, 2005 16433054

Granville-Grossman KL, Turner P: The effect of propranolol on anxiety. Lancet 1(7441):788–790, 1966 4159809

Gray SL, Dublin S, Yu O, et al: Benzodiazepine use and risk of incident dementia or cognitive decline: prospective population based study. BMJ 352:i90, 2016 26837813

Greenblatt DJ, Shader RI, Koch-Weser J: Pharmacokinetics in clinical medicine: oxazepam versus other benzodiazepines. Dis Nerv Syst 36(5 Pt. 2):6–13, 1975 1095326

Griffin CE 3rd, Kaye AM, Bueno FR, et al: Benzodiazepine pharmacology and central nervous system-mediated effects. Ochsner J 13(2):214–223, 2013 23789008

Grunze H, Vieta E, Goodwin GM, et al: The World Federation of Societies of Biological Psychiatry (WFSBP) guidelines for the biological treatment of bipolar
disorders: acute and long-term treatment of mixed states in bipolar disorder.
World J Biol Psychiatry 19(1):2–58, 2018 29098925

Guberman AH, Besag FM, Brodie MJ, et al: Lamotrigine-associated rash: risk/
benefit considerations in adults and children. Epilepsia 40(7):985–991, 1999
10403224

Guelen PJ, Janssen TJ, De Witte TC, et al: Bioavailability of lithium from lithium
citrate syrup versus conventional lithium carbonate tablets. Biopharm Drug
Dispos 13(7):503–511, 1992 1489941

Guglielmo R, Martinotti G, Quatrale M, et al: Topiramate in alcohol use disorders: review and update. CNS Drugs 29(5):383–395, 2015 25899459

Gupta S, Khastgir U: Drug information update. Lithium and chronic kidney disease: debates and dilemmas. BJPsych Bull 41(4):216–220, 2017

Gupta S, Gao JJ, Emmett M, et al: Topiramate and metabolic acidosis: an evolving
story. Hosp Pract (1995) 45(5):192–195, 2017 28828886

Haertling F, Mueller B, Bilke-Hentsch O: Effectiveness and safety of a long-acting,
once-daily, two-phase release formulation of methylphenidate (Ritalin LA) in
school children under daily practice conditions. Atten Defic Hyperact Disord
7(2):157–164, 2015 25346231

Hajek T, Alda M, Grof P: Discontinuation of lithium because of side effects. J Psychiatry Neurosci 36(6):E39–E40, 2011 22011562

Heal DJ, Smith SL, Gosden J, et al: Amphetamine, past and present—a pharmacological and clinical perspective. J Psychopharmacol 27(6):479–496, 2013 23539642

Heel RC, Brogden RN, Speight TM, et al: Temazepam: a review of its pharmacological properties and therapeutic efficacy as an hypnotic. Drugs 21(5):321–
340, 1981 6112127

Hellewell JS: Oxcarbazepine (Trileptal) in the treatment of bipolar disorders: a review
of efficacy and tolerability. J Affect Disord 72(suppl 1):S23–S34, 2002 12589900

Herring WJ, Connor KM, Snyder E, et al: Suvorexant in patients with insomnia:
pooled analyses of three-month data from phase-3 randomized controlled
clinical trials. J Clin Sleep Med 12(9):1215–1225, 2016 27397664

Heydorn WE: Zaleplon—a review of a novel sedative hypnotic used in the treatment of insomnia. Expert Opin Investig Drugs 9(4):841–858, 2000 11060714

Higgins A, Nash M, Lynch AM: Antidepressant-associated sexual dysfunction:
impact, effects, and treatment. Drug Healthc Patient Saf 2:141–150, 2010
21701626

Hirschfeld RM, Kasper S: A review of the evidence for carbamazepine and oxcarbazepine in the treatment of bipolar disorder. Int J Neuropsychopharmacol
7(4):507–522, 2004 15458610

Honigfeld G, Arellano F, Sethi J, et al: Reducing clozapine-related morbidity and
mortality: 5 years of experience with the Clozaril National Registry. J Clin
Psychiatry 59(suppl 3):3–7, 1998 9541331

Hoorn EJ, Zietse R: Diagnosis and treatment of hyponatremia: compilation of the
guidelines. J Am Soc Nephrol 28(5):1340–1349, 2017 28174217

Horwitz AV: Book review: Happy Pills in America: From Miltown to Prozac; The Age of Anxiety: A History of America's Turbulent Affair With Tranquilizers; Before Prozac: The Troubled History of Mood Disorders in Psychiatry. N Engl J Med 360:841–844, 2009

Houghton KT, Forrest A, Awad A, et al: Biological rationale and potential clinical use of gabapentin and pregabalin in bipolar disorder, insomnia and anxiety: protocol for a systematic review and meta-analysis. BMJ Open 7(3):e013433, 2017 28348186

Hsiao YT, Wei IH, Huang CC: Oxcarbazepine-related neutropenia: a case report. J Clin Psychopharmacol 30(1):94–95, 2010 20075666

Huffman JC, Stern TA: Neuropsychiatric consequences of cardiovascular medications. Dialogues Clin Neurosci 9(1):29–45, 2007 17506224

Huss M, Chen W, Ludolph AG: Guanfacine extended release: a new pharmacological treatment option in Europe. Clin Drug Investig 36(1):1–25, 2016 26585576

Huss M, Duhan P, Gandhi P, et al: Methylphenidate dose optimization for ADHD treatment: review of safety, efficacy, and clinical necessity. Neuropsychiatr Dis Treat 13:1741–1751, 2017 28740389

Hvolby A: Associations of sleep disturbance with ADHD: implications for treatment. Atten Defic Hyperact Disord 7(1):1–18, 2015 26585576

Ibrahim K, Donyai P: Drug holidays from ADHD medication: international experience over the past four decades. J Atten Disord 19(7):551–568, 2015 25253684

Ibrahim K, Donyai P: What stops practitioners discussing medication breaks in children and adolescents with ADHD? Identifying barriers through theory-driven qualitative research. Atten Defic Hyperact Disord 10(4):273–283, 2018 29982921

Ibrahim K, Vogt C, Donyai P: Caught in the eye of the storm: a qualitative study of views and experiences of planned drug holidays from methylphenidate in child and adolescent ADHD treatment. Child Adolesc Ment Health 21(4):192–200, 2016

Ichikawa J, Ishii H, Bonaccorso S, et al: 5-HT(2A) and D(2) receptor blockade increases cortical DA release via 5-HT(1A) receptor activation: a possible mechanism of atypical antipsychotic-induced cortical dopamine release. J Neurochem 76(5):1521–1531, 2001 11238736

Ingimarsson O, MacCabe JH, Haraldsson M, et al: Neutropenia and agranulocytosis during treatment of schizophrenia with clozapine versus other antipsychotics: an observational study in Iceland. BMC Psychiatry 16(1):441, 2016 27955666

Isojärvi JIT, Taubøll E, Tapanainen JS, et al: On the association between valproate and polycystic ovary syndrome: a response and an alternative view. Epilepsia 42(3):305–310, 2002 11442144

Jha KK, Chaudhary DP, Rijal T, et al: Delayed Stevens-Johnson syndrome secondary to the use of lamotrigine in bipolar mood disorder. Indian J Psychol Med 39(2):209–212, 2017 28515564

Jing E, Straw-Wilson K: Sexual dysfunction in selective serotonin reuptake inhibitors (SSRIs) and potential solutions: a narrative literature review. Ment Health Clin 6(4):191–196, 2016 29955469

Joe SH, Chang JS, Won S, et al: Feasibility of a slower lamotrigine titration schedule for bipolar depression: a naturalistic study. Int Clin Psychopharmacol 24(2):105–110, 2009 19190502

Joffe H, Cohen LS, Suppes T, et al: Longitudinal follow-up of reproductive and metabolic features of valproate-associated polycystic ovarian syndrome features: a preliminary report. Biol Psychiatry 60(12):1378–1381, 2006 16950230

Johnson FN (ed): Handbook of Lithium Therapy. Dordrecht, The Netherlands, Springer, 1980

Joseph A, Ayyagari R, Xie M, et al: Comparative efficacy and safety of attention-deficit/hyperactivity disorder pharmacotherapies, including guanfacine extended release: a mixed treatment comparison. Eur Child Adolesc Psychiatry 26(8):875–897, 2017 28258319

Judd LL, Akiskal HS, Schettler PJ, et al: The long-term natural history of the weekly symptomatic status of bipolar I disorder. Arch Gen Psychiatry 59(6):530–537, 2002 12044195

Kalk NJ, Lingford-Hughes AR: The clinical pharmacology of acamprosate. Br J Clin Pharmacol 77(2):315–323, 2014 23278595

Kane J, Honigfeld G, Singer J, et al: Clozapine for the treatment-resistant schizophrenic. A double-blind comparison with chlorpromazine. Arch Gen Psychiatry 45(9):789–796, 1988 3046553

Kane JM, Davis JM, Schooler N, et al: A multidose study of haloperidol decanoate in the maintenance treatment of schizophrenia. Am J Psychiatry 159(4):554–560, 2002 11925292

Kane JM, Detke HC, Naber D, et al: Olanzapine long-acting injection: a 24-week, randomized, double-blind trial of maintenance treatment in patients with schizophrenia. Am J Psychiatry 167(2):181–189, 2010 20008947

Katona C, Hansen T, Olsen CK: A randomized, double-blind, placebo-controlled, duloxetine-referenced, fixed-dose study comparing the efficacy and safety of Lu AA21004 in elderly patients with major depressive disorder. Int Clin Psychopharmacol 27(4):215–223, 2012 22572889

Katzman MA, Bleau P, Blier P, et al: Canadian clinical practice guidelines for the management of anxiety, posttraumatic stress and obsessive-compulsive disorders. BMC Psychiatry 14(suppl 1):S1, 2014 25081580

Kavoor AR, Mitra S, Mondal SK, et al: Risperidone-induced mania: an emergent complication of treatment. J Pharmacol Pharmacother 5(4):258–260, 2014 25422570

Keating GM, McClellan K, Jarvis B: Methylphenidate (OROS formulation). CNS Drugs 15(6):495–500, discussion 501–503, 2001 11524026

Kellner M: Drug treatment of obsessive-compulsive disorder. Dialogues Clin Neurosci 12(2):187–197, 2010 20623923

Kessing LV, Gerds TA, Feldt-Rasmussen B, et al: Use of lithium and anticonvulsants and the rate of chronic kidney disease: a nationwide population-based study. JAMA Psychiatry 72(12):1182–1191, 2015 26535805

King C, Voruganti LNP: What's in a name? The evolution of the nomenclature of antipsychotic drugs. J Psychiatry Neurosci 27(3):168–175, 2002 12066446

Kishi T, Matsunaga S, Oya K, et al: Memantine for Alzheimer's disease: an updated systematic review and meta-analysis. J Alzheimers Dis 60(2):401–425, 2017 28922160

Kishimoto T, Robenzadeh A, Leucht C, et al: Long-acting injectable vs oral antipsychotics for relapse prevention in schizophrenia: a meta-analysis of randomized trials. Schizophr Bull 40(1):192–213, 2014 23256986

Klein DF: Importance of psychiatric diagnosis in prediction of clinical drug effects. Arch Gen Psychiatry 16(1):118–126, 1967 5333776

Knopman DS, Petersen RC: Mild cognitive impairment and mild dementia: a clinical perspective. Mayo Clin Proc 89(10):1452–1459, 2014 25282431

Kocsis JH, Zisook S, Davidson J, et al: Double-blind comparison of sertraline, imipramine, and placebo in the treatment of dysthymia: psychosocial outcomes. Am J Psychiatry 154(3):390–395, 1997 9054788

Kolar D, Keller A, Golfinopoulos M, et al: Treatment of adults with attention-deficit/hyperactivity disorder. Neuropsychiatr Dis Treat 4(2):389–403, 2008 18728745

Komossa K, Rummel-Kluge C, Schwarz S, et al: Risperidone versus other atypical antipsychotics for schizophrenia. Cochrane Database Syst Rev (1):CD006626, 2011 21249678

Kopala LC, Good KP, Honer WG: Extrapyramidal signs and clinical symptoms in first-episode schizophrenia: response to low-dose risperidone. J Clin Psychopharmacol 17(4):308–313, 1997 9241011

Kramer PD: Listening to Prozac. New York, Viking Penguin, 1993

Kratochvil CJ, Newcorn JH, Arnold LE, et al: Atomoxetine alone or combined with fluoxetine for treating ADHD with comorbid depressive or anxiety symptoms. J Am Acad Child Adolesc Psychiatry 44(9):915–924, 2005 16113620

Kumar PNS, Gopalakrishnan A: Oxcarbazepine-induced hyponatremia in bipolar disorder: a report of two cases. Indian J Psychiatry 58(2):233–234, 2016 27385863

Lally MD, Kral MC, Boan AD: Not all generic Concerta is created equal: comparison of OROS versus non-OROS for the treatment of ADHD. Clin Pediatr (Phila) 55(13):1197–1201, 2016 26467563

Lambert PA, Borselli S, Marcou G, et al: Neuro-psychotropic properties of the Depamide: psychic action among epileptics and presenting direct disorders diseases [in French]. CR Congres de Psychiatrie et de Neurologie de Langue Francaise, Masson, Paris, 1966, pp 1034–1039

Lane HY, Lin YC, Chang WH: Mania induced by risperidone: dose related? J Clin Psychiatry 59(2):85–86, 1998 9501895

Lann MA, Molina DK: A fatal case of benzodiazepine withdrawal. Am J Forensic Med Pathol 30(2):177–179, 2009 19465812

Laver K, Dyer S, Whitehead C, et al: Interventions to delay functional decline in people with dementia: a systematic review of systematic reviews. BMJ Open 6(4):e010767, 2016 27121704

Leary E, Sheth RD, Gidal BE: Time course of reversal of valproate-mediated inhibition of lamotrigine. Seizure 57:76–79, 2018 29574285

Lee KC, Chen JJ: Transdermal selegiline for the treatment of major depressive disorder. Neuropsychiatr Dis Treat 3(5):527–537, 2007 19300583

Leggio L, Lee MR: Treatment of alcohol use disorder in patients with alcoholic liver disease. Am J Med 130(2):124–134, 2017 27984008

Leucht S, Cipriani A, Spineli L, et al: Comparative efficacy and tolerability of 15 antipsychotic drugs in schizophrenia: a multiple-treatments meta-analysis. Lancet 382(9896):951–962, 2013 23810019

Li L, Vlisides PE: Ketamine: 50 years of modulating the mind. Front Hum Neurosci 10:612, 2016 27965560

Li XB, Tang YL, Wang CY, et al: Clozapine for treatment-resistant bipolar disorder: a systematic review. Bipolar Disord 17(3):235–247, 2015 25346322

Licata SC, Mashhoon Y, Maclean RR, et al: Modest abuse-related subjective effects of zolpidem in drug-naive volunteers. Behav Pharmacol 22(2):160–166, 2011 21301324

Lindström L, Lindström E, Nilsson M, et al: Maintenance therapy with second generation antipsychotics for bipolar disorder—a systematic review and meta-analysis. J Affect Disord 213:138–150, 2017 28222360

Linssen AM, Sambeth A, Vuurman EF, et al: Cognitive effects of methylphenidate in healthy volunteers: a review of single dose studies. Int J Neuropsychopharmacol 17(6):961–977, 2014 24423151

Loebel A, Citrome L: Lurasidone: a novel antipsychotic agent for the treatment of schizophrenia and bipolar depression. BJPsych Bull 39(5):237–241, 2015 26755968

Lonergan MH, Olivera-Figueroa LA, Pitman RK, et al: Propranolol's effects on the consolidation and reconsolidation of long-term emotional memory in healthy participants: a meta-analysis. J Psychiatry Neurosci 38(4):222–231, 2013 23182304

López-Muñoz F, Ucha-Udabe R, Alamo C: The history of barbiturates a century after their clinical introduction. Neuropsychiatr Dis Treat 1(4):329–343, 2005 18568113

López-Muñoz F, Shen WW, D'Ocon P, et al: A history of the pharmacological treatment of bipolar disorder. Int J Mol Sci 19(7):2143, 2018 30041458

Lucki I, Rickels K, Geller AM: Chronic use of benzodiazepines and psychomotor and cognitive test performance. Psychopharmacology (Berl) 88(4):426–433, 1986 2871579

Maelicke A: Pharmacokinetic rationale for switching from donepezil to galantamine. Clin Ther 23(suppl A):A8–A12, 2001 11396871

Mahableshwarkar AR, Zajecka J, Jacobson W, et al: A randomized, placebo-controlled, active-reference, double-blind, flexible-dose study of the efficacy of vortioxetine on cognitive function in major depressive disorder. Neuropsychopharmacology 40(8):2025–2037, 2015 25687662

Mahmood S, Booker I, Huang J, et al: Effect of topiramate on weight gain in patients receiving atypical antipsychotic agents. J Clin Psychopharmacol 33(1):90–94, 2013 23277264

Mahone EM, Denckla MB: Attention-deficit/hyperactivity disorder: a historical neuropsychological perspective. J Int Neuropsychol Soc 23(9–10):916–929, 2017 29198277

Mark TL, Levit KR, Buck JA: Datapoints: psychotropic drug prescriptions by medical specialty. Psychiatr Serv 60(9):1167, 2009 19723729

Marken PA, Haykal RF, Fisher JN: Management of psychotropic-induced hyperprolactinemia. Clin Pharm 11(10):851–856, 1992 1341991

Markowitz JS, DeVane CL, Pestreich LK, et al: A comprehensive in vitro screening of d-, l-, and dl-threo-methylphenidate: an exploratory study. J Child Adolesc Psychopharmacol 16(6):687–698, 2006 17201613

Marrazzi MA, Wroblewski JM, Kinzie J, et al: High-dose naltrexone and liver function safety. Am J Addict 6(1):21–29, 1997 9097868

Mashiko H, Kurita M, Shirakawa H, et al: Case of bipolar disorder successfully stabilized with clonazepam, valproate and lithium after numerous relapses for 47 years. Psychiatry Clin Neurosci 58(3):340–341, 2004 15149305

Mason BL, Brown ES, Croarkin PE: Historical underpinnings of bipolar disorder diagnostic criteria. Behav Sci (Basel) 6(3):14, 2016 27429010

Massoud F, Desmarais JE, Gauthier S: Switching cholinesterase inhibitors in older adults with dementia. Int Psychogeriatr 23(3):372–378, 2011 21044399

Matsunaga S, Kishi T, Iwata N: Memantine monotherapy for Alzheimer's disease: a systematic review and meta-Analysis. PLoS One 10(4):e0123289, 2015

Mattei C, Rapagnani MP, Stahl SM: Ziprasidone hydrochloride: what role in the management of schizophrenia? J Cent Nerv Syst Dis 3:1–16, 2011 25860130

Mayo-Wilson E, Li T, Fusco N, et al: Cherry-picking by trialists and meta-analysts can drive conclusions about intervention efficacy. J Clin Epidemiol 91:95–110, 2017 28842290

McCloud TL, Caddy C, Jochim J, et al: Ketamine and other glutamate receptor modulators for depression in adults. Cochrane Database Syst Rev (9):CD011612, 2015 26415966

McIntyre RS, Lophaven S, Olsen CK: A randomized, double-blind, placebo-controlled study of vortioxetine on cognitive function in depressed adults. Int J Neuropsychopharmacol 17(10):1557–1567, 2014 24787143

McKnight RF, Adida M, Budge K, et al: Lithium toxicity profile: a systematic review and meta-analysis. Lancet 379(9817):721–728, 2012 22265699

McNamara PJ, Colburn WA, Gibaldi M: Time course of carbamazepine self-induction. J Pharmacokinet Biopharm 7(1):63–68, 1979 458557

Medicines and Healthcare Products Regulatory Agency: Reboxetine: a review of the benefits and risks. September 2011. Available at: http://www.mhra.gov.uk/home/groups/s-par/documents/websiteresources/con129107.pdf. Accessed September 29, 2019.

Meyer JM, Simpson GM: From chlorpromazine to olanzapine: a brief history of antipsychotics. Psychiatr Serv 48(9):1137–1139, 1997 9285972

Meyer JM, Ng-Mak DS, Chuang CC, et al: Weight changes before and after lurasidone treatment: a real-world analysis using electronic health records. Ann Gen Psychiatry 16:36, 2017 29075309

Michelson D, Bancroft J, Targum S, et al: Female sexual dysfunction associated with antidepressant administration: a randomized, placebo-controlled study of pharmacologic intervention. Am J Psychiatry 157(2):239–243, 2000 10671393

Milia A, Pilia G, Mascia MG: Oxcarbazepine-induced leukopenia. J Neuropsychiatry Clin Neurosci 20(4):502–503, 2008 19196947

Miller LG, Greenblatt DJ, Barnhill JG, et al: Chronic benzodiazepine administration. I. Tolerance is associated with benzodiazepine receptor downregulation and decreased gamma-aminobutyric acid-A receptor function. J Pharmacol Exp Ther 246(1):170–176, 1988 2839660

Ming X, Mulvey M, Mohanty S, et al: Safety and efficacy of clonidine and clonidine extended-release in the treatment of children and adolescents with attention deficit and hyperactivity disorders. Adolesc Health Med Ther 2:105–112, 2011 24600280

Minzenberg MJ, Carter CS: Modafinil: a review of neurochemical actions and effects on cognition. Neuropsychopharmacology 33(7):1477–1502, 2008 17712350

Mirza N, Marson AG, Pirmohamed M: Effect of topiramate on acid-base balance: extent, mechanism and effects. Br J Clin Pharmacol 68(5):655–661, 2009 19916989

Miyamoto S, Fleischhacker W: The use of long-acting injectable antipsychotics in schizophrenia. Curr Treat Options Psychiatry 4(2):117–126, 2017 28580230

Mock CM, Schwetschenau KH: Levocarnitine for valproic-acid-induced hyperammonemic encephalopathy. Am J Health Syst Pharm 69(1):35–39, 2012 22180549

Mockenhaupt M, Messenheimer J, Tennis P, et al: Risk of Stevens-Johnson syndrome and toxic epidermal necrolysis in new users of antiepileptics. Neurology 64(7):1134–1138, 2005 15824335

Modell JG, Katholi CR, Modell JD, et al: Comparative sexual side effects of bupropion, fluoxetine, paroxetine, and sertraline. Clin Pharmacol Ther 61(4):476–487, 1997 9129565

Montgomery KA: Sexual desire disorders. Psychiatry (Edgmont Pa) 5(6):50–55, 2008 19727285

Montgomery W, Treuer T, Karagianis J, et al: Orally disintegrating olanzapine review: effectiveness, patient preference, adherence, and other properties. Patient Prefer Adherence 6:109–125, 2012 22346347

Moore M, Yuen HM, Dunn N, et al: Explaining the rise in antidepressant prescribing: a descriptive study using the general practice research database. BMJ 339(7727):b3999, 2009 19833707

Morishita S: Clonazepam as a therapeutic adjunct to improve the management of depression: a brief review. Hum Psychopharmacol 24(3):191–198, 2009 19330803

Morishita S, Aoki S: Clonazepam augmentation of antidepressants: does it distinguish unipolar from bipolar depression? J Affect Disord 71(1–3):217–220, 2002 12167520

Moskal JR, Burch R, Burgdorf JS, et al: GLYX-13, an NMDA receptor glycine site functional partial agonist enhances cognition and produces antidepressant effects without the psychotomimetic side effects of NMDA receptor antagonists. Expert Opin Investig Drugs 23(2):243–254, 2014 24251380

Moskal JR, Burgdorf JS, Stanton PK, et al: The development of rapastinel (formerly GLYX-13): a rapid acting and long lasting antidepressant. Curr Neuropharmacol 15(1):47–56, 2017 26997507

Mousavi SG, Rostami H, Sharbafchi MR, et al: Onset of action of atypical and typical antipsychotics in the treatment of acute psychosis. J Res Pharm Pract 2(4):138–144, 2013 24991622

Munetz MR, Benjamin S: How to examine patients using the Abnormal Involuntary Movement Scale. Hosp Community Psychiatry 39(11):1172–1177, 1988 2906320

Murrough JW, Iosifescu DV, Chang LC, et al: Antidepressant efficacy of ketamine in treatment-resistant major depression: a two-site randomized controlled trial. Am J Psychiatry 170(10):1134–1142, 2013 23982301

Murrough JW, Soleimani L, DeWilde KE, et al: Ketamine for rapid reduction of suicidal ideation: a randomized controlled trial. Psychol Med 45(16):3571–3580, 2015 26266877

Muscatello MRA, Bruno A, Micali Bellinghieri P, et al: Sertindole in schizophrenia: efficacy and safety issues. Expert Opin Pharmacother 15(13):1943–1953, 2014 25084209

Najib J: The efficacy and safety profile of lisdexamfetamine dimesylate, a prodrug of d-amphetamine, for the treatment of attention-deficit/hyperactivity disorder in children and adults. Clin Ther 31(1):142–176, 2009 19243715

Nakagawa A, Watanabe N, Omori IM, et al: Milnacipran versus other antidepressive agents for depression. Cochrane Database Syst Rev (3):CD006529, 2009 19588396

National Institute of Diabetes and Digestive Diseases: Kidney disease statistics for the United States. December 2016. Available at: https://www.niddk.nih.gov/health-information/health-statistics/kidney-disease. Accessed September 30, 2019.

National Institutes of Health: Drug record: tacrine. LiverTox: Clinical and Research Information on Drug-Induced Liver Injury, October 30, 2018. Available at: https://www.livertox.nih.gov/Tacrine.htm. Accessed September 29, 2019.

Neubauer DN: A review of ramelteon in the treatment of sleep disorders. Neuropsychiatr Dis Treat 4(1):69–79, 2008 18728808

Ni HC, Shang CY, Gau SS, et al: A head-to-head randomized clinical trial of methylphenidate and atomoxetine treatment for executive function in adults with attention-deficit hyperactivity disorder. Int J Neuropsychopharmacol 16(9):1959–1973, 2013 23672818

Nierenberg AA, Adler LA, Peselow E, et al: Trazodone for antidepressant-associated insomnia. Am J Psychiatry 151(7):1069–1072, 1994 8010365

Nolan BP, Schulte JJ Jr: Mania associated with initiation of ziprasidone. J Clin Psychiatry 64(3):336, 2003 12716277

Norman JL, Anderson SL: Novel class of medications, orexin receptor antagonists, in the treatment of insomnia—critical appraisal of suvorexant. Nat Sci Sleep 8:239–247, 2016 27471419

Norn S, Permin H, Kruse E, et al: On the history of barbiturates [in Danish]. Dan Medicinhist Arbog 43:133–151, 2015 27086450

Nucifora FCJr, Mihaljevic M, Lee BJ, et al: Clozapine as a model for antipsychotic development. Neurotherapeutics 14(3):750–761, 2017 28653280

O'Brien JT, Holmes C, Jones M, et al: Clinical practice with anti-dementia drugs: a revised (third) consensus statement from the British Association for Psychopharmacology. J Psychopharmacol 31(2):147–168, 2017 28103749

Obata H: Analgesic mechanisms of antidepressants for neuropathic pain. Int J Mol Sci 18(11):2483, 2017 29160850

Okuma T, Kishimoto A: A history of investigation on the mood stabilizing effect of carbamazepine in Japan. Psychiatry Clin Neurosci 52(1):3–12, 1998 9682927

Orr C, Deshpande S, Sawh S, et al: Asenapine for the treatment of psychotic disorders. Can J Psychiatry 62(2):123–137, 2017 27481921

Orser BA, Pennefather PS, MacDonald JF: Multiple mechanisms of ketamine blockade of N-methyl-D-aspartate receptors. Anesthesiology 86(4):903–917, 1997 9105235

Otasowie J, Castells X, Ehimare UP, et al: Tricyclic antidepressants for attention deficit hyperactivity disorder (ADHD) in children and adolescents. Cochrane Database Syst Rev (9):CD006997, 2014 25238582

Palmer RH, Periclou A, Banerjee P: Milnacipran: a selective serotonin and norepinephrine dual reuptake inhibitor for the management of fibromyalgia. Ther Adv Musculoskelet Dis 2(4):201–220, 2010 22870448

Palpacuer C, Duprez R, Huneau A, et al: Pharmacologically controlled drinking in the treatment of alcohol dependence or alcohol use disorders: a systematic review with direct and network meta-analyses on nalmefene, naltrexone, acamprosate, baclofen and topiramate. Addiction 113(2):220–237, 2018 28940866

Pande AC, Davidson JR, Jefferson JW, et al: Treatment of social phobia with gabapentin: a placebo-controlled study. J Clin Psychopharmacol 19(4):341–348, 1999 10440462

Parker G: Development of an incipient Stevens-Johnson reaction while on a stable dose of lamotrigine. Australas Psychiatry 24(2):193–194, 2016 26498148

Parker G: Risks associated with lamotrigine prescription: a review and personal observations. Australas Psychiatry 26(6):640–642, 2018 29480028

Parker WF, Gorges RJ, Gao YN, et al: Association between groundwater lithium and the diagnosis of bipolar disorder and dementia in the United States. JAMA Psychiatry 75(7):751–754, 2018 29799907

Patrick KS, Straughn AB, Jarvi EJ, et al: The absorption of sustained-release methylphenidate formulations compared to an immediate-release formulation. Biopharm Drug Dispos 10(2):165–171, 1989 2706316

Patten SB: Propranolol and depression: evidence from the antihypertensive trials. Can J Psychiatry 35(3):257–259, 1990 2140288

Peabody CA: Trazodone withdrawal and formication. J Clin Psychiatry 48(9):385, 1987 3624211

Peña MS, Yaltho TC, Jankovic J: Tardive dyskinesia and other movement disorders secondary to aripiprazole. Mov Disord 26(1):147–152, 2011 20818603

Pétursson H: The benzodiazepine withdrawal syndrome. Addiction 89(11):1455–1459, 1994 7841856

Peuskens J, Pani L, Detraux J, et al: The effects of novel and newly approved antipsychotics on serum prolactin levels: a comprehensive review. CNS Drugs 28(5):421–453, 2014 24677189

Philip NS, Carpenter LL, Tyrka AR, et al: Augmentation of antidepressants with atypical antipsychotics: a review of the current literature. J Psychiatr Pract 14(1):34–44, 2008 18212601

Pichler EM, Hattwich G, Grunze H, et al: Safety and tolerability of anticonvulsant medication in bipolar disorder. Expert Opin Drug Saf 14(11):1703–1724, 2015 26359219

Pigott K, Galizia I, Vasudev K, et al: Topiramate for acute affective episodes in bipolar disorder in adults. Cochrane Database Syst Rev (9):CD003384, 2016 27591453

Pigott TA, Seay SM: A review of the efficacy of selective serotonin reuptake inhibitors in obsessive-compulsive disorder. J Clin Psychiatry 60(2):101–106, 1999 10084636

Plosker GL: Acamprosate: a review of its use in alcohol dependence. Drugs 75(11):1255–1268, 2015 26084940

Pohl R, Berchou R, Rainey JM Jr: Tricyclic antidepressants and monoamine oxidase inhibitors in the treatment of agoraphobia. J Clin Psychopharmacol 2(6):399–407, 1982 7174863

Pons G, Francoual C, Guillet P, et al: Zolpidem excretion in breast milk. Eur J Clin Pharmacol 37(3):245–248, 1989 2612539

Post RM: The new news about lithium: an underutilized treatment in the United States. Neuropsychopharmacology 43(5):1174–1179, 2018 28976944

Post RM, Uhde TW, Putnam FW, et al: Kindling and carbamazepine in affective illness. J Nerv Ment Dis 170(12):717–731, 1982 6754868

Post RM, Ketter TA, Uhde T, et al: Thirty years of clinical experience with carbamazepine in the treatment of bipolar illness: principles and practice. CNS Drugs 21(1):47–71, 2007 17190529

Pozzi R: True and presumed contraindications of beta blockers. Peripheral vascular disease, diabetes mellitus, chronic bronchopneumopathy [in Italian]. Ital Heart J Suppl 1(8):1031–1037, 2000 10993010

Preskorn S: The evolution of antipsychotic drug therapy: reserpine, chlorpromazine, and haloperidol. J Psychiatr Pract 13(4):253–257, 2007 17667738

Preskorn S, Macaluso M, Mehra DO, et al: Randomized proof of concept trial of GLYX-13, an N-methyl-D-aspartate receptor glycine site partial agonist, in major depressive disorder nonresponsive to a previous antidepressant agent. J Psychiatr Pract 21(2):140–149, 2015 25782764

Prichard BN, Walden RJ: The syndrome associated with the withdrawal of beta-adrenergic receptor blocking drugs. Br J Clin Pharmacol 13(suppl 2):337S–343S, 1982 6125186

Psychiatric Times: Psychotropic medications around the world. Psychiatric Times, April 1, 2004. Available at: https://www.psychiatrictimes.com/bipolar-disorder/psychotropic-medications-around-world. Accessed September 29, 2019.

Psychiatry and Behavioral Health Learning Network: Rapastinel fails to outperform placebo in Phase 3 studies. March 12, 2019. Available at: https://www.psychcongress.com/article/rapastinel-fails-outperform-placebo-phase-3-studies. Accessed February 27, 2020.

Pynnönen S, Frey H, Sillanpää M: The auto-induction of carbamazepine during long-term therapy. Int J Clin Pharmacol Ther Toxicol 18(6):247–252, 1980 7450925

Rabinovici GD, Stephens ML, Possin K: Executive dysfunction. Continuum (Minneap Minn) 21(3):646–659, 2015 26039846

Rachid F, Bertschy G, Bondolfi G, et al: Possible induction of mania or hypomania by atypical antipsychotics: an updated review of reported cases. J Clin Psychiatry 65(11):1537–1545, 2004 15554769

Ragguett RM, Rong C, Kratiuk K, et al: Rapastinel—an investigational NMDA-R modulator for major depressive disorder: evidence to date. Expert Opin Investig Drugs 28(2):113–119, 2019 30585524

Reimherr FW, Hedges DW, Strong RE, et al: Bupropion SR in adults with ADHD: a short-term, placebo-controlled trial. Neuropsychiatr Dis Treat 1(3):245–251, 2005 18568102

Remington G, Kapur S: D2 and 5-HT2 receptor effects of antipsychotics: bridging basic and clinical findings using PET. J Clin Psychiatry 60(suppl 10):15–19, 1999 10340683

Rho JM, Donevan SD, Rogawski MA: Barbiturate-like actions of the propanediol dicarbamates felbamate and meprobamate. J Pharmacol Exp Ther 280(3):1383–1391, 1997 9067327

Rhyne DN, Anderson SL: Suvorexant in insomnia: efficacy, safety and place in therapy. Ther Adv Drug Saf 6(5):189–195, 2015 26478806

Richa S, Yazbek JC: Ocular adverse effects of common psychotropic agents: a review. CNS Drugs 24(6):501–526, 2010 20443647

Riordan HJ, Antonini P, Murphy MF: Atypical antipsychotics and metabolic syndrome in patients with schizophrenia: risk factors, monitoring, and healthcare implications. Am Health Drug Benefits 4(5):292–302, 2011 25126357

Roehrs TA, Roth T: Hyperarousal in insomnia and hypnotic dose escalation. Sleep Med 23:16–20, 2016 27692272

Rösner S, Hackl-Herrwerth A, Leucht S, et al: Acamprosate for alcohol dependence. Cochrane Database Syst Rev (9):CD004332, 2010a 20824837

Rösner S, Hackl-Herrwerth A, Leucht S, et al: Opioid antagonists for alcohol dependence. Cochrane Database Syst Rev (12):CD001867, 2010b 20824837

Sachdeva A, Choudhary M, Chandra M: Alcohol withdrawal syndrome: benzodiazepines and beyond. J Clin Diagn Res 9(9):VE01–VE07, 2015 26500991

Sachs GS: Use of clonazepam for bipolar affective disorder. J Clin Psychiatry 51(suppl):31–34, discussion 50–53, 1990 1970815

Saivin S, Hulot T, Chabac S, et al: Clinical pharmacokinetics of acamprosate. Clin Pharmacokinet 35(5):331–345, 1998 9839087

Salvà P, Costa J: Clinical pharmacokinetics and pharmacodynamics of zolpidem. Therapeutic implications. Clin Pharmacokinet 29(3):142–153, 1995 8521677

Samuels JA, Franco K, Wan F, et al: Effect of stimulants on 24-h ambulatory blood pressure in children with ADHD: a double-blind, randomized, cross-over trial. Pediatr Nephrol 21(1):92–95, 2006 16254730

Sanacora G, Frye MA, McDonald W, et al: A consensus statement on the use of ketamine in the treatment of mood disorders. JAMA Psychiatry 74(4):399–405, 2017 28249076

Sanford AM: Mild cognitive impairment. Clin Geriatr Med 33(3):325–337, 2017 28689566

Santos C, Olmedo RE, Kim J: Sedative-hypnotic drug withdrawal syndrome: recognition and treatment [digest]. Emerg Med Pract 19(3):S1–S2, 2017 28745845

Savitz AJ, Haiyan X, Gopal S, et al: Efficacy and safety of paliperidone palmitate 3-month formulation for patients with schizophrenia: a randomized, multicenter, double-blind, noninferiority study. Int J Neuropsychopharmacol 19(7):pyw018, 2016 26902950

Schatzberg AF, Haddad P, Kaplan EM, et al: Serotonin reuptake inhibitor discontinuation syndrome: a hypothetical definition. Discontinuation Consensus panel. J Clin Psychiatry 58(suppl 7):5–10, 1997 9219487

Schatzberg AF, Blier P, Delgado PL, et al: Antidepressant discontinuation syndrome: consensus panel recommendations for clinical management and additional research. J Clin Psychiatry 67(suppl 4):27–30, 2006 16683860

Schmidt D, Krämer G: The new anticonvulsant drugs. Implications for avoidance of adverse effects. Drug Saf 11(6):422–431, 1994 7727052

Schwabe L, Nader K, Pruessner JC: Beta-adrenergic blockade during reactivation reduces the subjective feeling of remembering associated with emotional episodic memories. Biol Psychol 92(2):227–232, 2013 23131614

Schwartz JR, Nelson MT, Schwartz ER, et al: Effects of modafinil on wakefulness and executive function in patients with narcolepsy experiencing late-day sleepiness. Clin Neuropharmacol 27(2):74–79, 2004 15252267

Schwienteck KL, Li G, Poe MM, et al: Abuse-related effects of subtype-selective GABA-A receptor positive allosteric modulators in an assay of intracranial self-stimulation in rats. Psychopharmacology (Berl) 234(14):2091–2101, 2017 28365836

Seager H: Drug-delivery products and the Zydis fast-dissolving dosage form. J Pharm Pharmacol 50(4):375–382, 1998 9625481

Seedat YK: Clonidine and guanfacine—comparison of their effects on haemodynamics in hypertension. S Afr Med J 67(14):557–559, 1985 3887593

Shader RI, Greenblatt DJ: Use of benzodiazepines in anxiety disorders. N Engl J Med 328(19):1398–1405, 1993 8292115

Shapiro DA, Renock S, Arrington E, et al: Aripiprazole, a novel atypical antipsychotic drug with a unique and robust pharmacology. Neuropsychopharmacology 28(8):1400–1411, 2003 12784105

Sheehan V: Ziprasidone mesylate (Geodon for injection): the first injectable atypical antipsychotic medication. Proc Bayl Univ Med Cent 16(4):497–501, 2003 16278769

Shelton RC: Serotonin and norepinephrine reuptake inhibitors, in Antidepressants: From Biogenic Amines to New Mechanisms of Action. Edited by Macaluso M, Preskorn SH. Handbook of Experimental Pharmacology book series (HEP, Vol 250). Berlin, Springer, 2018, pp 145–180

Shen WW: A history of antipsychotic drug development. Compr Psychiatry 40(6):407–414, 1999 10579370

Shorter E: The history of lithium therapy. Bipolar Disord 11(suppl 2):4–9, 2009 19538681

Shyu YC, Lee SY, Yuan SS, et al: Seasonal patterns of medications for treating attention-deficit/hyperactivity disorder: comparison of methylphenidate and atomoxetine. Clin Ther 38(3):595–602, 2016 26874787

Silberstein SD: Topiramate in migraine prevention: a 2016 perspective. Headache 57(1):165–178, 2017 27902848

Singh H, Thangaraju P, Natt NK: Sleep-walking a rarest side effect of zolpidem. Indian J Psychol Med 37(1):105–106, 2015 25722525

Singh LK, Nizamie SH, Akhtar S, et al: Improving tolerability of lithium with a once-daily dosing schedule. Am J Ther 18(4):288–291, 2011 20592663

Sommer BR, Mitchell EL, Wroolie TE: Topiramate: effects on cognition in patients with epilepsy, migraine headache and obesity. Ther Adv Neurol Disorder 6(4):211–227, 2013 23858325

Steenen SA, van Wijk AJ, van der Heijden GJMG, et al: Propranolol for the treatment of anxiety disorders: systematic review and meta-analysis. J Psychopharmacol 30(2):128–139, 2016 26487439

Steinert T, Fröscher W: Epileptic seizures under antidepressive drug treatment: systematic review. Pharmacopsychiatry 51(4):121–135, 2018 28850959

Stevens JC, Pollack MH: Benzodiazepines in clinical practice: consideration of their long-term use and alternative agents. J Clin Psychiatry 66(suppl 2):21–27, 2005 15762816

Stevenson RD, Wolraich ML: Stimulant medication therapy in the treatment of children with attention deficit hyperactivity disorder. Pediatr Clin North Am 36(5):1183–1197, 1989 2677938

Stewart SA: The effects of benzodiazepines on cognition. J Clin Psychiatry 66(suppl 2):9–13, 2005 15762814

Stoner SC, Worrel JA, Vlach D, et al: Retrospective analysis of serum valproate levels and need for an antidepressant drug. Pharmacotherapy 21(7):850–854, 2001 11444581

Stowe CD, Gardner SF, Gist CC, et al: 24-hour ambulatory blood pressure monitoring in male children receiving stimulant therapy. Ann Pharmacother 36(7–8):1142–1149, 2002 12086544

Strohl MP: Bradley's Benzedrine studies on children with behavioral disorders. Yale J Biol Med 84(1):27–33, 2011 21451781

Subramanian S, Rummel-Kluge C, Hunger H, et al: Zotepine versus other atypical antipsychotics for schizophrenia. Cochrane Database Syst Rev (10):CD006628, 2010 20927748

Suppes T: Review of the use of topiramate for treatment of bipolar disorders. J Clin Psychopharmacol 22(6):599–609, 2002 12454560

Sutton EL: Profile of suvorexant in the management of insomnia. Drug Des Devel Ther 9:6035–6042, 2015 26648692

Swanson J, Gupta S, Lam A, et al: Development of a new once-a-day formulation of methylphenidate for the treatment of attention-deficit/hyperactivity disorder: proof-of-concept and proof-of-product studies. Arch Gen Psychiatry 60(2):204–211, 2003 12578439

Swearingen D, Aronoff GM, Ciric S, et al: Pharmacokinetics of immediate release, extended release, and gastric retentive gabapentin formulations in healthy adults? Int J Clin Pharmacol Ther 56(5):231–238, 2018 29633699

Tandon R, Cucchiaro J, Phillips D, et al: A double-blind, placebo-controlled, randomized withdrawal study of lurasidone for the maintenance of efficacy in patients with schizophrenia. J Psychopharmacol 30(1):69–77, 2016 26645209

Tannenbaum C, Paquette A, Hilmer S, et al: A systematic review of amnestic and non-amnestic mild cognitive impairment induced by anticholinergic, antihistamine, GABAergic and opioid drugs. Drugs Aging 29(8):639–658, 2012 22812538

Thielking M: A STAT investigation: ketamine gives hope to patients with severe depression. But some clinics stray from the science and hype its benefits. STAT, September 24, 2018. Available at: https://www.statnews.com/2018/09/24/ketamine-clinics-severe-depression-treatment/. Accessed October 2, 2019.

Thompson JW Jr, Ware MR, Blashfield RK: Psychotropic medication and priapism: a comprehensive review. J Clin Psychiatry 51(10):430–433, 1990 2211542

Thorén P, Asberg M, Cronholm B, et al: Clomipramine treatment of obsessive-compulsive disorder. I. A controlled clinical trial. Arch Gen Psychiatry 37(11):1281–1285, 1980 7436690

Tian Y, Du J, Spagna A, et al: Venlafaxine treatment reduces the deficit of executive control of attention in patients with major depressive disorder. Sci Rep 6:28028, 2016 27306061

Tom SE, Wickwire EM, Park Y, et al: Nonbenzodiazepine sedative hypnotics and risk of fall-related injury. Sleep (Basel) 39(5):1009–1014, 2016 26943470

Tschoner A, Engl J, Rettenbacher M, et al: Effects of six second generation antipsychotics on body weight and metabolism—risk assessment and results from a prospective study. Pharmacopsychiatry 42(1):29–34, 2009 19153944

Turner P: Therapeutic uses of beta-adrenoceptor blocking drugs in the central nervous system in man. Postgrad Med J 65(759):1–6, 1989 2571143

Upadhyaya HP, Desaiah D, Schuh KJ, et al: A review of the abuse potential assessment of atomoxetine: a nonstimulant medication for attention-deficit/hyperactivity disorder. Psychopharmacology (Berl) 226(2):189–200, 2013 23397050

U.S. Food and Drug Administration: Label for Cylert. December 2002. Available at: https://www.accessdata.fda.gov/drugsatfda_docs/label/2003/016832s022_017703s018lbl.pdf. Accessed September 29, 2019.

U.S. Food and Drug Administration: Label for risperidone. July 2009. Available at: https://www.accessdata.fda.gov/drugsatfda_docs/label/2009/020272s056, 020588s044,021346s033,021444s03lbl.pdf. Accessed September 29, 2019.

U.S. Food and Drug Administration: Label for Celexa. March 19, 2012. Available at: https://www.accessdata.fda.gov/drugsatfda_docs/label/2012/020822s042, 021046s019lbl.pdf. Accessed September 29, 2019.

U.S. Food and Drug Administration: FDA drug safety communication: FDA approves new label changes and dosing for zolpidem products and a recommendation to avoid driving the day after using Ambien CR. January 10, 2013. Available at: http://www.fda.gov/Drugs/DrugSafety/ucm352085.htm. Accessed September 29, 2019.

U.S. Food and Drug Administration: Clozapine REMS, updated January 23, 2020. Available at: https://www.clozapinerems.com/CpmgClozapineUI/home.u##. Accessed February 15, 2020.

U.S. Food and Drug Administration: Label for Adzenys XR-ODT. Updated January 2017. Available at: https://www.accessdata.fda.gov/drugsatfda_docs/label/2017/204326s002lbl.pdf. Accessed September 29, 2019.

U.S. Food and Drug Administration: Breakthrough therapy. January 4, 2018. Available at: https://www.fda.gov/forpatients/approvals/fast/ucm405397.htm. Accessed September 29, 2019.

U.S. Food and Drug Administration: FDA approves new nasal spray medication for treatment-resistant depression; available only at a certified doctor's office or clinic. March 7, 2019. Available at: https://www.fda.gov/NewsEvents/Newsroom/PressAnnouncements/ucm632761.htm. Accessed September 29, 2019.

Vasile RG, Shelton RP: Alleviating gastrointestinal side effects of lithium carbonate by substituting lithium citrate. J Clin Psychopharmacol 2(6):420–423, 1982 6816839

Vasilescu AN, Schweinfurth N, Borgwardt S, et al: Modulation of the activity of N-methyl-d-aspartate receptors as a novel treatment option for depression: current clinical evidence and therapeutic potential of rapastinel (GLYX-13). Neuropsychiatr Dis Treat 13:973–980, 2017 28408831

Vasudev A, Macritchie K, Watson S, et al: Oxcarbazepine in the maintenance treatment of bipolar disorder. Cochrane Database Syst Rev (1):CD005171, 2008 18254071

Vasudev A, Macritchie K, Vasudev K, et al: Oxcarbazepine for acute affective episodes in bipolar disorder. Cochrane Database Syst Rev (12):CD004857, 2011 22161387

Vázquez M, Fagiolino P, Maldonado C, et al: Hyperammonemia associated with valproic acid concentrations. Biomed Res Int 2014:217269, 2014 24868521

Verbeeck W, Bekkering GE, Van den Noortgate W, et al: Bupropion for attention deficit hyperactivity disorder (ADHD) in adults. Cochrane Database Syst Rev (10):CD009504, 2017 28965364

Veronese A, Garatti M, Cipriani A, et al: Benzodiazepine use in the real world of psychiatric practice: low-dose, long-term drug taking and low rates of treatment discontinuation. Eur J Clin Pharmacol 63(9):867–873, 2007 17619867

Vieta E, Manuel Goikolea J, Martínez-Arán A, et al: A double-blind, randomized, placebo-controlled, prophylaxis study of adjunctive gabapentin for bipolar disorder. J Clin Psychiatry 67(3):473–477, 2006 16649836

Vozeh S: Pharmacokinetic of benzodiazepines in old age [in German]. Schweiz Med Wochenschr 111(47):1789–1793, 1981 6118950

Wagner AK, Zhang F, Soumerai SB, et al: Benzodiazepine use and hip fractures in the elderly: who is at greatest risk? Arch Intern Med 164(14):1567–1572, 2004 15277291

Waln O, Jankovic J: An update on tardive dyskinesia: from phenomenology to treatment. Tremor Other Hyperkinet Mov (NY) 3, 2013 23858394

Wang SM, Han C, Lee SJ, et al: Modafinil for the treatment of attention-deficit/ hyperactivity disorder: a meta-analysis. J Psychiatr Res 84:292–300, 2017 27810669

Warner CH, Bobo W, Warner C, et al: Antidepressant discontinuation syndrome. Am Fam Physician 74(3):449–456, 2006 16913164

Warner MD, Dorn MR, Peabody CA: Survey on the usefulness of trazodone in patients with PTSD with insomnia or nightmares. Pharmacopsychiatry 34(4):128–131, 2001 11518472

Watanabe N, Omori IM, Nakagawa A, et al: Mirtazapine versus other antidepressive agents for depression. Cochrane Database Syst Rev (12):CD006528, 2011 22161405

Wehry AM, Beesdo-Baum K, Hennelly MM, et al: Assessment and treatment of anxiety disorders in children and adolescents. Curr Psychiatry Rep 17(7):52, 2015 25980507

Weisler RH: Carbamazepine extended-release capsules in bipolar disorder. Neuropsychiatr Dis Treat 2(1):3–11, 2006 19412441

Weisler RH, Calabrese JR, Bowden CL, et al: Discovery and development of lamotrigine for bipolar disorder: a story of serendipity, clinical observations, risk taking, and persistence. J Affect Disord 108(1–2):1–9, 2008 18001843

Westover AN, Halm EA: Do prescription stimulants increase the risk of adverse cardiovascular events?: A systematic review. BMC Cardiovasc Disord 12:41, 2012 22682429

Wick JY: The history of benzodiazepines. Consult Pharm 28(9):538–548, 2013 24007886

Wilens TE, Haight BR, Horrigan JP, et al: Bupropion XL in adults with attention-deficit/hyperactivity disorder: a randomized, placebo-controlled study. Biol Psychiatry 57(7):793–801, 2005a 15820237

Wilens TE, Hammerness PG, Biederman J, et al: Blood pressure changes associated with medication treatment of adults with attention-deficit/hyperactivity disorder. J Clin Psychiatry 66(2):253–259, 2005b 15705013

Willcutt EG, Doyle AE, Nigg JT, et al: Validity of the executive function theory of attention-deficit/hyperactivity disorder: a meta-analytic review. Biol Psychiatry 57(11):1336–1346, 2005 15950006

Winans E: Aripiprazole. Am J Health Syst Pharm 60(23):2437–2445, 2003 14686220

Wood S, Sage JR, Shuman T, et al: Psychostimulants and cognition: a continuum of behavioral and cognitive activation. Pharmacol Rev 66(1):193–221, 2013 24344115

Worrel JA, Marken PA, Beckman SE, et al: Atypical antipsychotic agents: a critical review. Am J Health Syst Pharm 57(3):238–255, 2000 10674777

Worthington JJ 3rd, Pollack MH, Otto MW, et al: Long-term experience with clonazepam in patients with a primary diagnosis of panic disorder. Psychopharmacol Bull 34(2):199–205, 1998 9641001

Zaccara G, Messori A, Moroni F: Clinical pharmacokinetics of valproic acid— 1988. Clin Pharmacokinet 15(6):367–389, 1988 3149565

Zafrir B, Amir O: Beta blocker therapy, decompensated heart failure, and inotropic interactions: current perspectives. Isr Med Assoc J 14(3):184–189, 2012 22675861

Zarate CAJr, Singh JB, Carlson PJ, et al: A randomized trial of an N-methyl-D-aspartate antagonist in treatment-resistant major depression. Arch Gen Psychiatry 63(8):856–864, 2006 16894061

Zhang JC, Li SX, Hashimoto K: R (-)-ketamine shows greater potency and longer lasting antidepressant effects than S (+)-ketamine. Pharmacol Biochem Behav 116:137–141, 2014 24316345

Zhang JP, Gallego JA, Robinson DG, et al: Efficacy and safety of individual second-generation vs first-generation antipsychotics in first episode psychosis: a systematic review and meta-analysis. Int J Neuropsychopharmacol 16(6):1205–1218, 2013 23199972

Zimbroff DL, Allen MH, Battaglia J, et al: Best clinical practice with ziprasidone IM: update after 2 years of experience. CNS Spectr 10(9):1–15, 2005 16247923

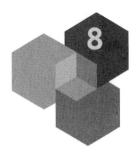

Supplements

Their Role in Helping and Not Helping

In many ways, the history of pharmacology is the history of herbal medicine. Remedies for a myriad of disorders began as folk medicines and eventually were isolated into active chemicals that were verified for safety, tolerability, and efficacy. Along the way, however, many popular treatments were also found to be ineffective, after all. Rational pharmacology is open to new treatments from the natural world, but only after they have survived scientific scrutiny. To skip these critical steps is to mislead ourselves—and, worse, our patients—on how to stay safe and function better. "First, do no harm."

Despite our significant progress in clinical psychopharmacology over the past near century, some patients ideologically still prefer nonprescription treatments. Even those who are open to prescription medication may, at times, still be influenced to consider questionable alternatives by friends, family, nonmedical clinicians, popular press, social media, and advertising. When something more (or other) than psychotherapy is indicated, individuals may consider dietary supplements or nutraceuticals rather than medications approved by the FDA or supported in randomized controlled trials (RCTs). While working to support the therapeutic alliance, clinicians will want to fully hear and understand such requests or demands but remain rational about the feasibility of such a treatment working or assisting or of it even being harmful. A strong knowledge of these often-called herbal or complementary treatments is not only essential in effective treatment planning but also may convince patients they have been heard, that you take their concerns seriously and are giving them the very best advice.

195

It also increases the chances they will disclose complementary treatments they are considering.

A discussion of what "natural" really means might be helpful. Much of psychiatric pharmacology utilizes molecules that are either natural or derived from nature with better efficacy, safety, or tolerability. Also, many naturally occurring elements or molecules, such as arsenic, are not desirable. Instead of linking the word *natural* to "safe, healthy, and effective," use the word *proven*, because patients will often consider alternative treatments to have been "proven" by someone. Focus on RCTs that convincingly demonstrate treatments to be safe, tolerable, and effective.

The cost of nutraceuticals may be as or more alarming than that of prescription medications. Local and national health food stores, and even some pharmacies, may charge patients hundreds of dollars monthly for an unproven supplement when older, proven, generic psychiatric medications may be only a fraction of that cost. Furthermore, governmental bodies such as the FDA and European Union monitor marketing claims from pharmaceutical manufacturers as well as the quality of the medicine dispensed. No such review for efficacy or safety is done for nutraceuticals until egregious overpromising occurs; one may even purchase a product that does not actually contain the labeled ingredient.

"Alternative" treatments are so labeled because they are not mainstream, usually meaning that they have not been subjected to sufficient RCTs or clinical review for safety or efficacy. It might be pointed out that treatments cease to be labeled alternative when they pass the tests of safety, tolerability, and efficacy and are widely adopted. To restrict choice to alternative treatments is to never take advantage of those that are safest, best tolerated, and most likely to be effective.

Discussion of nutritional supplements treating or curing mental illness is reminiscent of the mid-twentieth century orthomolecular movement, which hoped to treat schizophrenia and other disorders through the correction of *localized cerebral deficiency diseases* (Pauling 1968). This practice was denounced by the American Psychiatric Association due to a lack of data (Lipton et al. 1973), and concern was also raised that patients and families would reject tested treatments in favor of unproven promises. Certain localized deficiencies have since been detected in some patients with treatment-resistant illness (Pan et al. 2017); locating and correcting these deficiencies can provide invaluable treatments to our patients. However, oversimplification and generalization must also be avoided; there is no substitute for good science.

This chapter discusses some of the most popular supplements you may encounter with your patients. Keep in mind that the quality of supplements is not regulated, and counterfeit preparations are a significant problem; some purchases may contain the substance in very small amounts or not at all, and worse, may sometimes contain undisclosed ingredients that may be allergens or bring other health risks. Certification of manufacturing processes has been attempted, but sometimes this has been counterfeited as well. *Caveat emptor:* buyer beware.

St. John's Wort (*Hypericum perforatum*)

Sparked by unfortunately biased research in the mid-1980s, *Hypericum perforatum*, known as St. John's wort (SJW), became a popular alternative treatment to traditional antidepressants (Shelton 2009). Its availability in the United States without a prescription also widened its use; patients and nonpatients tried it without the filter of review from professionals. Well-performed RCTs and meta-analyses have convincingly shown that SJW has not demonstrated efficacy in major depression (Asher et al. 2017; Grobler et al. 2014). Adverse events with solo use are usually not severe, including gastrointestinal symptoms, confusion, dizziness, sedation, or tiredness (Ernst et al. 1998). However, SJW is not benign, and it carries a risk of drug–drug interactions that every clinician should know and share with patients. SJW is a selective serotonin uptake inhibitor (SSRI), although to a degree that is insufficient for clinical response, and its concomitant use with other SSRIs, serotonin-norepinephrine reuptake inhibitors (SNRIs), triptans, or any other medication with similar effects on serotonin may provoke serotonin syndrome (see Chapter 11, "Serotonin Syndrome"). Its induction of CYP3A4 lowers serum levels of oral contraceptives, HIV protease inhibitors, HIV nonnucleoside reverse transcriptase inhibitors, cyclosporin, and anticonvulsants (e.g., carbamazepine, phenobarbital, and phenytoin), and its induction of CYP1A2 lowers levels of oral contraceptives as well as theophylline. SJW lowers warfarin and digoxin levels through induction of CYP2C9 and transport protein P-glycoprotein, respectively (Henderson et al. 2002). Similarly, stopping SJW may raise the levels of these medications (Baede-van Dijk et al. 2000). Patients should be warned that even occasional use of SJW, on their own, to supplement traditional treatments can be dangerous.

SAMe (*S*-Adenosyl-L-Methionine)

Another popular over-the-counter (OTC) self-treatment for major depression has been *S*-adenosyl-L-methionine (SAMe). A rare inherited error of metabolism leads to lower levels of folate and vitamin B_{12}, co-factors in the synthesis of SAMe. This causes a deficiency to develop in the CNS, inter-

fering with myelination and the biosynthesis of monoamine neurotransmitters and resulting in dementia and depression. Although oral doses of
SAMe are often well tolerated, nausea, vomiting, abdominal discomfort,
and diarrhea appear to be the most common side effects. Some patients
have reported anxiety, agitation, and insomnia; hypomania and mania
have been seen in patients with bipolar disorder. Evidence for drug–drug
interactions such as serotonin syndrome is not strong but remains under
study (Sharma et al. 2017).

As with SJW, public acceptance and use of SAMe has also outpaced
scientific review and confirmation. Data to date are not as indicative of
failed efficacy as they are of insufficient rigor to demonstrate utility (Asher
et al. 2017; De Berardis et al. 2016). One meta-analysis was more favorable for SAMe but reviewed only four studies of adjunctive treatment,
three of which were open label, with doses of 800 or 1,600 mg, and judged
the results in combination with other one-carbon cycle nutraceuticals: folic acid and vitamins B_6 and B_{12} (Ducker and Rabinowitz 2017; Sarris et
al. 2016). A double-blind study included in this meta-analysis did show
promising benefit for adding SAMe to an SSRI for treatment of depression
but encouraged replication (Papakostas et al. 2010).

L-Tryptophan

L-Tryptophan was popular among clinicians in the 1980s as a soporific that
would avoid risks such as addiction, withdrawal, and tolerance (Schneider-
Helmert and Spinweber 1986). In 1989, however, it became associated with
the sudden appearance of eosinophilia-myalgia syndrome (EMS) in the
United States. The FDA and many countries placed a ban on L-tryptophan
in 1990 that was only fully lifted in 2005. It later became clear that this outbreak of EMS was linked to an impurity from one large manufacturer that
resulted from a change in their production process, not from L-tryptophan
itself (Mayeno and Gleich 1994). Public concern and the ban, however,
have significantly reversed the use of L-tryptophan. Some interest has been
shown in its use for the treatment of depression, both unipolar and bipolar, because it is a precursor of serotonin and low levels have been associated with major depression (Boman 1988; Ogawa et al. 2014; Thomson
et al. 1982). Reliable evidence supporting this indication, however, is not
available (Sarris et al. 2016; Shaw et al. 2002).

L-Tryptophan is also a precursor, via serotonin, to another popular
OTC agent used for sleep: melatonin (N-acetyl-5-methoxytryptamine), an
endogenous hormone released by the pineal gland. It has been shown in
RCTs to help with initial (or delayed-phase) insomnia, although support
for broader application, such as for jet lag and shift-work sleep disorder,

appears weaker (Auld et al. 2017; Costello et al. 2014; Ferracioli-Oda et al. 2013; Sletten et al. 2018). Short-term dosing in RCTs usually ranges from 0.3 to 5.0 mg at bedtime, but great variation exists in the quality of melatonin preparations, especially in the United States, where it is unregulated and not standardized in all RCTs.

Although tolerated short term, because its sedative effects are desirable, long-term safety of melatonin has not been established. As an endogenous hormone, it has many delicately balanced effects, and its secretion, normally linked to darkness in the day/night schedule, is inhibited by exogenous dosing. Patients and nonpatients often determine their own doses and schedules, so the risks of various doses and long-term use need better assessment; use is not suggested for children or adolescents or during pregnancy or breastfeeding (Andersen et al. 2016; Claustrat and Leston 2015; Kennaway 2015).

L-Methylfolate

L-Methylfolate became popular with many practitioners in the twenty-first century, when manufacturers received FDA approval and aggressively marketed this supplement (as Deplin) for treatment-resistant major depression. Based on observations that these patients sometimes have low levels of folate in their serum or cerebrospinal fluid, some success was achieved with oral replacement of either folinic acid or L-methylfolate (Fava et al. 1997; Ghadirian et al. 1980; Wesson et al. 1994). Usually, dietary folic acid is converted in the CNS to L-methylfolate by methylenetetrahydrofolate reductase (*MTHFR*) which, in turn, facilitates the manufacture of the cofactor tetrahydrobiopterin (BH_4), which is necessary for the activation of tryptophan hydroxylase and tyrosine hydroxylase, rate-limiting enzymes for synthesis of monoamine neurotransmitters serotonin, norepinephrine, and dopamine (Papakostas et al. 2012). A polymorphism of this enzyme labeled 677C>T has been theorized to block this conversion, resulting in insufficient monoamine neurotransmission and thus in depression that is also less amenable to treatment with SSRIs and SNRIs (Kelly et al. 2004). Oral administration of L-methylfolate, which crosses the blood–brain barrier, is intended to correct this inborn error of metabolism and allow treatment response to traditional antidepressants. Doses of 15 mg added to an SSRI for patients with treatment-resistant depression have shown significant improvement over 30 days, whereas doses of 7.5 mg have not (Papakostas et al. 2012). Response to this strategy has also shown sustained results over a 12-month period (Zajecka et al. 2016). L-Methylfolate, therefore, is always taken as a supplement to antidepressant treatment, never as monotherapy (Roberts et al. 2018).

The use of L-methylfolate for schizophrenia, in general, shows no clinical benefit. However, a subpopulation with at least one copy of the *MTHFR* polymorphism did show improvement in negative symptoms, and a similar finding was reported for the combination of folate with vitamin B_{12} (Hill et al. 2011; Roffman et al. 2013).

Testing for 677C>T or 1298A>C defects (also referred to as *MTHFR* polymorphisms) is available but actually not reliable for treatment guidance. In the general population, 60%–70% have at least one of these alterations, and 10% of the population will be heterozygous or compound homozygous for both. *MTHFR* testing for other disorders, psychiatric and nonpsychiatric, has also been determined *not indicated* and might be misinterpreted (Camp and Trujillo 2014; Cohen-Woods et al. 2010; Hickey et al. 2013; Lok et al. 2014; Long and Goldblatt 2016; Moorthy et al. 2012; Wilcken et al. 2003). Marketers for testing and supplement sales, along with many clinicians, suggest going ahead and adding L-methylfolate in cases of treatment-resistant depression to see if it will help. Originally, L-methylfolate was thought to be well tolerated and safe when taken above recommended daily amounts; however, new data are demonstrating adverse events, such as cognitive impairment and possible tumor growth, from high serum folate levels (Mudryj et al. 2016).

The use of L-methylfolate supplementation in patients with treatment-resistant depression and normal serum folate levels has yielded only modest response (Alpert et al. 2002). Not all patients have low serum levels of folate at the time of depression (Wolfersdorf and König 1995), and the measurement of folate in serum or erythrocytes is not sufficient to detect cerebral folate deficiency (Hyland et al. 2010). L-Methylfolate may be useful in treating depressed patients with the *MTHFR* polymorphism, but not for cerebral folate deficiency, and its use will distort measurements of folate in the cerebrospinal fluid such that testing for cerebral folate deficiency must take place prior to L-methylfolate administration.

In the small sample examined so far, a significant number of patients with treatment-resistant depression have inborn errors of metabolism that are not easily detected by conventional laboratory techniques. Once these are identified, however, correction leads to improvement; replacement of low BH_4 with the analogue sapropterin plus 5-hydroxytryptophan and carbidopa showed response in one patient, and cerebral folate deficiency has been corrected with positive clinical results in one-third of these patients (Pan et al. 2011, 2017).

Clinicians must be thoughtful in approaching evaluation of treatment-resistant depression. The example of folate deficiency illustrates that the routine or impulsive use of supplements can obscure the actual pathway to treatment success (Mathew and Lijffijt 2017). Although genetic testing is popular with many patients, rational psychopharmacologists will need to explore with them what the data actually indicate so that expensive, unnecessary, and potentially misleading tests do not interfere with good treatment planning or the therapeutic alliance (see Chapter 6, "Pharmacogenomics").

Vitamin B_{12} (Cyanocobalamin)

Cyanocobalamin (vitamin B_{12}) deficiency is recognized as contributing to cognitive impairment and, in some cases, depressed mood (Köbe et al. 2016; Mikkelsen et al. 2016; Moorthy et al. 2012). As with the other one-carbon cycle agents, B_{12} is essential for methylation of monoamines (Sarris et al. 2016). Awareness of the link between folate (vitamin B_9) and B_{12} levels is important for practitioners (Table 8–1), because low serum folate levels may lead to falsely low measurements of B_{12}. Additionally, the generally accepted *normal* levels of serum B_{12} have been shown inadequate for half of the population, particularly older patients. A finding of elevated methylmalonic acid or homocysteine levels may help clarify B_{12} deficiency when levels are in the standard range, although the former is more specific: homocysteine also rises if folate is low (Oh and Brown 2003; Sobczynska-Malefora and Harrington 2018). Studies have not supported the addition of B_{12} to treat depression or impaired cognitive function acutely, although some have indicated that long-term use might help reduce the recurrence of major depression (Almeida et al. 2015; Ford et al. 2008; Hvas et al. 2004).

Vitamin D

Vitamin D levels have concerned many clinicians during the past two decades; literature has suggested that low levels are associated with cardiovascular disease, stroke, type 2 diabetes mellitus, and colorectal cancer (in addition to already recognized rickets, osteopenia, and osteoporosis [Holick 2004]). Despite the lack of confirmatory evidence that supplementation might reduce mortality and morbidity from these conditions (Allan et al. 2016; Autier et al. 2017), these associations mobilized many, particularly in primary care and internal medicine, to test and supplement patients (Wacker and Holick 2013).

Mental health concerns about vitamin D deficiency include mood, psychosis, eating disorders, and cognitive function in psychosis and aging. Low levels of vitamin D have been associated with depression (Anglin et al. 2013); a study in the United Kingdom found a positive correlation with levels in the warmer months (with presumably greater ultraviolet B expo-

TABLE 8–1. Vitamin B_{12} and folate serum level guide

Vitamin B_{12}	Folate	MMA	Homocysteine	Action/Result
Low	Low			Replace folate, repeat tests
Low	Normal			B_{12} deficiency
Low normal	Low	Normal	High	Replace folate, repeat tests
Low normal	Normal		High	B_{12} deficiency
Low normal	Normal	High		B_{12} deficiency
Low normal	Normal	Normal	Normal	No B_{12} deficiency

Note. MMA=methylmalonic acid.

sure) and a negative correlation with parathyroid hormone levels in patients with psychosis compared with healthy control subjects (Adamson et al. 2017). Evidence has shown that developmental exposure to low levels of vitamin D may lead to dopaminergic transmission alterations, but this mechanism is not clarified (Cui et al. 2015). Patients with anorexia nervosa who had the same dietary intake of vitamin D as healthy control subjects showed substantially lower serum levels (Veronese et al. 2015).

Of course, correlation is not necessarily causation, and efforts to supplement pharmacological treatment of psychotic disorders with vitamin D have so far fallen short; major depression and mental well-being studies are also insufficient to show improvement, once corrected for bias (Allan et al. 2016; Li et al. 2014). One RCT showed that annual fall/winter dosing fails to alter the course of depressive symptoms, despite raising serum levels above the levels of control subjects (Sanders et al. 2011). Although cross-sectional and longitudinal studies appear to show a protective effect for vitamin D against various forms of dementia, including vascular and Alzheimer's disease, this has not been confirmed by RCTs. Low levels are associated with poor cognition, but replacement is not observed to be clinically effective for improvement; a possible window for this therapeutic intervention has been proposed but not demonstrated (Anastasiou et al. 2014; Goodwill and Szoeke 2017).

Vitamin D deficiency has been found to be global, in all age groups, despite most industrialized countries supplementing endogenous production with fortified foods, usually containing plant-based ergocalciferol (vitamin D_2) (Palacios and Gonzalez 2014). Otherwise, dietary sources of vitamin D are weak, except fatty fish, which contains cholecalciferol (vitamin D_3). D_3 also is produced in human skin when 7-dehydrocholesterol is altered by ultraviolet B radiation and heat. This step is limited by environmental ultraviolet B exposure, clothing, sunscreen, and the degree of melanin in the skin. Vitamin D_2 has less affinity for metabolism by the liver into 25-hydroxyvitamin D (25[OH]D) and exits the body more quickly, resulting in the need for its daily replacement, unlike D_3. 25(OH)D is then enzymatically converted in the kidneys to 1,25(OH)$_2$D, the active form of vitamin D—a process regulated by the parathyroid hormone and levels of calcium and phosphorus (Bikle 2014).

There is some disagreement on the sufficient levels of circulating vitamin D. Patients' vitamin D status is best assessed by measuring 25(OH)D, the major circulating form (Saida et al. 2015). Uncertainty still exists as to whether total or bioavailable free 25(OH)D offers the better choice, although good arguments have been made for measuring the latter (Chun et al. 2014; Shieh et al. 2016). The Institute of Medicine determined that total 25(OH)D levels of 20 ng/mL (50 nmol/L) would be sufficient for more than 97% of the U.S. population. The Endocrine Society defines deficiency as less than that level and insufficiency as 21–29 ng/mL (52.5–72.5 nmol/L), recommending treatment with vitamin D_2 or D_3, in most cases, to correct or prevent deficiency (Holick et al. 2011).

Should replacement be considered, early recommendations stressed no clinical difference between D_2 and D_3, but most authors have found vitamin D_3 to be superior in the elevation of serum levels, particularly free 25(OH)D (Shieh et al. 2016). Either may be given orally at 50,000 IU twice weekly, weekly, or monthly or at 2,000–4,000 IU daily until levels reach these standards. Once the public became aware of the potential risks of low vitamin D and began self-treating without monitoring, the Institute of Medicine convened a panel to determine what level of supplementation might be safe without testing serum levels (recommended daily allowances); their conclusion was a daily dose of 600 IU for adults 19–70 years of age and 800 IU for adults older than 70 years (Ross et al. 2011).

Even though a U.S. federal task force has recommended against routine screening (LeFevre 2015), patients who take supplemental vitamin D above the amount referenced by the Institute of Medicine should be monitored. Always recall that vitamins A, D, E, and K are fat soluble and build up in adipose tissue, unlike the hydrophilic B vitamins (less so with D_2 due to limited human metabolism, resulting in a shorter half-life, as noted earlier). Toxicity from high total serum levels (>50 ng/mL [125 nmol/L]) may result in kidney stones (especially if calcium is also taken), hypercalcemia, and hypercalciuria. These latter two conditions may present as polyuria, cardiac ectopy, gastrointestinal distress, vascular calcification, depression, lethargy, confusion, and hallucinations (Malihi et al. 2016; Sarris et al. 2016; Tebben et al. 2016). Vitamin D sensitivity, distinct from toxicity, may develop from primary hyperparathyroidism, granulomatous diseases, and some cancers (Alshahrani and Aljohani 2013).

Omega-3

The possible use of omega-3 long chain polyunsaturated fatty acids (LC-PUFAs) in preventing and treating major and perinatal depression represents a compelling theory seeking confirmation. Cell membranes require these lipids for proper function. The necessary fatty acid α-linolenic acid is converted to eicosapentaenoic acid (EPA) and then to docosahexaenoic acid (DHA), although conversion in humans is limited and further influenced by genetic polymorphisms (Levant 2011). Ingestion of fatty fish may supplement levels.

Western diets are typically lower in omega-3 than omega-6 LC-PUFAs. A negative correlation exists between national fish consumption and the incidence of major depression, as well as between maternal fish consumption and postpartum depression; neither correlation, however, may be causal (Hibbeln 1998, 2002). High ratios of omega-6 to omega-3 have been shown to reversibly alter serotonergic and dopaminergic transmission, including during lactation, at least in animal models (Chalon 2006). Mothers divert DHA to the fetus during pregnancy, and replenishment may not occur even after 6 months, particularly in women with multiple pregnancies (Al et al. 1997; Holman et al. 1991). Low serum levels of omega-3 relative to omega-6 have been associated with major and perinatal depression (Adams et al. 1996; Rees et al. 2009). These observations led to the hypothesis that supplementation with omega-3 as EPA or DHA might either prevent the development of mood disorders, especially peripartum, or assist in recovery.

Open-label studies were often encouraging, followed by conflicting results in RCTs. Early meta-analysis was promising for use in unipolar and bipolar depression but not in schizophrenia (Freeman et al. 2006). Initial studies often utilized flax oil as the source for omega-3; due to individual variations in ability to convert this form to EPA, however, the use of fish oil eventually became the standard (Gracious et al. 2010). Given the high dosages often used, up to 10 g daily, study participants often reported burping a fishy smell, which was hardly practical and made the double blind more difficult to manage (Damico et al. 2002).

Subsequent meta-analysis has revealed that the indiscriminate use of omega-3 to prevent or treat these depressive illnesses is not justified (Bloch and Hannestad 2012), although separating the EPA from DHA and distinguishing use in patients who are depressed versus those who are not depressed shows a significant treatment effect. EPA (ethyl-EPA, specifically) as monotherapy or supplemental to antidepressants is significantly superior to DHA, but only in patients who actually meet the criteria for major depression (Hallahan et al. 2016; Mocking et al. 2016; Sarris et al. 2016). Any omega-3 used for major depression should have a higher proportion of EPA than DHA. Supplementation and monotherapy with omega-3 in peripartum depression (cases of DHA depletion) has not been successful in a small number of open-label studies and RCTs (Borja-Hart and Marino 2010; Levant 2011; Marangell et al. 2004). Analysis of a small number of studies in dementia showed some possible benefit for mild cognitive impairment but not Alzheimer's disease (Burckhardt et al. 2016; La Rosa et al. 2018). The addition of omega-3 has not shown symptom reduction in children and adolescents with ADHD (Abdullah et al. 2019). Other mental disorders, including schizophrenia, OCD, autism, and anxiety, lack sufficient RCTs with omega-3 to determine its efficacy (Bozzatello et al. 2016).

Many patients take omega-3 for cardiac reasons, prescribed or not. Indications for broad benefit (against stroke, heart failure, diabetes mellitus, and prediabetes) are weak, although it may help patients with existing atherosclerotic cardiovascular disease (Burke et al. 2017; Goel et al. 2018). Mercury levels in fish may represent a risk of toxicity (Smith and Sahyoun 2005); due to geographic variation of fish species, mercury levels, and dietary habits, some local recommendations for dietary consumption have been published (Persson et al. 2018; Raimann et al. 2014). With supplements, this issue is complicated by the lack of standard recommended doses. Most estimates are that levels are low enough in supplements and fish servings that, except for pregnant and nursing women, this should not influence omega-3 consumption (Wenstrom 2014). Some concerns have surfaced about omega-3 increasing the risk of prostate cancer while, at the same time, it has been touted for treatment of the same. Meta-analyses of both fish-based dietary and supplement intake so far can confirm neither effect (Aucoin et al. 2017). It is rational to suggest that patients taking supplemental fatty acids without prescription or clinical direction identify a clear indication before continuing.

Other Herbal Preparations

Valerian (*Valeriana officinalis*) has been used for centuries for sleep, although contemporary meta-analyses have not found it particularly effective and recommend it only for improvement of the subjective experience of sleep. A few conflicting studies have been published regarding its use for anxiety, but toxicity is not apparent (Baek et al. 2014).

Kava kava (*Piper methysticum*) is a drink from Pacific island communities that is used in cultural ceremonies, but it is also available in extract, capsule, and pill form (National Center for Complementary and Integrative Health 2016). It has been studied for the treatment of anxiety, and short-term use has been found somewhat helpful. However, due to severe liver toxicity, kava kava is inferior to traditional medications for treatment lasting longer than 8 weeks (Pittler and Ernst 2016; Smith and Leiras 2018).

Ginkgo biloba has enjoyed public acceptance for prevention of cognitive impairment, yet large, long-term RCTs have not demonstrated any preventive effect on progression into dementia for those with normal cognitive function or mild cognitive impairment (DeKosky et al. 2008; Vellas et al. 2012). Worse, this tree-based extract has been reported to lower levels of the anticonvulsants phenytoin and valproic acid through induction of CYP2C19 and to lead to hemorrhagic consequences, particularly when combined with anticoagulants and platelet aggregation inhibitors. Additionally, it is now listed as a possible carcinogen (Di Lorenzo et al. 2015; Mei et al. 2017).

Ginseng is popular around in the world; more than 10 different varieties or imitators exist. Journal articles most often refer to Oriental ginseng (*Panax ginseng*), although American wild or cultivated ginseng (*P. quinquefolius*), grown in the United States and Canada, is also widely available. White ginseng is unprocessed, and red ginseng, preserved with heat and steam, is purported to be of higher potency (New York State Department of Environmental Conservation 2019). Ginseng is often taken with the intention of fighting fatigue. Evidence has shown that high doses or long-term use may lead to insomnia and nervousness. Although ginseng has not boosted mood in healthy young adults (Cardinal and Engels 2001), mania resulting from its use has been reported (Bostock et al. 2018; Joshi and Faubion 2005).

Practitioners may also encounter patients using zinc, vitamin C, inositol, mixed amino acids, creatine, or acai (and other South American) berries. Unfortunately, insufficient evidence for these is available (Sarris et al. 2016; Schreckinger et al. 2010). Be aware of every substance your patients are taking, including nutraceuticals, herbs, and complementary and alternative treatments; query them at every visit (see Chapters 3, 9, and 12). New promises for nutrients and nutraceuticals are always appearing, and rational psychopharmacologists must approach evaluation of their safety and efficacy in the same manner they would any prescription medication. Clinicians familiar with each new candidate are more likely to influence patients than are those who reject the idea with little discussion. Patient education about supplements is as important as it is for prescription medications, because patients' use of supplements does not require a practitioner's approval or even knowledge.

Summary

Herbal treatments are popular, but they are poorly regulated and often inadequately studied for safety, efficacy, and drug–drug interactions. SJW has been found ineffective for major depression, and its addition to standard treatment may lead to serotonin syndrome and interfere with many nonpsychiatric medical treatments. SAMe might be helpful for major depression in rare cases of an inherited metabolism disorder, but it may also provoke mania in susceptible patients. L-Tryptophan is reliable only as a mild soporific, as is melatonin for initial insomnia, although patients taking melatonin should be cautious given its multiple effects as an endogenous hormone.

L-Methylfolate may be helpful at certain doses as a supplement to antidepressants in cases of *MTHFR* polymorphism and treatment-resistant depression but not for cerebral folate deficiency, which might be obscured by use of the supplement prior to testing. Commercial testing for *MTHFR* polymorphism is not specific enough to guide practice. Accurate testing of vitamin B_{12} levels will involve folate and possibly methylmalonic acid or homocysteine levels. Although B_{12} deficiency is associated with some cognitive impairments and depression, its replacement has demonstrated little clinical benefit other than possibly reducing recurrence of major depression.

Vitamin D deficiency is endemic, but widespread claims of its contribution to a number of mental and nonpsychiatric health problems may not be accurate. Supplementation with oral doses >600 IU daily (800 IU for geriatric patients) warrants testing; levels <20 ng/mL (50 nmol/L) are deficient and those >50 ng/mL (125 nmol/L) are toxic. Vitamin D_3 has some advantages over D_2. The EPA form of omega-3 LC-PUFA may be effective in treating some cases of major depression.

Valerian may only enhance the subjective evaluation of sleep. Kava kava is hepatotoxic and should not be used for anxiety for more than 8 weeks. *Ginkgo biloba* has failed to demonstrate efficacy in the prevention and treatment of cognitive impairment. It may lower serum levels of anticonvulsants, promote bleeding in patients taking anticoagulants or platelet aggregation inhibitors, and is a possible carcinogen. Ginseng, used for fatigue, may lead to insomnia, anxiety, or mania. Evidence for other popular supplements is insufficient. Encourage patients to discuss any plans they have for unilateral use of supplements and inquire about use at every visit. Clinician knowledge about these alternative treatments will enhance the therapeutic alliance and guard patient safety.

Key Points

■ Use the word *proven* to discuss treatments so that the term *natural* is not equated with safe and effective.

■ Treatments cease to be "alternative" once they pass tests of tolerability, safety, and efficacy.

■ Supplements are not regulated by governments for quality or safety unless egregious practices are discovered.

■ Serum testing for folate polymorphisms is unreliable for clinical guidance.

■ Practitioners must always know every substance a patient is taking, including nutraceuticals.

Self-Assessment

1. Mania has been reported with the use of

   A. SAMe
   B. St. John's wort
   C. Ginseng
   D. All of the above

2. Some anticonvulsant levels may be lowered by (choose all that apply)

   A. St. John's wort
   B. Ginseng
   C. SAMe
   D. Ginkgo biloba

3. Oral L-methylfolate may

   A. Correct central folate deficiency
   B. Assist in the treatment of treatment-resistant depression at dosages of 15 mg/day
   C. Assist in the treatment of treatment-resistant depression at dosages of 7.5 mg/day
   D. Be helpful if one or more *MTHFR* polymorphisms is detected

4. Vitamin D (choose all that apply)

   A. Is best measured by determining the 25(OH)D serum level
   B. Deficiency is defined as levels <20 ng/mL (50 nmol/L)
   C. Levels must be measured for daily doses >600 IU (800 IU for geriatric use)
   D. Is fat soluble

5. Omega-3 long chain polyunsaturated fatty acid (LC-PUFA) (choose all that apply)

   A. Levels are more negatively associated with depression than omega-6 LC-PUFA
   B. Is diverted to the fetus during pregnancy, with replacement taking months
   C. Replacement in the docosahexaenoic acid (DHA) form is effective in the treatment of major depression
   D. Replacement is effective in the treatment of mood in general

Discussion Topics

1. A patient requests supplementation with vitamin D. How would you assess the indication, interaction with ultraviolet B exposure and diet, and likelihood of success? What form of vitamin D might you prescribe, and what dosing schedule? What toxicities would you be concerned about, and how would you monitor for them?

2. A patient with mild cognitive impairment asks for an evaluation. What role can supplements play in evaluation and treatment, acute and long term?

Additional Reading

Lake JH, Spiegel D (eds): Complementary and Alternative Treatments in Mental Health Care. Washington, DC, American Psychiatric Publishing, 2007
(Chapters 5–8 most directly address the use of supplements in psychiatry.)
Mischoulon D (ed): Complementary and integrative medicine. Focus 16(1), 2018

References

Abdullah M, Jowett B, Whittaker PJ, et al: The effectiveness of omega-3 supplementation in reducing ADHD associated symptoms in children as measured by the Conners' rating scales: a systematic review of randomized controlled trials. J Psychiatr Res 110:64–73, 2019 30594823

Adams PB, Lawson S, Sanigorski A, et al: Arachidonic acid to eicosapentaenoic acid ratio in blood correlates positively with clinical symptoms of depression. Lipids 31(1, pt 2 suppl):S157–S161, 1996 8729112

Adamson J, Lally J, Gaughran F, et al: Correlates of vitamin D in psychotic disorders: a comprehensive systematic review. Psychiatry Res 249:78–85, 2017 28081455

Al MD, van Houwelingen AC, Hornstra G: Relation between birth order and the maternal and neonatal docosahexaenoic acid status. Eur J Clin Nutr 51(8):548–553, 1997 11248881

Allan GM, Cranston L, Lindblad A, et al: Vitamin D: a narrative review examining the evidence for ten beliefs. J Gen Intern Med 31(7):780–791, 2016 26951286

Almeida OP, Ford AH, Flicker L: Systematic review and meta-analysis of randomized placebo-controlled trials of folate and vitamin B12 for depression. Int Psychogeriatr 27(5):727–737, 2015 25644193

Alpert JE, Mischoulon D, Rubenstein GE, et al: Folinic acid (Leucovorin) as an adjunctive treatment for SSRI-refractory depression. Ann Clin Psychiatry 14(1):33–38, 2002 12046638

Alshahrani F, Aljohani N: Vitamin D: deficiency, sufficiency and toxicity. Nutrients 5(9):3605–3616, 2013 24067388

Anastasiou CA, Yannakoulia M, Scarmeas N: Vitamin D and cognition: an update of the current evidence. J Alzheimers Dis 42(suppl 3):S71–S80, 2014 24820017

Andersen LP, Gögenur I, Rosenberg J, et al: The safety of melatonin in humans. Clin Drug Investig 36(3):169–175, 2016 26692007

Anglin RE, Samaan Z, Walter SD, et al: Vitamin D deficiency and depression in adults: systematic review and meta-analysis. Br J Psychiatry 202:100–107, 2013 23377209

Asher GN, Gartlehner G, Gaynes BN, et al: Comparative benefits and harms of complementary and alternative medicine therapies for initial treatment of major depressive disorder: systematic review and meta-analysis. J Altern Complement Med 23(12):907–919, 2017 28700248

Aucoin M, Cooley K, Knee C, et al: Fish-derived omega-3 fatty acids and prostate cancer: a systematic review. Integr Cancer Ther 16(1):32–62, 2017 27365385

Auld F, Maschauer EL, Morrison I, et al: Evidence for the efficacy of melatonin in the treatment of primary adult sleep disorders. Sleep Med Rev 34:10–22, 2017 28648359

Autier P, Mullie P, Macacu A, et al: Effect of vitamin D supplementation on non-skeletal disorders: a systematic review of meta-analyses and randomised trials. Lancet Diabetes Endocrinol 5(12):986–1004, 2017 29102433

Baede-van Dijk PA, van Galen E, Lekkerkerker JF: Drug interactions of Hypericum perforatum (St. John's wort) are potentially hazardous [in Dutch]. Ned Tijdschr Geneeskd 144(17):811–812, 2000 10800553

Baek JH, Nierenberg AA, Kinrys G: Clinical applications of herbal medicines for anxiety and insomnia; targeting patients with bipolar disorder. Aust NZ J Psychiatry 48(8):705–715, 2014 24947278

Bikle DD: Vitamin D metabolism, mechanism of action, and clinical applications. Chem Biol 21(3):319–329, 2014 24529992

Bloch MH, Hannestad J: Omega-3 fatty acids for the treatment of depression: systematic review and meta-analysis. Mol Psychiatry 17(12):1272–1282, 2012 21931319

Boman B: l-Tryptophan: a rational anti-depressant and a natural hypnotic? Aust N Z J Psychiatry 22(1):83–97, 1988 3285826

Borja-Hart NL, Marino J: Role of omega-3 fatty acids for prevention or treatment of perinatal depression. Pharmacotherapy 30(2):210–216, 2010 20099994

Bostock E, Kirkby K, Garry M, et al: Mania associated with herbal medicines, other than cannabis: a systematic review and quality assessment of case reports. Front Psychiatry 9:280, 2018 30034348

Bozzatello P, Brignolo E, De Grandi E, et al: Supplementation with omega-3 fatty acids in psychiatric disorders: a review of literature data. J Clin Med 5(8):67, 2016 27472373

Burckhardt M, Herke M, Wustmann T, et al: Omega-3 fatty acids for the treatment of dementia. Cochrane Database Syst Rev (4):CD009002, 2016 2747237

Burke MF, Burke FM, Soffer DE: Review of cardiometabolic effects of prescription omega-3 fatty acids. Curr Atheroscler Rep 19(12):60, 2017 29116404

Camp KM, Trujillo E: Position of the Academy of Nutrition and Dietetics: nutritional genomics. J Acad Nutr Diet 114(2):299–312, 2014 24439821

Cardinal BJ, Engels H-J: Ginseng does not enhance psychological well-being in healthy, young adults: results of a double-blind, placebo-controlled, randomized clinical trial. J Am Diet Assoc 101(6):655–660, 2001 11424544

Chalon S: Omega-3 fatty acids and monoamine neurotransmission. Prostaglandins Leukot Essent Fatty Acids 75(4–5):259–269, 2006 16963244

Chun RF, Peercy BE, Orwoll ES, et al: Vitamin D and DBP: the free hormone hypothesis revisited. J Steroid Biochem Mol Biol 144(pt A):132–137, 2014 24095930

Claustrat B, Leston J: Melatonin: Physiological effects in humans. Neurochirurgie 61(2–3):77–84, 2015 25908646

Cohen-Woods S, Craig I, Gaysina D, et al: The Bipolar Association Case-Control Study (BACCS) and meta-analysis: no association with the 5,10-methylenetetrahydrofolate reductase gene and bipolar disorder. Am J Med Genet B Neuropsychiatr Genet 153B(7):1298–1304, 2010 20552676

Costello RB, Lentino CV, Boyd CC, et al: The effectiveness of melatonin for promoting healthy sleep: a rapid evidence assessment of the literature. Nutr J 13:106, 2014 25380732

Cui X, Gooch H, Groves NJ, et al: Vitamin D and the brain: key questions for future research. J Steroid Biochem Mol Biol 148:305–309, 2015 25448739

Damico KE, Stoll AL, Marangell LB, et al: How blind is double-blind? A study of fish oil versus placebo. Prostaglandins Leukot Essent Fatty Acids 66(4):393–395, 2002 12054908

De Berardis D, Orsolini L, Serroni N, et al: A comprehensive review on the efficacy of S-adenosyl-L-methionine in major depressive disorder. CNS Neurol Disord Drug Targets 15(1):35–44, 2016 26295824

DeKosky ST, Williamson JD, Fitzpatrick AL, et al: Ginkgo biloba for prevention of dementia: a randomized controlled trial. JAMA 300(19):2253–2262, 2008 19017911

Di Lorenzo C, Ceschi A, Kupferschmidt H, et al: Adverse effects of plant food supplements and botanical preparations: a systematic review with critical evaluation of causality. Br J Clin Pharmacol 79(4):578–592, 2015 25251944

Ducker GS, Rabinowitz JD: One-carbon metabolism in health and disease. Cell Metab 25(1):27–42, 2017

Ernst E, Rand JI, Barnes J, et al: Adverse effects profile of the herbal antidepressant St. John's wort (Hypericum perforatum L.). Eur J Clin Pharmacol 54(8):589–594, 1998 9860144

Fava M, Borus JS, Alpert JE, et al: Folate, vitamin B12, and homocysteine in major depressive disorder. Am J Psychiatry 154(3):426–428, 1997 9054796

Ferracioli-Oda E, Qawasmi A, Bloch MH: Meta-analysis: melatonin for the treatment of primary sleep disorders. PLoS One 8(5):e63773, 2013 23691095

Ford AH, Flicker L, Thomas J, et al: Vitamins B12, B6, and folic acid for onset of depressive symptoms in older men: results from a 2-year placebo-controlled randomized trial. J Clin Psychiatry 69(8):1203–1209, 2008 18557664

Freeman MP, Hibbeln JR, Wisner KL, et al: Omega-3 fatty acids: evidence basis for treatment and future research in psychiatry. J Clin Psychiatry 67(12):1954–1967, 2006 17194275

Ghadirian AM, Ananth J, Engelsmann F: Folic acid deficiency and depression. Psychosomatics 21(11):926–929, 1980 7433596

Goel A, Pothineni NV, Singhal M, et al: Fish, fish oils and cardio protection: promise or fish tale? Int J Mol Sci 19(12):3703, 2018 30469489

Goodwill AM, Szoeke C: A systematic review and meta-analysis of the effect of low vitamin D on cognition. J Am Geriatr Soc 65(10):2161–2168, 2017 28758188

Gracious BL, Chirieac MC, Costescu S, et al: Randomized, placebo-controlled trial of flax oil in pediatric bipolar disorder. Bipolar Disord 12(2):142–154, 2010 20402707

Grobler AC, Matthews G, Molenberghs G: The impact of missing data on clinical trials: a re-analysis of a placebo controlled trial of Hypericum perforatum (St Johns wort) and sertraline in major depressive disorder. Psychopharmacology (Berl) 231(9):1987–1999, 2014 24232445

Hallahan B, Ryan T, Hibbeln JR, et al: Efficacy of omega-3 highly unsaturated fatty acids in the treatment of depression. Br J Psychiatry 209(3):192–201, 2016 27103682

Henderson L, Yue QY, Bergquist C, et al: St John's wort (Hypericum perforatum): drug interactions and clinical outcomes. Br J Clin Pharmacol 54(4):349–356, 2002 12392581

Hibbeln JR: Fish consumption and major depression. Lancet 351(9110):1213, 1998 9643729

Hibbeln JR: Seafood consumption, the DHA content of mothers' milk and prevalence rates of postpartum depression: a cross-national, ecological analysis. J Affect Disord 69(1–3):15–29, 2002 12103448

Hickey SE, Curry CJ, Toriello HV: ACMG practice guideline: lack of evidence for MTHFR polymorphism testing. Genet Med 15(2):153–156, 2013 23288205

Hill M, Shannahan K, Jasinski S, et al: Folate supplementation in schizophrenia: a possible role for MTHFR genotype. Schizophr Res 127(1–3):41–45, 2011 21334854

Holick MF: Vitamin D: importance in the prevention of cancers, type 1 diabetes, heart disease, and osteoporosis. Am J Clin Nutr 79(3):362–371, 2004 14985208

Holick MF, Binkley NC, Bischoff-Ferrari HA, et al: Evaluation, treatment, and prevention of vitamin D deficiency: an Endocrine Society clinical practice guideline. J Clin Endocrinol Metab 96(7):1911–1930, 2011 21646368

Holman RT, Johnson SB, Ogburn PL: Deficiency of essential fatty acids and membrane fluidity during pregnancy and lactation. Proc Natl Acad Sci USA 88(11):4835–4839, 1991 2052562

Hvas AM, Juul S, Lauritzen L, et al: No effect of vitamin B-12 treatment on cognitive function and depression: a randomized placebo controlled study. J Affect Disord 81(3):269–273, 2004 15337331

Hyland K, Shoffner J, Heales SJ: Cerebral folate deficiency. J Inherit Metab Dis 33(5):563–570, 2010 20668945

Joshi KG, Faubion MD: Mania and psychosis associated with St. John's wort and ginseng. Psychiatry (Edgmont Pa) 2(9):56–61, 2005 21120109

Kelly CB, McDonnell AP, Johnston TG, et al: The MTHFR C677T polymorphism is associated with depressive episodes in patients from Northern Ireland. J Psychopharmacol 18(4):567–571, 2004 15582924

Kennaway DJ: Potential safety issues in the use of the hormone melatonin in paediatrics. J Paediatr Child Health 51(6):584–589, 2015 25643981

Köbe T, Witte AV, Schnelle A, et al: Vitamin B-12 concentration, memory performance, and hippocampal structure in patients with mild cognitive impairment. Am J Clin Nutr 103(4):1045–1054, 2016 26912492

La Rosa F, Clerici M, Ratto D, et al: The gut-brain axis in Alzheimer's disease and omega-3. A critical overview of clinical trials. Nutrients 10(9):1267, 2018 30205543

LeFevre ML: Screening for vitamin D deficiency in adults: U.S. Preventive Services Task Force recommendation statement. Ann Intern Med 162(2):133–140, 2015 25419853

Levant B: N-3 (omega-3) fatty acids in postpartum depression: implications for prevention and treatment. Depress Res Treat 2011:467349, 2011 21151517

Li G, Mbuagbaw L, Samaan Z, et al: Efficacy of vitamin D supplementation in depression in adults: a systematic review. J Clin Endocrinol Metab 99(3):757–767, 2014 24423304

Lipton MA, Ban TA, Kane FJ, et al: Task Force Report 7: Megavitamin and Orthomolecular Therapy in Psychiatry. Washington, DC, American Psychiatric Association, 1973

Lok A, Mocking RJ, Assies J, et al: The one-carbon-cycle and methylenetetrahydrofolate reductase (MTHFR) C677T polymorphism in recurrent major depressive disorder; influence of antidepressant use and depressive state? J Affect Disord 166:115–123, 2014 25012419

Long S, Goldblatt J: MTHFR genetic testing: controversy and clinical implications. Aust Fam Physician 45(4):237–240, 2016 27052143

Malihi Z, Wu Z, Stewart AW, et al: Hypercalcemia, hypercalciuria, and kidney stones in long-term studies of vitamin D supplementation: a systematic review and meta-analysis. Am J Clin Nutr 104(4):1039–1051, 2016 27604776

Marangell LB, Martinez JM, Zboyan HA, et al: Omega-3 fatty acids for the prevention of postpartum depression: negative data from a preliminary, open-label pilot study. Depress Anxiety 19(1):20–23, 2004 14978781

Mathew SJ, Lijffijt M: Neurometabolic abnormalities in treatment-resistant depression. Am J Psychiatry 174(1):3–5, 2017 28041002

Mayeno AN, Gleich GJ: Eosinophilia-myalgia syndrome and tryptophan production: a cautionary tale. Trends Biotechnol 12(9):346–352, 1994 7765187

Mei N, Guo X, Ren Z, et al: Review of ginkgo biloba–induced toxicity, from experimental studies to human case reports. J Environ Sci Health C Environ Carcinog Ecotoxicol Rev 35(1):1–28, 2017 28055331

Mikkelsen K, Stojanovska L, Apostolopoulos V: The effects of vitamin B in depression. Curr Med Chem 23(38):4317–4337, 2016 27655070

Mocking RJ, Harmsen I, Assies J, et al: Meta-analysis and meta-regression of omega-3 polyunsaturated fatty acid supplementation for major depressive disorder. Transl Psychiatry 15(6):e756, 2016 26978738

Moorthy D, Peter I, Scott TM, et al: Status of vitamins B-12 and B-6 but not of folate, homocysteine, and the methylenetetrahydrofolate reductase C677T polymorphism are associated with impaired cognition and depression in adults. J Nutr 142(8):1554–1560, 2012 22739363

Mudryj AN, de Groh M, Aukema HM, et al: Folate intakes from diet and supplements may place certain Canadians at risk for folic acid toxicity. Br J Nutr 116(7):1236–1245, 2016 27609220

National Center for Complementary and Integrative Health: Kava. National Institutes of Health, Updated September 2016. Available at: https://nccih.nih.gov/health/kava. Accessed October 2, 2019.

New York State Department of Environmental Conservation: Ginseng varieties and glossary. Albany, NY, Department of Environmental Conservation, 2019. Available at: https://www.dec.ny.gov/animals/7474.html. Accessed October 2, 2019.

Ogawa S, Fujii T, Koga N, et al: Plasma L-tryptophan concentration in major depressive disorder: new data and meta-analysis. J Clin Psychiatry 75(9):e906–e915, 2014 25295433

Oh R, Brown DL: Vitamin B12 deficiency. Am Fam Physician 67(5):979–986, 2003 12643357

Palacios C, Gonzalez L: Is vitamin D deficiency a major global public health problem? J Steroid Biochem Mol Biol 144(Pt A):138–145, 2014 26978738

Pan L, McKain BW, Madan-Khetarpal S, et al: GTP-cyclohydrolase deficiency responsive to sapropterin and 5-HTP supplementation: relief of treatment-refractory depression and suicidal behaviour. BMJ Case Rep 2011:bcr0320113927, 2011 22691588

Pan LA, Martin P, Zimmer T, et al: Neurometabolic disorders: potentially treatable abnormalities in patients with treatment-refractory depression and suicidal behavior. Am J Psychiatry 174(1):42–50, 2017 27523499

Papakostas GI, Mischoulon D, Shyu I, et al: S-adenosyl methionine (SAMe) augmentation of serotonin reuptake inhibitors for antidepressant nonresponders with major depressive disorder: a double-blind, randomized clinical trial. Am J Psychiatry 167(8):942–948, 2010 20595412

Papakostas GI, Shelton RC, Zajecka JM, et al: l-Methylfolate as adjunctive therapy for SSRI-resistant major depression: results of two randomized, double-blind, parallel-sequential trials. Am J Psychiatry 169(12):1267–1274, 2012 23212058

Pauling P: Vitamin therapy: treatment for the mentally ill. Science 160(3833):1181–1182, 1968 5648257

Persson M, Fagt S, Nauta MJ: Personalised fish intake recommendations: the effect of background exposure on optimisation. Br J Nutr 120(8):946–957, 2018 30168411

Pittler MH, Ernst E: Kava extract for treating anxiety. Cochrane Database Syst Rev (1):CD003383, 2016 12535473

Raimann X, Rodríguez OL, Chávez P, et al: Mercury in fish and its importance in health [in Spanish]. Rev Med Chil 142(9):1174–1180, 2014 25517058

Rees AM, Austin MP, Owen C, et al: Omega-3 deficiency associated with perinatal depression: case control study. Psychiatry Res 166(2–3):254–259, 2009 19268372

Roberts E, Carter B, Young AH: Caveat emptor: folate in unipolar depressive illness, a systematic review and meta-analysis. J Psychopharmacol 32(4):377–384, 2018 29442609

Roffman JL, Lamberti JS, Achtyes E, et al: Randomized multicenter investigation of folate plus vitamin B12 supplementation in schizophrenia. JAMA Psychiatry 70(5):481–489, 2013 23467813

Ross AC, Manson JE, Abrams SA, et al: The 2011 report on dietary reference intakes for calcium and vitamin D from the Institute of Medicine: what clinicians need to know. J Clin Endocrinol Metab 96(1):53–58, 2011 21118827

Saida FB, Chen X, Tran K, et al: First 25-hydroxyvitamin D assay for general chemistry analyzers. Expert Rev Mol Diagn 15(3):313–323, 2015 25434745

Sanders KM, Stuart AL, Williamson EJ, et al: Annual high-dose vitamin D3 and mental well-being: randomised controlled trial. Br J Psychiatry 198(5):357–364, 2011 21525520

Sarris J, Murphy J, Mischoulon D, et al: Adjunctive nutraceuticals for depression: a systematic review and meta-analyses. Am J Psychiatry 173(6):575–587, 2016 27113121

Schneider-Helmert D, Spinweber CL: Evaluation of L-tryptophan for treatment of insomnia: a review. Psychopharmacology (Berl) 89(1):1–7, 1986 3090582

Schreckinger ME, Lotton J, Lila MA, et al: Berries from South America: a comprehensive review on chemistry, health potential, and commercialization. J Med Food 13(2):233–246, 2010 20170356

Sharma A, Gerbarg P: Bottiglieri T, et al: S-adenosylmethionine (SAMe) for neuropsychiatric disorders: a clinician-oriented review of research. J Clin Psychiatry 78(6):e656–e667, 2017 28682528

Shaw K, Turner J, Del Mar C: Tryptophan and 5-hydroxytryptophan for depression. Cochrane Database Syst Rev (1):CD003198, 2002 11869656

Shelton RC: St John's wort (Hypericum perforatum) in major depression. J Clin Psychiatry 70(suppl 5):23–27, 2009 19909690

Shieh A, Chun RF, Ma C, et al: Effects of high-dose vitamin D2 versus D3 on total and free 25-hydroxyvitamin D and markers of calcium balance. J Clin Endocrinol Metab 101(8):3070–3078, 2016 27192696

Sletten TL, Magee M, Murray JM, et al: Efficacy of melatonin with behavioural sleep-wake scheduling for delayed sleep-wake phase disorder: a double-blind, randomised clinical trial. PLoS Med 15(6):e1002587, 2018 29912983

Smith K, Leiras C: The effectiveness and safety of kava kava for treating anxiety symptoms: a systematic review and analysis of randomized clinical trials. Complement Ther Clin Pract 33:107–117, 2018 30396607

Smith KM, Sahyoun NR: Fish consumption: recommendations versus advisories, can they be reconciled? Nutr Rev 63(2):39–46, 2005 15762087

Sobczynska-Malefora A, Harrington DJ: Laboratory assessment of folate (vitamin B9) status. J Clin Pathol 71(11):949–956, 2018 30228213

Tebben PJ, Singh RJ, Kumar R: Vitamin D-mediated hypercalcemia: mechanisms, diagnosis, and treatment. Endocr Rev 37(5):521–547, 2016 27588937

Thomson J, Rankin H, Ashcroft GW, et al: The treatment of depression in general practice: a comparison of L-tryptophan, amitriptyline, and a combination of L-tryptophan and amitriptyline with placebo. Psychol Med 12(4):741–751, 1982 7156248

Vellas B, Coley N, Ousset PJ, et al: Long-term use of standardised Ginkgo biloba extract for the prevention of Alzheimer's disease (GuidAge): a randomised placebo-controlled trial. Lancet Neurol 11(10):851–859, 2012 22959217

Veronese N, Solmi M, Rizza W, et al: Vitamin D status in anorexia nervosa: a meta-analysis. Int J Eat Disord 48(7):803–813, 2015 25445242

Wacker M, Holick MF: Sunlight and vitamin D: a global perspective for health. Dermatoendocrinol 5(1):51–108, 2013 24494042

Wenstrom KD: The FDA's new advice on fish: it's complicated. Am J Obstet Gynecol 211(5):475.e1–478.e1, 2014 25072735

Wesson VA, Levitt AJ, Joffe RT: Change in folate status with antidepressant treatment. Psychiatry Res 53(3):313–322, 1994 7870851

Wilcken B, Bamforth F, Li Z, et al: Geographical and ethnic variation of the 677C>T allele of 5,10 methylenetetrahydrofolate reductase (MTHFR): findings from over 7000 newborns from 16 areas world wide. J Med Genet 40(8):619–625, 2003 12920077

Wolfersdorf M, König F: Serum folic acid and vitamin B12 in depressed inpatients. A study of serum folic acid with radioimmunoassay in 121 depressed inpatients [in German]. Psychiatr Prax 22(4):162–164, 1995 7675908

Zajecka JM, Fava M, Shelton RC, et al: Long-term efficacy, safety, and tolerability of l-methylfolate calcium 15 mg as adjunctive therapy with selective serotonin reuptake inhibitors: a 12-month, open-label study following a placebo-controlled acute study. J Clin Psychiatry 77(5):654–660, 2016 27035404

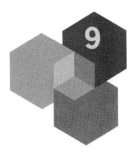

Critical Lifestyle Supports to Successful Clinical Psychopharmacology

Our focus as clinical psychopharmacologists is to determine whether patients may be helped with prescribed medication and to help them choose the best medication and then use it safely and effectively. To accomplish this, however, we must consider the milieu in which the medicine will be attempting to have its effects. A brain stressed by sleep deprivation, stimulant abuse (legal and illegal), CNS depressants, or other influences may not respond in the desired manner. Therefore, assessing, monitoring, and correcting any compromising lifestyle interferences, before and during prescription of medicines, is essential to achieving a positive outcome.

Sleep

As discussed in Chapter 3, sleep is not only, arguably, the most important symptom for diagnosis but also one of the most powerful nonpharmacological interventions. Many psychiatric disorders include impaired sleep, but we must also be certain that patients' lifestyle choices are not worsening their symptoms. Although prescribing a soporific to rapidly improve sleep—on top of an otherwise hopeful pharmacological plan—is not necessary, our goal of treatment is good, healthy, restorative sleep, and we must be certain patients are taking steps to allow this to happen.

You should thus include, at every session, an assessment of and discussion about adequate sleep. The amount of necessary sleep appears to be between 7 and 9 hours in the healthy adult population; evidence shows that 8–8.5 hours is essential for adults and 7–8 hours for older adults (outliers from genetic mutation being so rare as to not be worth taking into consideration [He et al. 2009]). The National Sleep Foundation also recommends 10–13 hours for preschoolers, 9–11 hours for school-age children, and 8–10 hours for teenagers (Hirshkowitz et al. 2015). During this time, the unencumbered brain can perform all of the necessary maintenance it requires.

In addition to the adult patient target of 8–8.5 hours of sleep every night, this sleep must take place at the same time every day and during the traditional nighttime or dark hours. Although we can expect that no one will follow this plan perfectly, we do need to urge patients to remain as close to this goal as possible. Encourage them to not vary the amount of sleep more than 1 hour each day, to go to bed at the same time every evening and get up at the same time every morning, even on days off from work or school. Predict for them that they will feel more energy by getting up on weekends than by sleeping in. Offering to allow 1 more hour on days off can be a tool to improve compliance, but actual data show that even this leads to impairment. Data on shifts into daylight saving time in both the northern and southern hemispheres show clear mental and physical risks from even 1 hour of sleep change (Manfredini et al. 2018; Robb and Barnes 2018; Sipilä et al. 2016).

Decades of research have shown that shift workers experience cognitive impairments, increased mood instability, and even increased cancer and dementia risk (Stryjewski et al. 2016). They are at such risk that some conditions, such as unstable mood, cannot be fully treated due to a 20% effect on stability from even fixed shift work. Advocate for your patients to obtain daytime shifts based on health necessity once you are both sure this will not threaten their job security. If night shifts cannot be changed, encourage patients to remain on a fixed schedule and to not attempt to change their day/night schedule back and forth, such as staying awake at night while working and during the day when off work. Although it may allow more time with family and for socializing, this alternating schedule is so damaging to their health that it cannot be effectively sustained with good mental and physical health results. Patients in such a situation might seek alternative employment, if possible.

Much has been published in the literature and lay media about blue light from light-emitting diode (LED) displays on electronic screens (large and small) interfering with sleep; many phones and other devices now have easy-to-use evening settings that minimize exposure. Encourage your patients to employ this feature, because even low levels significantly reduce endogenous melatonin release. They should minimize the amount of bright light in the evening and maximize it in the morning, being sure to take proper protection from ultraviolet radiation (Bedrosian et al. 2016; Rahman et al. 2017; West et al. 2011).

A drop in body temperature also may be necessary for initiation of sleep (Murphy and Campbell 1997), so keeping the bedroom cooler may help. Scientists recommend a room temperature of 68°–70°F (20°–21°C) on average, allowing for clothing and bedclothes (Harding et al. 2019). Patients should use their beds only for sleep and sex and not for lounging or studying, if possible. Foam earplugs may be helpful if noise is a problem; important noises such as cries of children are usually heard through these (although patients should test purchases). Clearly, any medical interferences with sleep, such as nocturia, sleep apnea, and narcolepsy, must be diagnosed and treated effectively.

For some patients, you may need to discuss the natural daily rhythm of sleep. Occasionally, patients seem to think they should go about their day actively until "struck down" by sleep. Teach them that healthy sleep is a decision that is made on a schedule: allowing time for slowing down prior to getting into bed, adjusting to reduced and indirect light, closing their eyes, and telling themselves that now is the time to sleep. Setting an alarm for 8–8.5 hours later is an option if they cannot wake naturally after that time. Discourage use of "snooze alarms" because body and brain physiology react poorly to repeated sudden awakenings (Lo et al. 2012; Wilkinson and Stretton 1971).

Napping should generally be discouraged unless a patient is compelled by symptomatology of the primary disorder, such as the hypersomnia of bipolar depression. Naps, although sometimes innocuous, often make it more difficult to sleep at night, distorting healthy physiology. Afternoon naps appear more damaging than morning naps.

Eating or exercising within 3 hours of bedtime is likely to impair sleep, as are alcohol and caffeine (including decaffeinated products and chocolate). Studies show that caffeine use even in the morning may compromise sleep later that night (Landolt et al. 1995). Alcohol in the bloodstream is always destructive to healthy sleep, limiting rapid eye movement (REM) sleep and deep non-REM (NREM) sleep. Like other interferences with REM and NREM sleep, the use of stimulants, alcohol, and some sedatives will predispose patients to a greater risk of memory problems, infections, cancers, and often, shorter lives (Mazzotti et al. 2014).

A very serious clinical example of how sleep is an important part of patients' prescription is found in the management of postpartum depression, which is most commonly attributable to bipolar disorder or major depression (Sharma et al. 2017). When planning ahead of delivery to minimize the risk of an episode, protecting the mother's sleep is one of the most important steps, just as it is in treating bipolar disorder. Waking a mother to feed or soothe a crying baby is likely to provoke mood symptoms, leading to postpartum depression or psychosis. Patients and their entire support system must be informed of this and understand that an uninterrupted night's sleep is essential. The family or support team must plan for the mother to not be awakened during the night, and certainly not exposed to bright lights if accidentally awakened. Partners and other significant others will have to arrange for feeding and caring for the infant during the night. The reverse is true, of course, if only the partner carries the risk of mood episodes (Dennis and Ross 2005; Krawczak et al. 2016; Park et al. 2013).

To obtain good psychopharmacological outcomes, insist on initiating treatment only in the context of good sleep hygiene. Patients' brains and bodies must be in sync with efforts to restore natural psychoneurological and endocrine function via pharmacological and somatic treatments. Emphasize to patients that we are attempting to allow their brains to work better. "Sleep hygiene" has now been repackaged as cognitive-behavioral therapy for insomnia, which is more akin to the list of lifestyle requirements for healthy sleep listed earlier than to classical cognitive-behavioral therapy. Whatever you choose to call it, as you work with your patients to employ these imperatives, they will enjoy greater success and come to understand sleep is an important tool of assessment as well as a focus of treatment.

Exercise

Some patients are convinced of the healing attributes of exercise and may wish this to be a major focus of their treatment plan. Others will have no interest. A large number of studies have attempted to link regular exercise with both a reduced incidence of depressive and anxious symptoms and therapeutic efficacy (Blumenthal et al. 2007; Schuch et al. 2016). Although these studies often associate exercise with symptom improvement, many also have methodological problems. A causal link has yet to be confirmed, but genetic factors influencing mood and anxiety symptoms and voluntary exercise may be involved (De Moor et al. 2008). Recent work identifying brain-derived neurotrophic factor as being depleted in patients with major depression but enhanced by moderate, prescribed, regular aerobic exercise may possibly determine a therapeutic mechanism (Ieraci et al. 2016; Mata et al. 2010; Phillips 2017).

The type of exercise was once thought to be important, especially in patients with anxiety disorders; now we recognize that the fitness of the patient or the severity of the anxiety disorder is more important than the anaerobic exercise producing oxygen debt that may worsen symptoms. Early studies in the pathogenesis and treatment of panic disorder utilized lactate infusions to provoke symptoms in willing volunteers (Cowley and Arana 1990); subsequent research sought to delineate the mechanism (Esquivel et al. 2010; Johnson et al. 2008; Maddock et al. 2013). Anerobic exercise was once thought solely responsible for a buildup of lactate in muscles, but we now know that lactate is also produced through aerobic metabolism. Excessive exercise with inadequate training or acclimatization to altitude nevertheless causes arterial lactate levels to rise, and lactate does cross the blood–brain barrier (Brooks 2009; Brooks et al. 1991).

Excessive respiration (Lum 1981) and heart rate (Ehlers and Breuer 1996) have also been documented to provoke panic episodes; more than a few conflicting studies have shown aerobic exercise to either provoke or ameliorate panic symptoms in patients with panic disorder (O'Connor et al. 2000). Currently, only a minority of these patients appear to have symptoms provoked by exercise, and these are likely the patients less conditioned to regular exercise. Explain this to your patients and help them identify a workout regimen that avoids sudden bursts in physical activity for which they have not adequately prepared with regular exercise and progressive training methods (Lattari et al. 2018). These methods allow increased metabolism of lactate by the mitochondria of liver, kidney, and heart cells. Most patients will understand and accept the recommendation.

Although physicians certainly support healthy exercise done in moderation (taking the patient's physical condition into account), help your patients understand that exercise should replace indicated pharmacological treatment (which it may support) only with good reason. A strong therapeutic alliance will allow respect for the patient's wish to employ exercise as part of treatment while still maximizing the chances for treatment success. As already mentioned, encourage your patients to not exercise within 3 hours of attempting to fall asleep, explaining that the body will still be in exercise mode while they are attempting to sleep. Remind them that some supplements they think will help them with exercise may actually prevent them from achieving success with medication.

Weight and Diet

Diet is important in terms of lifestyle choices, although it may also be influenced by symptoms. Patients may not be in full control of their weight

TABLE 9–1.   Adult body mass index calculation

Scale	Formula
U.S. customary	Weight [lb]/(height [in])$^2 \times 703$
Metric	Weight (kg)/(height [m])^2
Imperial	Converting to metric:
	(weight [stone]$\times 6.35$)/(height [m])^2
	Converting to English:
	(weight [stone]$\times 14$)/(height [in])$^2 \times 703$

and hunger; optimal dietary choices may be difficult to make, especially early in treatment. In this section, I do not discuss specific treatment for eating disorders but consider the appetite effects of other diagnoses and weight effects of some treatments and how these might be addressed by dietary planning. The goal is a healthy, moderate appetite and weight in a range that will not lead to additional health problems.

Because you assess appetite and calculate patients' body mass index (BMI) at every visit, you will have a working knowledge of how their weight may be a problem. BMI calculators (Table 9–1) are included in many electronic medical records, websites, and phone applications; the National Institutes of Health (NIH) offers a useful page (U.S. Department of Health and Human Services 2019a). BMI is not a perfect measure and can overestimate body fat in extreme athletes, those with excessive muscle mass (e.g., bodybuilders), and pregnant women and underestimate it in geriatric patients and those with muscle wasting (Prentice and Jebb 2001). BMI is not valid in children and adolescents unless corrected for age and sex (Centers for Disease Control and Prevention 2001) nor in patients with eating disorders. For most adult psychiatric patients seen in the office, however, BMI can be a useful tool (Flegal and Graubard 2009) and is certainly better than using weight alone.

Unless adult patients' BMI is between 18.5 and 24.9 (Table 9–2), dietary planning to change their weight should be addressed. Data appear to demonstrate that mild increases above 25 are not harmful, especially in older patients, but these findings have been argued to stem from altered muscle mass, leading back to the original normal range as safest for patients (Abramowitz et al. 2018). Educating patients with tools for maintaining a reasonable BMI should be part of a treatment plan.

Reducing the discussion to simple arithmetic and bypassing motivation and excuses may be helpful. Traditionally, a change in 1 lb (0.454 kg) of body weight has been assumed to represent a net change in 3,500 kcal (ex-

TABLE 9–2.   Adult body mass index range

Normal range	Underweight	Overweight	Obese	Severely obese
18.5–24.9	<18.5	25–29.9	30–40	>40

plain that these are colloquially called *calories*) (Wishnofsky 1958). If a body retains 3,500 kcal more than it had before, a pound is gained. If a body uses 3,500 kcal more, or ingests that amount less than usual, a pound is lost. Therefore, the simple math is that a daily reduction of 500 kcal, either via dietary restriction or exercise, should result in an average weight loss of 1 lb in 1 week (Guth 2014). Similarly, a daily increase of 500 kcal through intake or less exercise will add 1 lb per week. More recent research has shown that although this is a rough estimate for moderate weight loss, it can be distorted by sex differences, the original amount of body fat versus lean body weight, and metabolic changes that occur during the weight loss process. For these reasons, actual weight loss might take longer or even stall, the latter more commonly resulting from waning patient compliance over long periods of time (Chow and Hall 2014; Hall 2008).

Work through BMI with your patients so they learn to do it themselves, using one of many online calculators that determine how many calories they must consume daily to maintain their current body weight (given a certain activity level, sex, and age). The NIH's Body Weight Planner is one helpful source (Hall et al. 2011; U.S. Department of Health and Human Services 2019b). You can then calculate together how long it will take for them to reach a BMI of 18.5–24.9 with an average change of 1 lb a week from changing net "calorie" intake by 500 kcal daily. Stress that *average* means that they may not see a 1 lb change every week, but over 5 weeks might expect to see a 5-lb change. Suggest that they mark the date for each expected 5 lb change on a calendar so that they do not become unrealistically discouraged within the first 2 weeks. Help patients understand that this is a long-term project that should lead to permanent lifestyle change. Explain that larger weight changes may take even longer due to the conditions mentioned. Additionally, although increasing exercise is equally likely to produce results as changing kcal intake, many patients find it easier to manipulate dietary intake than exercise, and diet offers more opportunities for change than activity.

As science continues to work to identify an improved weight loss equation, strengthening the locus of control for dietary intake will provide a useful skill for your patients. Using methods such as this can help them realize they do have some say over their weight, once they adopt a long-term view, with relatively small daily changes. Groups such as Weight Watchers, a behavioral and support method, and Overeaters Anonymous, a 12-step program, may also be helpful for certain patients who require additional support. *Mindless Eating* by Wansink (2006) can be an eye-opener into behavioral patterns that can be consciously interrupted.

Alcohol

As discussed in Chapters 3 and 12, assess patients' alcohol use at every visit, because alcohol's presence in the body is likely to complicate symptoms and pharmacological success. Alcohol is, of course, a well-known CNS depressant, although initial disinhibition of impulse control from the frontal lobe may lead some patients to think of it as a stimulant. Use of alcohol within the 14 days preceding evaluation complicates accurate assessment of mood and diagnosis of mood disorders. Alcohol can block patients' response to antidepressants; prolonged use may lead to severe and permanent cognitive impairment; and severe and chronic use can lead to symptoms of psychosis. Most of your patients will not have severe alcohol use problems, but their consumption of even small amounts will affect their treatment response.

Ideally, all pharmacological treatment would take place in a milieu devoid of alcohol. Honestly, this must be our best recommendation to patients, because we can never assure them that any use of alcohol will not have negative consequences. Some patients will accept this suggestion, but others will not, and negotiation may be necessary (unless the patient has a diagnosable substance abuse disorder that requires eventual total sobriety). Assess patients' intake of alcohol and make sure that any suggestion of reducing or ceasing their intake will not provoke a serious alcohol withdrawal condition. Alcohol use may usually be reduced by as much as 20% per day in patients without history of severe withdrawals or withdrawal seizures, although a slower rate is more practical for outpatient management. Propose their use be reduced by 25% a week, with reassessment in 5 weeks, or 2 weeks after use is stopped, making it clear that you mean *absolutely no alcohol* should be consumed over that final 14-day period; otherwise, your assessment will be invalid. If a patient has recently ceased alcohol use prior to his or her visit with you, assess for clinical symptoms of withdrawal (e.g., sweating, tachycardia, hypertension, nausea, tremor, cognitive impairment, delusions, hallucinations) and, as always, take the patient's blood pressure. Initiate treatment for withdrawal if indicated. If not, describe these symptoms to the patient so that he or she can report their occurrence between sessions to you for immediate intervention.

Once the issue of withdrawal is addressed, suggest to patients who refuse to cease all alcohol that an intermediate step might be consuming no more than 1 oz (30 mL) of alcohol twice a week, and not on the same day, after the 14-day washout period for diagnosis has been completed. This 1-oz quantity equals one standard beer, one standard mixed drink, or one 8-oz glass of wine. Some people believe the alcohol content of beer and even wine is less than that of hard liquor, and educating them is important. Explore other beverages they might enjoy substituting for alcohol so that they feel less deprived, such as a special sparkling water or juice, but nothing that will also complicate treatment, such as caffeinated products. Many patients who are unwilling to give up alcohol may accept this compromise and eventually limit their alcohol use to rare as they begin to appreciate the benefits of the changes you have achieved together. Remind patients who improve with this plan that it must be continued to sustain response or remission.

Drugs

I hope it is obvious that as we attempt to improve patients' brain function through lifestyle and pharmacological methods, their use of recreational psychoactive substance is likely to interfere. As mentioned in Chapters 3 and 12, questions about use of illegal or recreational substances should be made with each patient at each visit, monitoring for any interference with the treatment plan. Even long-term patients of any age and background may surprise you. Also, as mentioned in Chapter 3, alert patients that cannabis is often available in food form as well. Not all patients will appreciate this importance or agree with the risk, but attempting psychopharmacological intervention while patients are using these other substances not only may be dangerous but also is likely to fail.

Just as some people incorrectly minimize the effects of beer compared with other forms of alcohol, others may minimize the effects of cannabis. Whether you and the patient believe it should be legal, illegal, or decriminalized, research shows that its effect on the brain and body affects successful treatment (Guttmannova et al. 2017; Hall and Degenhardt 2014; Volkow et al. 2016; Weinstein et al. 2016). Although cannabis has been legalized for medical use in many U.S. states, most commonly for the treatment of cancer pain, glaucoma, HIV/AIDS, cachexia, severe chronic pain, severe nausea, seizures, and severe muscle spasms (Hoffmann and Weber 2010), studies of its efficacy remain equivocal (Allan et al. 2018; Wilkinson 2013). Additionally, claims of benefits from cannabis in psychiatric, developmental, and neurodegenerative disorders are poorly substantiated (Hadland et al. 2015; Lim et al. 2017).

A large group of synthetic cannabinoids is available to provide medical benefit without the psychoactive motivation that leads to recreational use or abuse; most of these have not received adequate study. Two are legally approved in the United States and United Kingdom: dronabinol and nabilone for refractory nausea and emesis during chemotherapy. The former is also used for anorexia in HIV cases. Nabiximols is available in Europe, the United Kingdom, and Canada for treating neuropathic pain, spasticity, overactive bladder, and other symptoms of multiple sclerosis. Clinicians should still heed the paucity of studies demonstrating the safety and efficacy of these synthetics and be aware of the data available on adverse reactions and intoxication (Papaseit et al. 2018).

Assess whether patients are using cannabis or other psychoactive drugs outside of your treatment plan to help alleviate symptoms (correctly or incorrectly) or whether they are truly doing it for enjoyment or escape (Haug et al. 2017). For example, patients with social phobia may rely on cannabis or alcohol to mute daily symptoms and allow functional interaction with others. Patients tapering their use of these substances while you initiate a safer and more effective pharmacological treatment for them is a reasonable compromise.

If patients have a diagnosable substance abuse disorder, make the diagnosis and prescribe appropriate treatment prior to initiating any treatment of comorbid conditions (unless urgent safety concerns with this plan arise). As mentioned in Chapter 3, many cases that appear to be adult ADHD clear up completely once cannabis has left the body. Reassess comorbid diagnoses after the offending substances are no longer present. This necessitates learning the half-lives of commonly used psychoactive substances (Table 9–3) so that their exit from the body can be accurately assessed. Cannabis is stored in body fat cells and released after about 12 months. Weight loss during that time may provoke spikes in the serum level. Waiting 12 months to initiate treatment for a mood or thought disorder may not be feasible, but this knowledge will allow you to calibrate the residual effects of confounding factors as treatment proceeds.

Again, stress that every intervention in the treatment plan should support brain health, allowing the brain to function as well as it can and lead to symptom resolution. Some clinicians insist on written contracts about compliance with patients, random urine or serum blood screenings, or even documentation of 12-step meeting attendance. A healthy therapeutic alliance, however, does not place the clinician in the authoritarian role, which may encourage patients to resist; rather, we should be working in agreement, side by side, to solve the same problems for the sole benefit of the patients. If this therapeutic alliance is not functioning, it should be addressed psychotherapeutically before proceeding.

TABLE 9–3. Half-lives of common psychoactive substances

Heroin	30 minutes
Cocaine	1 hour or less
Opiate analgesics	3–12 hours
MDMA (Ecstasy)	8 hours
Methamphetamine	12 hours
Phencyclidine (PCP)	21 hours
Cannabis	67 days (in chronic users)

TABLE 9–4. Caffeine content

Product	Caffeine content, *mg*
Average soft drink with caffeine	30–40
Green or black tea	30–50
Coffee (8 oz)	80–100
Energy drink (8 oz)	40–250
Dark chocolate (per oz)	5–20
Milk chocolate	3.5–6
White chocolate	Check ingredients to see if added

Caffeine and Other Stimulants

Inquire about patients' use of caffeine, and remember that our society consumes it in many forms: coffee, tea, energy drinks, some soft drinks, and all chocolate, including many forms of commercially produced white chocolate (Table 9–4). It is also included in a few prescription analgesics (Fioricet, Norgesic) and some over-the-counter (OTC) medications (e.g., pain relievers such as BC Powder, Midol, Anacin, Goody's [Headache] Powder, and most forms of Excedrin; weight loss preparations such as Dexatrim; and cold remedies such as Dristan). Determine their use of other stimulants, such as prescription and OTC decongestants, particularly those containing pseudoephedrine. Again, elicit specific amounts of each source consumed and the frequency.

Decaffeinated products still contain caffeine: the average decaffeinated coffee contains about 10% of the original amount of caffeine, less in a decaffeinated darker roast, such as French or espresso, although individual servings might vary greatly (McCusker et al. 2006). *Herbal* tea has become a marketing term and does not necessarily denote the absence of caffeine;

look for *caffeine free* instead. Teas promising to help with sleep are often caffeine free. Determine whether soft drinks being consumed contain caffeine (e.g., Mountain Dew, Dr. Pepper, Coke Zero, Big Red, Sunkist Orange, A&W cream soda) or not (e.g., A&W and Mug root beers, ginger ale, Sprite, Fanta, Diet Rite Cola, Fresca, Sierra Mist) and explain that although decaffeinated products have the caffeine *partially* removed, caffeine-free products never contained it and would be a better choice. Not all root beers are caffeine free, and patients should check labels each time they consider consuming soft drinks, because companies do alter formulas. Note that so-called zero soft drinks are referring to calories, not caffeine, and that a single brand may have both caffeinated and caffeine-free products (e.g., A&W's cream soda and root beer).

Many people believe that green tea is low in caffeine when, in fact, it contains a substantial amount, similar to other teas and more than some soft drinks (Heckman et al. 2010). Patients seeking increased physical energy may be attracted to OTC preparations claiming to boost this, such as ginseng (see Chapter 8). Since the U.S. ban of ephedra in 2004, the strongest way for U.S. OTC products to offer stimulation is through caffeine, often poorly disguised in ingredients as "green tea extract." Energy drinks have become very popular with younger patients, but their effects on mental health and health in general are concerning (Sankararaman et al. 2018). Encourage patients to avoid this strong caffeine source.

Caffeine is widely distributed throughout the body and largely metabolized by cytochrome P450 1A2 (CYP1A2), although xanthine oxidase and N-acetyltransferase 2 also influence its rate of metabolism. The half-life of the parent compound ranges from 2 to 12 hours and that of its major psychoactive metabolites, paraxanthine and theobromine, from 2 to 12 and 8 to 12 hours, respectively. Levels of paraxanthine often rise 8–10 hours after ingestion (Cappelletti et al. 2015).

CYP1A2 also metabolizes many antidepressants, including duloxetine, imipramine, amitriptyline, and clomipramine, in addition to the atypical antipsychotics clozapine and olanzapine (Table 9–5; see also Table 6–1 in Chapter 6). Fluvoxamine is a strong inhibitor of this enzyme, as clinicians learned when it was released and marketed in the United States for OCD. Patients receiving this medication began to show increased anxiety not reported in clinical trials (where caffeine was limited); prescribers quickly associated the significant delay in caffeine metabolism with this side effect and learned to significantly restrict caffeine use in patients prescribed fluvoxamine. Fluvoxamine was increasing circulating caffeine by a factor of five, leading to caffeine intoxication (Jeppesen et al. 1996). Verapamil is also a strong inhibitor. This is only one example of the importance of con-

TABLE 9–5. Caffeine effects through CYP1A2

Caffeine increases levels of	Caffeine level is increased by
Asenapine	Fluvoxamine
Theophylline	Disulfiram
Riluzole	Ciprofloxacin
Clozapine	Verapamil
Acetaminophen	Estrogens

sidering caffeine use when planning and monitoring the use of many, particularly psychoactive, medications (Carrillo and Benitez 2000).

The use of legal stimulants will have implications not only for diagnosis but also for successful treatment outcomes. Serious concern has been raised about caffeine provoking anxiety (Bergin and Kendler 2012) and bipolar disorder symptoms (Baethge et al. 2009; Rizkallah et al. 2011); its total effect on mental and physical health should be considered for each patient (Temple et al. 2017). Similarly, the use of pseudoephedrine has been linked to the provocation of bipolar symptoms (Dalton 1990; Stuer and Claes 2007). Some pharmacological failures may, therefore, be attributed to the unfettered use of stimulants. Controlling and, often, eliminating their use is an important part of most treatment plans, particularly those targeting anxiety and unstable mood.

When helping patients cease caffeine use, remember that a significant withdrawal syndrome may develop that is uncomfortable and never clinically necessary (Silverman et al. 1992). Suggest that they cut their total caffeine use in half for 1 week before stopping it completely. This will usually allow a comfortable taper without withdrawal symptoms. Heaviest users may need to halve use twice, for 1 week each time (i.e., over 2 weeks). Discourage enthusiastic patients from stopping abruptly and predict for them the expected results (e.g., headaches, fatigue, anxiety, irritability, mood changes, tachycardia, tachypnea) so that these will not be confused with primary symptoms or medication side effects.

Patients often complain in advance that giving up caffeine will leave them devoid of the focus and energy they need to complete daily tasks. Educate them that tolerance develops to its effects on mental alertness, which are also offset by induced anxiety (Rogers et al. 2013); that daily administration of caffeine in well-conducted physiological studies has not demonstrated beneficial effects (Sigmon et al. 2009); and that only their subjective perceptions of fatigue may improve while taking it, because caffeine has no positive effect on power (Hahn et al. 2018). Demonstrate that clenched muscles will tire more easily and predict that after about 1 month off caffeine, when supervised physiological withdrawal is complete, they may be surprised to find more physical energy than they had while using it, probably largely due to enhanced sleep benefits and reduced anxiety and tension.

Patients may no doubt inquire about studies reported in the media promoting the use of caffeine for health. In addition to educating them on the scientific evaluation of data, including the sponsorship of such studies, inform them that early data have shown that some components of coffee (e.g., chlorogenic acid, quinic acid, caffeic acid, quercetin, and phenylindane) may inhibit amyloid-β or tau aggregation associated with dementia—phenylindane appearing to be the only potential dual inhibitor so far (Mancini et al. 2018). Further studies are needed to determine the veracity of this claim, but studies also clearly indicate that the potentially neuroprotective effects against dementia have not been found to be induced by caffeine itself (Trinh et al. 2010).

Nicotine

All health care practitioners are likely to be aware of the health risks of smoking and nicotine use, but clinical psychopharmacologists must also be aware of how these factors may alter symptoms and successful treatment. This is particularly important because the percentage of patients diagnosed with psychiatric disorders who smoke is twice that of the percentage of smokers in the U.S. general population: 41% compared with 20% (Lasser et al. 2000). A variety of new nicotine delivery methods were introduced in the 2010s, so practitioners must remain current on these and the data regarding their use.

Nicotine is metabolized by CYP1A2 and CYP2A6; the enzymatic induction produced through polycyclic aromatic hydrocarbons in smoke lowers the levels of antidepressants and antipsychotic medications also utilizing these enzymes. Changes in smoking, then, must be monitored in patients using these medications (Table 9–6) to follow rises and falls in serum levels (Desai et al. 2001; Hukkanen et al. 2011).

Evidence has linked nicotine use and dependence with ADHD, anxiety disorders, and depression. In many studies, nicotine appears to be associated with mild therapeutic effects on these disorders, and cessation of use, not withdrawal, is associated with a return of these same symptoms (Kutlu et al. 2015). Depression in major depression and mood instability in bipolar disorder might be provoked by nicotine reduction or cessation, again apart from nicotine withdrawal, although ultimately mood improvement might be seen (Glassman 1993; Thomson et al. 2015). For this reason, nicotine should usually be tapered cautiously and often slowly, over several

TABLE 9–6.   Smoking and psychiatric medications

Smoking lowers levels of

Caffeine	Olanzapine
Clomipramine	Ramelteon
Clozapine	Ropinirole
Duloxetine	Tacrine
Mirtazapine	Zolpidem

months, in these patients. In some cases, any reduction provokes symptoms so severe that the costs and benefits must be weighed, at least temporarily.

The very high percentage of patients with schizophrenia receiving major tranquilizers who also smoke (60%–80%) is well documented, and the amount they smoke is higher than that of average smokers in the population (Dickerson et al. 2013; Glassman 1993). Some of this may be attributable to underlying pathology (de Leon and Diaz 2005), but other authors have suggested it is linked to medication side effects. Lower levels of extrapyramidal symptoms and akathisia have been observed in treated patients who smoke, mediated through lower serum levels of antipsychotic medications from enzymatic induction; higher nicotine use is found in patients treated with first-generation antipsychotics than with atypical antipsychotics (Barnes et al. 2006; Winterer 2010). Schizophrenia has been linked to chromosomal abnormalities leading to deficient P50 gating, and increasing evidence shows that a least a subgroup of patients with schizophrenia experience neurocognitive deficits linked to associated nicotinic acetylcholinergic receptor dysregulation; these deficits improved with nicotinic agents in the short term, although long-term use remained deleterious (Depp et al. 2015; Mackowick et al. 2014; Pal and Balhara 2016).

Whether psychiatric patients' heavy nicotine use is mediated through common disease pathways, intuitive attempts at self-treatment, or social milieu, the overarching amount of data still support nicotine cessation as a primary public health goal for these patients. Some smokers tend to use electronic (e-)cigarettes to slowly taper their nicotine content, allowing them to eventually cease use altogether; some data support this plan (Bullen et al. 2013). Others, however, continue with regular use. In fact, many nicotine users continue to use both traditional cigarettes and "vape" with e-cigarettes; the Centers for Disease Control and Prevention (2020) recently alerted that in the United States, youths are vaping to an alarming degree without the intention of reducing nicotine intake. Patients should be made aware that e-cigarettes may not be safer than traditional cigarettes and at time of this writing have been banned in at least 10 U.S. states until the FDA can provide further answers about the safely and regulation of these devices. They still contain toxins, are not proven cessation devices, and in the United States have been recently linked with more than 2,700 cases of hospitalization for e-cigarette, or vaping, product use–associated lung injury and 64 deaths (Centers for Disease Control and Prevention 2020; Grana et al. 2014).

Particularly dangerous in vaping fluids are flavorings (including benzaldehyde and vanillin) that are either aldehydes or decompose into them and represent a toxicity risk when inhaled, although they are safe when taken orally (Behar et al. 2014, 2016; Khlystov and Samburova 2016; Kosmider et al. 2016; Tierney et al. 2015). Patients should be informed of these risks and advised to refrain from e-cigarettes until more is known about their effect on lung function and health in general. Those patients over age 21 who choose to continue vaping should be strongly warned to completely avoid aldehyde-related flavorings. They should also discuss this toxicity issue with the vendor of their product and change sources if ingredient information is not readily available for them.

Other treatments for nicotine cessation may present their own psychopharmacological challenges (Aubin et al. 2012). Bupropion (see Chapter 7) is well documented as an aid in smoking cessation, but although it might be a useful tool, it is also an antidepressant and should not be used when that class of medication might worsen symptoms, such as in bipolar disorder or, in some cases, combined with other antidepressants (Giasson-Gariépy and Jutras-Aswad 2013). Not surprisingly, response is dose dependent; 300 mg/day is more effective than 150 mg/day, but the lower dose does offer some benefit (Hurt et al. 1997).

Varenicline has adequate data supporting its use in nicotine cessation, but given early reports of it worsening mental health symptoms in psychiatric patients (Freedman 2007; Kohen and Kremen 2007; Popkin 2008), governmental warnings have been issued in the United States and United Kingdom. Subsequent studies of varying quality have since been performed and found little concern, along with good evidence of efficacy. The most thorough meta-analysis of these studies to date found no increase in suicide, suicidality, or depression with its use but did find evidence for an increase in insomnia and abnormal dreams (Thomas et al. 2015). Full consideration and discussion with patients and their families, along with careful monitoring, appear wise if varenicline is their first choice.

Nicotine taper using a transdermal nicotine patch appears relatively safe, well tolerated, and potentially effective with motivated patients (Greenland et al. 1998). Early reports of sudden death from combining the use of patches with smoking led to concerns, although subsequent studies have shown that use as recommended—while not smoking—represents no additional cardiovascular risk (Benowitz et al. 2018; Kimmel et al. 2001). The half-life of nicotine is 2 hours. To maximize safety, suggest that patients wait 2 hours after using nicotine before putting on the patch and a similar 2 hours to use any nicotine after removing it. Remind them that the goal is to use the transdermal patch for 24 hours, in place of any other nicotine. The patch is available in 21-mg, 14-mg, and 7-mg strengths. Trials of higher-dose patches for patients who smoke more than 20 cigarettes per day have yet to demonstrate safety or greater efficacy, although this finding is largely due to inadequate study design (Brokowski et al. 2014).

Suggest that patients use the appropriate starting strength for their daily use: 21 mg for 20 or more cigarettes per day, 14 mg for 10–19 cigarettes, and 7 mg for fewer than 10 cigarettes. They should use that strength daily for 28–42 days, then step down to the next lower strength for 28–42 days, with the final strength being used for 14–42 days. Again, with bipolar disorder and other mood disorders, a much slower taper may be preferable. Moving the patch to different locations each day may reduce skin irritation.

Efficacy has been found for each form of nicotine replacement (e.g., gum, nasal spray, lozenges [Wadgave and Nagesh 2016]), but the clear endpoint with patch use often produces effective results for motivated patients. A handful of studies have investigated combining patches with these supplemental shorter-term deliveries of nicotine and found it to be helpful and safe (Shah et al. 2008); however, consider the total amount of nicotine patients are consuming and their individual medical status. Prescriptions of varenicline or bupropion with a nicotine patch would not present this same risk.

Summary

The best psychopharmacological interventions may not be effective when up against inadequate sleep, abnormal weight, or alcohol, stimulant, nicotine, and drug use. Clarifying these factors before initiating pharmacotherapy not only will lead to safer interventions but also will improve the overall health of patients and empower them to take greater responsibly for their health over the long term.

Target 8–8.5 hours of sleep during the dark hours as the goal for patients, and educate them on adequate sleep hygiene. Healthy exercise may complement, rather than replace, treatment, but only if an adequate progressive training period is allowed. Use dietary calculators to teach patients how to alter their weight with rational dietary planning, equating 1 lb with 3,500 kcal and targeting a BMI of 18.5–24.9, with the exceptions noted earlier. Ideally, patients will not consume alcohol while receiving psychopharmacological treatment, and initial diagnosis, especially for mood disorders, must occur only after at least 14 days of abstinence. Cannabis may interfere with symptoms and treatments and should be ceased, allowing for a very long elimination period. Treatment for substance use and abuse disorders must allow for safe taper or detoxification, as indicated. It is rational to safely eliminate use of a substance, when possible, before confirming other diagnoses or initiating treatment for them.

Identify all stimulants, legal and illegal, patients are using, because these may negatively impact symptoms and treatment and may be included in other prescribed or OTC medical treatments. Assess patients' caffeine use and educate them as to common sources of caffeine in their diet. With certain diagnoses and treatments, caffeine may interfere with outcome and tolerability, and it almost always has some impact on sleep. Decaffeinated products still contain some caffeine; caffeine-free products do not. Psychiatric patients are twice as likely to smoke nicotine as the general population, with ultimately adverse consequences. Vaping has not been adequately evaluated for safety, and flavorings with benzaldehyde and vanillin are toxic when inhaled. Nicotine patches, in particular, may represent a useful method for assisting nicotine withdrawal and discontinuation when used safely.

Addressing these matters will increase the chances that any successful pharmacological treatment may provide sustained results. Working with patients to establish a healthy therapeutic alliance that encourages and supports these lifestyle changes is the job of the rational psychopharmacologist.

Key Points

- Good sleep hygiene should always be prescribed.
- Gradually progressive exercise may support, but not replace, indicated psychopharmacological treatment.
- Teach patients simple calculations to manage their weight.
- Unfettered use of stimulants, both prescribed and over-the-counter, may lead to treatment failure.
- Use of alcohol and recreational drugs may compromise diagnosis and treatment success.
- In whatever way nicotine may influence symptoms and side effects, in the long term, patients are better off not using it in any form.

Self-Assessment

1. Which of the following statements is true?

   A. Shift work has no impact on mental and physical health.
   B. Patients may easily catch up on missed sleep by sleeping longer on days off.
   C. Warmer rooms are better for sleep.
   D. Daytime napping can assist in healthy sleep hygiene.

2. Exercise

   A. Should be avoided 3 hours prior to bedtime
   B. May provoke anxiety symptoms in cases of inadequate training or acclimatization
   C. Benefits for major depression may have a genetic basis for some patients
   D. All of the above

3. Body mass index (choose all that apply)

   A. May overestimate body fat in extreme athletes, pregnant women, and bodybuilders
   B. Is valid in patients with eating disorders
   C. May underestimate body fat in geriatric patients
   D. Is valid, uncorrected, for children and adolescents

4. Which of the following is true? (Choose all that apply)

   A. One standard mixed drink, one beer, and one 8-oz glass of wine all contain about 1 oz of alcohol.
   B. Claims of cannabis' benefits in psychiatric, developmental, and neurodegenerative disorders are poorly substantiated.
   C. Cannabis is stored in body fat cells and released after about 12 months.
   D. The half-life of MDMA is 4 hours.

5. Caffeine (choose all that apply)

   A. Serum levels are elevated by the use of fluvoxamine and verapamil
   B. Is low in green and herbal teas

    C. May provoke anxiety and bipolar disorder symptoms

    D. Is the central factor from coffee in the inhibition of amyloid-β or tau aggregation associated with dementia

6. Which of following are reasonable pharmacological options for nicotine addiction treatment? (Choose all that apply)

    A. Nicotine taper using transdermal nicotine patches, as long as patients do not smoke while using them

    B. Nicotine transdermal patches with varenicline or bupropion

    C. Varenicline alone

    D. Bupropion alone

Discussion Topics

1. A patient comes to you complaining of severe social anxiety that he has been managing with alcohol and cannabis in order to socialize at all with others. What steps would you take to confirm his diagnosis and evaluate the possibility of substance abuse disorders? Develop treatment plans that could transition him from these agents to safer and effective medications to control his symptoms. How would you handle removing the use of alcohol and cannabis?

2. A patient in your practice is highly motivated to take responsibility for her own health while you treat her for bipolar disorder. In addition to taking your medication, she goes to bed by midnight but awakens each morning at 6 A.M. so she can run 3 miles. She has cut back, but not eliminated, caffeine and uses herbal supplements containing ginseng, firmly believing in their health-promoting qualities. Although she has not had a manic or severe depressive episode in 24 months, she does exhibit mild periods of depression and hypomania that you have been unable to fully control with various pharmacological interventions. Given your knowledge of medicine and psychopharmacology, discuss what lifestyle recommendations you would make. How would you utilize your therapeutic alliance to achieve further progress in her symptom control?

Additional Reading

Johnson PL, Federici LM, Shekhar A: Etiology, triggers and neurochemical circuits associated with unexpected, expected, and laboratory-induced panic attacks. Neurosci Biobehav Rev 46(Pt 3):429–454, 2014

Riske L, Thomas RK, Baker GB, et al: Lactate in the brain: an update on its relevance to brain energy, neurons, glia and panic disorder. Ther Adv Psychopharmacol 7(2):85–89, 2017

Sarris J, Moylan S, Camfield DA, et al: Complementary medicine, exercise, meditation, diet, and lifestyle modification for anxiety disorders: a review of current evidence. Evid Based Complement Alternat Med 2012(809653), 2012

Sharma P, Murthy P, Bharath MMS: Chemistry, metabolism, and toxicology of cannabis: clinical implications. Iran J Psychiatry 7(4):149–156, 2012

U.S. Department of Health and Human Services: Managing overweight and obesity in adults: systematic evidence review from the obesity expert panel. November 2013. Available at: https://www.nhlbi.nih.gov/health-topics/managing-overweight-obesity-in-adults. Accessed October 3, 2019.

Webb D: Farewell to the 3,500-calorie rule. Today's Dietitian 26(11):36, 2014

Suggested Reading for Patients

Walker M: Why We Sleep: Unlocking the Power of Sleep and Dreams. New York, Scribner, 2017

Wansink B: Mindless Eating: Why We Eat More Than We Think. New York, Bantam, 2006

References

Abramowitz MK, Hall CB, Amodu A, et al: Muscle mass, BMI, and mortality among adults in the United States: a population-based cohort study. PLoS One 13(4):e0194697, 2018 29641540

Allan GM, Finley CR, Ton J, et al: Pain, nausea and vomiting, spasticity, and harms. Can Fam Physician 64(2):e78–e94, 2018 29449262

Aubin H-J, Rollema H, Svensson TH, et al: Smoking, quitting, and psychiatric disease: a review. Neurosci Biobehav Rev 36(1):271–284, 2012 21723317

Baethge C, Tondo L, Lepri B, et al: Coffee and cigarette use: association with suicidal acts in 352 Sardinian bipolar disorder patients. Bipolar Disord 11(5):494–503, 2009 19624388

Barnes M, Lawford BR, Burton SC, et al: Smoking and schizophrenia: is symptom profile related to smoking and which antipsychotic medication is of benefit in reducing cigarette use? Aust N Z J Psychiatry 40(6–7):575–580, 2006 16756583

Bedrosian TA, Fonken LK, Nelson RJ: Endocrine effects of circadian disruption. Annu Rev Physiol 78:109–131, 2016 26208951

Behar RZ, Davis B, Wang Y, et al: Identification of toxicants in cinnamon-flavored electronic cigarette refill fluids. Toxicol In Vitro 28(2):198–208, 2014 24516877

Behar RZ, Luo W, Lin SC, et al: Distribution, quantification and toxicity of cinnamaldehyde in electronic cigarette refill fluids and aerosols. Tob Control 25(suppl 2):ii94–ii102, 2016 27633763

Benowitz NL, Pipe A, West R, et al: Cardiovascular safety of varenicline, bupropion, and nicotine patch in smokers: a randomized clinical trial. JAMA Intern Med 178(5):622–631, 2018 29630702

Bergin JE, Kendler KS: Common psychiatric disorders and caffeine use, tolerance, and withdrawal: an examination of shared genetic and environmental effects. Twin Res Hum Genet 15(4):473–482, 2012 22854069

Blumenthal JA, Babyak MA, Doraiswamy PM, et al: Exercise and pharmacotherapy in the treatment of major depressive disorder. Psychosom Med 69(7):587–596, 2007 17846259

Brokowski L, Chen J, Tanner S: High-dose transdermal nicotine replacement for tobacco cessation. Am J Health Syst Pharm 71(8):634–638, 2014 24688036

Brooks GA: Cell-cell and intracellular lactate shuttles. J Physiol 587(pt 23):5591–5600, 2009 19805739

Brooks GA, Butterfield GE, Wolfe RR, et al: Decreased reliance on lactate during exercise after acclimatization to 4,300 m. J Appl Physiol (1985) 71(1):333–341, 1991 1917759

Bullen C, Howe C, Laugesen M, et al: Electronic cigarettes for smoking cessation: a randomised controlled trial. Lancet 382(9905):1629–1637, 2013 24029165

Cappelletti S, Piacentino D, Sani G, et al: Caffeine: cognitive and physical performance enhancer or psychoactive drug? Curr Neuropharmacol 13(1):71–88, 2015 26074744

Carrillo JA, Benitez J: Clinically significant pharmacokinetic interactions between dietary caffeine and medications. Clin Pharmacokinet 39(2):127–153, 2000 10976659

Centers for Disease Control and Prevention: Data table of BMI-for-age charts. August 23, 2001. Available at: https://www.cdc.gov/growthcharts/html_charts/bmiagerev.htm#males. Accessed October 3, 2019.

Centers for Disease Control and Prevention: Outbreak of lung injury associated with the use of e-cigarette, or vaping, products. Atlanta, GA, Centers for Disease Control and Prevention, 2020. Available at: https://www.cdc.gov/tobacco/basic_information/e-cigarettes/severe-lung-disease.html. Accessed February 15, 2020.

Chow CC, Hall KD: Short and long-term energy intake patterns and their implications for human body weight regulation. Physiol Behav 134:60–65, 2014 24582679

Cowley DS, Arana GW: The diagnostic utility of lactate sensitivity in panic disorder. Arch Gen Psychiatry 47(3):277–284, 1990 2407210

Dalton R: Mixed bipolar disorder precipitated by pseudoephedrine hydrochloride. South Med J 83(1):64–65, 1990 2300837

de Leon J, Diaz FJ: A meta-analysis of worldwide studies demonstrates an association between schizophrenia and tobacco smoking behaviors. Schizophr Res 76(2–3):135–157, 2005 15949648

De Moor MHM, Boomsma DI, Stubbe JH, et al: Testing causality in the association between regular exercise and symptoms of anxiety and depression. Arch Gen Psychiatry 65(8):897–905, 2008 18678794

Dennis CL, Ross L: Relationships among infant sleep patterns, maternal fatigue, and development of depressive symptomatology. Birth 32(3):187–193, 2005 16128972

Depp CA, Bowie CR, Mausbach BT, et al: Current smoking is associated with worse cognitive and adaptive functioning in serious mental illness. Acta Psychiatr Scand 131(5):333–341, 2015 25559296

Desai HD, Seabolt J, Jann MW: Smoking in patients receiving psychotropic medications: a pharmacokinetic perspective. CNS Drugs 15(6):469–494, 2001 11524025

Dickerson F, Stallings CR, Origoni AE, et al: Cigarette smoking among persons with schizophrenia or bipolar disorder in routine clinical settings, 1999–2011. Psychiatr Serv 64(1):44–50, 2013 23280457

Ehlers A, Breuer P: How good are patients with panic disorder at perceiving their heartbeats? Biol Psychol 42(1–2):165–182, 1996 8770377

Esquivel G, Schruers KR, Maddock RJ, et al: Acids in the brain: a factor in panic? J Psychopharmacol 24(5):639–647, 2010 19460873

Flegal KM, Graubard BI: Estimates of excess deaths associated with body mass index and other anthropometric variables. Am J Clin Nutr 89(4):1213–1219, 2009 19190072

Freedman R: Exacerbation of schizophrenia by varenicline. Am J Psychiatry 164(8):1269, 2007 17671295

Giasson-Gariépy K, Jutras-Aswad D: A case of hypomania during nicotine cessation treatment with bupropion. Addict Sci Clin Pract 8(1):22, 2013 24359680

Glassman AH: Cigarette smoking: implications for psychiatric illness. Am J Psychiatry 150(4):546–553, 1993 8465868

Grana R, Benowitz N, Glantz SA: E-cigarettes: a scientific review. Circulation 129(19):1972–1986, 2014 24821826

Greenland S, Satterfield MH, Lanes SF: A meta-analysis to assess the incidence of adverse effects associated with the transdermal nicotine patch. Drug Saf 18(4):297–308, 1998 9565740

Guth E: JAMA patient page. Healthy weight loss. JAMA 312(9):974, 2014 25182116

Guttmannova K, Kosterman R, White HR, et al: The association between regular marijuana use and adult mental health outcomes. Drug Alcohol Depend 179:109–116, 2017 28763778

Hadland SE, Knight JR, Harris SK: Medical marijuana: review of the science and implications for developmental-behavioral pediatric practice. J Dev Behav Pediatr 36(2):115–123, 2015 25650954

Hahn CJ, Jagim AR, Camic CL, et al: Acute effects of a caffeine-containing supplement on anaerobic power and subjective measurements of fatigue in recreationally active men. J Strength Cond Res 32(4):1029–1035, 2018 29337831

Hall KD: What is the required energy deficit per unit weight loss? Int J Obes 32(3):573–576, 2008 17848938

Hall KD, Sacks G, Chandramohan D, et al: Quantification of the effect of energy imbalance on bodyweight. Lancet 378(9793):826–837, 2011 21872751

Hall W, Degenhardt L: The adverse health effects of chronic cannabis use. Drug Test Anal 6(1–2):39–45, 2014 23836598

Harding EC, Franks NP, Wisden W: The temperature dependence of sleep. Front Neurosci 13:336, 2019 31105512

Haug NA, Padula CB, Sottile JE, et al: Cannabis use patterns and motives: a comparison of younger, middle-aged, and older medical cannabis dispensary patients. Addict Behav 72:14–20, 2017 28340421

He Y, Jones CR, Fujiki N, et al: The transcriptional repressor DEC2 regulates sleep length in mammals. Science 325(5942):866–870, 2009 19679812

Heckman MA, Weil J, Gonzalez de Mejia E: Caffeine (1,3,7-trimethylxanthine) in foods: a comprehensive review on consumption, functionality, safety, and regulatory matters. J Food Sci 75(3):R77–R87, 2010 20492310

Hirshkowitz M, Whiton K, Albert SM, et al: National Sleep Foundation's updated sleep duration recommendations: final report. Sleep Health 1(4):233–243, 2015 29073398

Hoffmann DE, Weber E: Medical marijuana and the law. N Engl J Med 362(16):1453–1457, 2010 20410512

Hukkanen J, Jacob P 3rd, Peng M, et al: Effect of nicotine on cytochrome P450 1A2 activity. Br J Clin Pharmacol 72(5):836–838, 2011 21599724

Hurt RD, Sachs DPL, Glover ED, et al: A comparison of sustained-release bupropion and placebo for smoking cessation. N Engl J Med 337(17):1195–1202, 1997 9337378

Ieraci A, Madaio AI, Mallei A, et al: Brain-derived neurotrophic factor Val66Met human polymorphism impairs the beneficial exercise-induced neurobiological changes in mice. Neuropsychopharmacology 41(13):3070–3079, 2016 27388329

Jeppesen U, Loft S, Poulsen HE, et al: A fluvoxamine-caffeine interaction study. Pharmacogenetics 6(3):213–222, 1996 8807660

Johnson PL, Truitt WA, Fitz SD, et al: Neural pathways underlying lactate-induced panic. Neuropsychopharmacology 33(9):2093–2107, 2008 18059441

Khlystov A, Samburova V: Flavoring compounds dominate toxic aldehyde production during e-cigarette vaping. Environ Sci Technol 50(23):13080–13085, 2016 27934275

Kimmel SE, Berlin JA, Miles C, et al: Risk of acute first myocardial infarction and use of nicotine patches in a general population. J Am Coll Cardiol 37(5):1297–1302, 2001 11300438

Kohen I, Kremen N: Varenicline-induced manic episode in a patient with bipolar disorder. Am J Psychiatry 164(8):1269–1270, 2007 17671294

Kosmider L, Sobczak A, Prokopowicz A, et al: Cherry-flavoured electronic cigarettes expose users to the inhalation irritant, benzaldehyde. Thorax 71(4):376–377, 2016 26822067

Krawczak EM, Minuzzi L, Simpson W, et al: Sleep, daily activity rhythms and postpartum mood: a longitudinal study across the perinatal period. Chronobiol Int 33(7):791–801, 2016 27097327

Kutlu MG, Parikh V, Gould TJ: Nicotine addiction and psychiatric disorders. Int Rev Neurobiol 124:171–208, 2015 26472530

Landolt H-P, Werth E, Borbély AA, et al: Caffeine intake (200 mg) in the morning affects human sleep and EEG power spectra at night. Brain Res 675(1–2):67–74, 1995 7796154

Lasser K, Boyd JW, Woolhandler S, et al: Smoking and mental illness: a population-based prevalence study. JAMA 284(20):2606–2610, 2000 11086367

Lattari E, Budde H, Paes F, et al: Effects of aerobic exercise on anxiety symptoms and cortical activity in patients with panic disorder: a pilot study. Clin Pract Epidemiol Ment Health 14:11–25, 2018 29515644

Lim K, See YM, Lee J: A systematic review of the effectiveness of medical cannabis for psychiatric, movement and neurodegenerative disorders. Clin Psychopharmacol Neurosci 15(4):301–312, 2017 29073741

Lo JC, Groeger JA, Santhi N, et al: Effects of partial and acute total sleep deprivation on performance across cognitive domains, individuals and circadian phase. PLoS One 7(9):e45987, 2012 23029352

Lum LC: Hyperventilation and anxiety state. J R Soc Med 74(1):1–4, 1981 6780688

Mackowick KM, Barr MS, Wing VC, et al: Neurocognitive endophenotypes in schizophrenia: modulation by nicotinic receptor systems. Prog Neuropsychopharmacol Biol Psychiatry 52:79–85, 2014 23871750

Maddock RJ, Buonocore MH, Miller AR, et al: Abnormal activity-dependent brain lactate and glutamate + glutamine responses in panic disorder. Biol Psychiatry 73(11):1111–1119, 2013 23332354

Mancini RS, Wang Y, Weaver DF: Phenylindanes in brewed coffee inhibit amyloid-beta and tau aggregation. Front Neurosci 12:735, 2018 30369868

Manfredini R, Fabbian F, De Giorgi A, et al: Daylight saving time and myocardial infarction: should we be worried? A review of the evidence. Eur Rev Med Pharmacol Sci 22(3):750–755, 2018 29461606

Mata J, Thompson RJ, Gotlib IH: BDNF genotype moderates the relation between physical activity and depressive symptoms. Health Psychol 29(2):130–133, 2010 20230085

Mazzotti DR, Guindalini C, Moraes WA, et al: Human longevity is associated with regular sleep patterns, maintenance of slow wave sleep, and favorable lipid profile. Front Aging Neurosci 6:134, 2014 25009494

McCusker RR, Fuehrlein B, Goldberger BA, et al: Caffeine content of decaffeinated coffee. J Anal Toxicol 30(8):611–613, 2006 17132260

Murphy PJ, Campbell SS: Nighttime drop in body temperature: a physiological trigger for sleep onset? Sleep 20(7):505–511, 1997 9322266

O'Connor PJ, Smith JC, Morgan WP: Physical activity does not provoke panic attacks in patients with panic disorder: a review of the evidence. Anxiety Stress Coping 13(4):333–353, 2000

Pal A, Balhara YP: A review of impact of tobacco use on patients with co-occurring psychiatric disorders. Tob Use Insights 9:7–12, 2016 26997871

Papaseit E, Pérez-Mañá C, Pérez-Acevedo AP, et al: Cannabinoids: from pot to lab. Int J Med Sci 15(12):1286–1295, 2018 30275754

Park EM, Meltzer-Brody S, Stickgold R: Poor sleep maintenance and subjective sleep quality are associated with postpartum maternal depression symptom severity. Arch Women Ment Health 16(6):539–547, 2013 23733081

Phillips C: Brain-derived neurotrophic factor, depression, and physical activity: making the neuroplastic connection. Neural Plast 2017:7260130, 2017 28928987

Popkin MK: Exacerbation of recurrent depression as a result of treatment with varenicline. Am J Psychiatry 165(6):774, 2008 18519539

Prentice AM, Jebb SA: Beyond body mass index. Obes Rev 2(3):141–147, 2001 12120099

Rahman SA, St Hilaire MA, Lockley SW: The effects of spectral tuning of evening ambient light on melatonin suppression, alertness and sleep. Physiol Behav 177:221–229, 2017 28472667

Rizkallah E, Bélanger M, Stavro K, et al: Could the use of energy drinks induce manic or depressive relapse among abstinent substance use disorder patients with comorbid bipolar spectrum disorder? Bipolar Disord 13(5–6):578–580, 2011 22017226

Robb D, Barnes T: Accident rates and the impact of daylight saving time transitions. Accid Anal Prev 111:193–201, 2018 29223028

Rogers PJ, Heatherley SV, Mullings EL, et al: Faster but not smarter: effects of caffeine and caffeine withdrawal on alertness and performance. Psychopharmacology (Berl) 226(2):229–240, 2013 23108937

Sankararaman S, Syed W, Medici V, et al: Impact of energy drinks on health and well-being. Curr Nutr Rep 7(3):121–130, 2018 29982915

Schuch FB, Deslandes AC, Stubbs B, et al: Neurobiological effects of exercise on major depressive disorder: a systematic review. Neurosci Biobehav Rev 61:1–11, 2016 26657969

Shah SD, Wilken LA, Winkler SR, et al: Systematic review and meta-analysis of combination therapy for smoking cessation. J Am Pharm Assoc (2003) 48(5):659–665, 2008 18826906

Sharma V, Doobay M, Baczynski C: Bipolar postpartum depression: an update and recommendations. J Affect Disord 219:105–111, 2017 28535448

Sigmon SC, Herning RI, Better W, et al: Caffeine withdrawal, acute effects, tolerance, and absence of net beneficial effects of chronic administration: cerebral blood flow velocity, quantitative EEG, and subjective effects. Psychopharmacology (Berl) 204(4):573–585, 2009 19241060

Silverman K, Evans SM, Strain EC, et al: Withdrawal syndrome after the double-blind cessation of caffeine consumption. N Engl J Med 327(16):1109–1114, 1992 1528206

Sipilä JOT, Ruuskanen JO, Rautava P, et al: Changes in ischemic stroke occurrence following daylight saving time transitions. Sleep Med 27–28:20–24, 2016 27938913

Stryjewski PJ, Kuczaj A, Domal-Kwiatkowska D, et al: Night work and shift work: effects on the health of workers. Przegl Lek 73(7):513–515, 2016 29677423

Stuer K, Claes S: Mania following the use of a decongestant [in Dutch]. Tijdschr Psychiatr 49(2):125–129, 2007 17290343

Temple JL, Bernard C, Lipshultz SE, et al: The safety of ingested caffeine: a comprehensive review. Front Psychiatry 8:80, 2017 28603504

Thomas KH, Martin RM, Knipe DW, et al: Risk of neuropsychiatric adverse events associated with varenicline: systematic review and meta-analysis. BMJ 350:h1109, 2015 25767129

Thomson D, Berk M, Dodd S, et al: Tobacco use in bipolar disorder. Clin Psychopharmacol Neurosci 13(1):1–11, 2015 25912533

Tierney PA, Karpinski CD, Brown JE, et al: Flavour chemicals in electronic cigarette fluids. Tob Control 25(e1):e10–e15, 2016 25877377

Trinh K, Andrews L, Krause J, et al: Decaffeinated coffee and nicotine-free tobacco provide neuroprotection in Drosophila models of Parkinson's disease through an NRF2-dependent mechanism. J Neurosci 30(16):5525–5532, 2010 20410106

U.S. Department of Health and Human Services: Calculate your body mass index. Washington, DC, U.S. Department of Health and Human Services, 2019a. Available at: https://www.nhlbi.nih.gov/health/educational/lose_wt/BMI/bmicalc.htm. Accessed October 3, 2019.

U.S. Department of Health and Human Services: Research behind the body weight planner. Washington, DC, U.S. Department of Health and Human Services, 2019b. Available at: https://www.niddk.nih.gov/research-funding/at-niddk/labs-branches/LBM/integrative-physiology-section/research-behind-body-weight-planner/Pages/default.aspx. Accessed October 3, 2019.

Volkow ND, Swanson JM, Evins AE, et al: Effects of cannabis use on human behavior, including cognition, motivation, and psychosis: a review. JAMA Psychiatry 73(3):292–297, 2016 26842658

Wadgave U, Nagesh L: Nicotine replacement therapy: an overview. Int J Health Sci (Qassim) 10(3):425–435, 2016 27610066

Wansink B: Mindless Eating: Why We Eat More Than We Think. New York, Bantam, 2006

Weinstein A, Livny A, Weizman A: Brain imaging studies on the cognitive, pharmacological and neurobiological effects of cannabis in humans: evidence from studies of adult users. Curr Pharm Des 22(42):6366–6379, 2016 27549374

West KE, Jablonski MR, Warfield B, et al: Blue light from light-emitting diodes elicits a dose-dependent suppression of melatonin in humans. J Appl Physiol (1985) 110(3)619–626, 2011 21164152

Wilkinson RT, Stretton M: Performance after awakening at different times of night. Psychonomic Science 23(4):283–285, 1971

Wilkinson ST: Medical and recreational marijuana: commentary and review of the literature. Mo Med 110(6):524–528, 2013 24564006

Winterer G: Why do patients with schizophrenia smoke? Curr Opin Psychiatry 23(2):112–119, 2010 20051860

Wishnofsky M: Caloric equivalents of gained or lost weight. Am J Clin Nutr 6(5):542–546, 1958 13594881

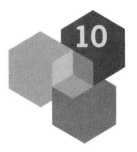

Nonpharmacological Somatic Treatments in Current Use

Although this book concerns pharmacotherapy, knowledge of competing or supplemental somatic treatments available to patients will assist you in treatment planning. This chapter reviews five somatic treatments, chosen for their demonstrated utility, popular use, or promise. As with medications, their use must be guided by outcomes of randomized controlled trials (RCTs) rather than theory.

Convulsive Therapies

Today, we consider electroconvulsive therapy (ECT) to be the only convulsive option, yet the history of convulsive therapies precedes the use of electricity. In the early twentieth century, an erroneous observation was made that patients with epilepsy were less likely to have schizophrenia (another example of the difficulty of realizing evidence-based medicine). Theorizing that seizures protected these patients from psychosis, clinicians began inducing seizures in schizophrenic patients, most commonly with chemicals such as camphor and pentylenetetrazol (Cooper and Fink 2014). In 1938, electricity was demonstrated to provide an easier route to seizure induction (Faedda et al. 2010). This practice caught on, but hypoglycemic convulsions induced by insulin were also commonly used until the 1960s (Brannon and Graham 1955). Some clinicians anecdotally insisted this "insulin shock" conferred greater efficacy than ECT, although the seizure, not its cause, is thought to be the source of the benefit (Fink 2014a). Eventually, practical factors led to ECT replacing insulin and other chemically induced convulsions (Van Mensvoort et al. 2012).

Not only did the form of convulsive treatment change but also the indication for it. Physicians quickly realized that schizophrenia, as it was then defined, did not usually respond to this treatment as well as melancholia (depression). This awareness developed decades before any pharmacological treatments for mood disorders had been discovered. Convulsive therapies, eventually as ECT, became the gold standard for treating mood disorders, including depression (unipolar and bipolar), mania, and mixed bipolar states (Kellner et al. 2015; UK ECT Review Group 2003). Recent data also have suggested that ECT may potentiate pharmacotherapy in treatment-resistant psychosis, after all (Sanghani et al. 2018).

The middle and late twentieth century saw stepwise improvements in administering and utilizing ECT, such as inducing brief paralysis to prevent broken limbs from violent motor convulsions, previously a common side effect; brief sedation to prevent the emotional distress from the paralysis; pretreatment with atropine to reduce cardiovascular events during treatment; unilateral versus bilateral electrode placement, reflecting better tolerability versus greater efficacy; electroencephalographic monitoring to confirm and quantify seizure activity in a paralyzed patient; and brief-pulse wave technology, which has largely replaced sine-wave constant voltage and constant energy devices, decreasing the cognitive side effects of ECT (Gálvez et al. 2017; Leiknes et al. 2012; Squire and Zouzounis 1986). Oddly, evidence-based recommendations for dosing ECT, particularly the length of treatment, were not developed until the latter part of the twentieth century.

Like antidepressants before arrival of selective serotonin reuptake inhibitors (see Chapter 7, "Medications to Treat Major Depression"), ECT was used acutely, discontinued, and then restarted following recurrence of mood symptoms (which were usually recurrent or cyclical). Research beginning in the 1990s revealed that the condition was more likely to recur when the treatment was not continued, which led to improved protocols (Bourgon and Kellner 2000). ECT treatment was then divided into acute, continuation, and maintenance phases. Originally, "continuation" meant the first few months after acute treatment, and "maintenance" referred to periods longer than that. The distinction remained arbitrary, so most contemporary authors use continuation ECT (C-ECT) to mean all treatment after acute. Once C-ECT was shown to be helpful, clinicians responded by adopting a clinically based strategy: 5–10 acute treatments were given over 2–3 weeks, and the interval between treatments was slowly increased until symptoms recurred. The longest interval that still prevented a recurrence became that patient's dose, whether it was once a week, biweekly, monthly, quarterly, and so on. C-ECT is much more successful than the previous approach, yet additional symptom-based adjustments to this fixed schedule, such as the Symptom-Titrated, Algorithm-Based Longitudinal ECT (STABLE) strategy, are leading to further progress (Fink 2014b; Gagné et al. 2000; Kellner et al. 2006, 2015; Lisanby et al. 2008; Petrides et al. 1994).

Many patients receiving ECT are referred because of failed responses to medication. The bulk of the literature has recommended continuing these failed medications during and following ECT, although the rationale for this practice may not be fully satisfied (Sackeim et al. 1990). The prophylactic use of medication alone, following ECT, appears equally effective to that of C-ECT alone but is more effective when the two treatments are combined (Gagné et al. 2000; Jelovac et al. 2013; Kellner et al. 2016). Concerns have been raised about the toxicity of combining ECT with medications such as lithium and monoamine oxidase inhibitors (MAOIs). Stimulants may prolong seizures and elevate cardiovascular risk, whereas anticonvulsants may inhibit the very seizures considered therapeutic (Naguib and Koorn 2002).

ECT has never relinquished its role as the fastest, cheapest, and safest treatment for affective disorders, but many patients and families find the idea distasteful, and some, abhorrent. This may be due to films such as 1975's *One Flew Over the Cuckoo's Nest* (winner of the 1976 Academy Award for Best Picture), which, among other things, confuses the effects of ECT (depicted inaccurately) with those of psychosurgery (McDonald and Walter 2009; Sienaert 2016). The "shock treatment/shock therapy" parlance in popular culture is stigmatizing; the persistence of the unsubstantiated belief that the short-term delirium and amnesia resulting from treatment leads to long-term memory impairment also discourages patients (Brus et al. 2017; Semkovska and McLoughlin 2010).

Therefore, although patterns differ around the world, referral for ECT is often limited to the urgent need for a quick response, such as with catatonia, treatment-resistant mania, and depression when the patient is refusing fluids and food. ECT may also be discussed as an option when two or more trials of medication have failed (Leiknes et al. 2012). In many communities, a small number of psychiatrists will provide ECT for the rest of the psychiatric community, keeping up their skills and maintaining a treatment team and facility current on standards.

Transcranial Magnetic Stimulation

Despite its efficacy, the awkwardness of administering ECT led to a search for alternative somatic treatments that would be equally effective and safe yet easier to employ. Transcranial magnetic stimulation (TMS) was developed in the 1980s (Barker et al. 1985). It consists of using a magnetic field to influence discrete neural circuits in the cerebral cortex. Whereas single stimulations may help localize brain function and connectivity as a research tool, repetitive stimulations are given for clinical purposes.

Unlike ECT, no hospitalization or medication is necessary with TMS. Treatment can be given in an office once the expensive machine is leased or purchased. Treatments are usually given 5 days a week for 3–6 weeks. Like ECT, the indication is most often a failure to achieve adequate response from medication in the treatment of major depression. Repetitive TMS (rTMS) may also be used to supplement inadequate medication responses rather than replace the medication. In 2008, the FDA approved rTMS for treating major depression in patients who have not responded to one or more trials of medication, largely based on a 2007 study (O'Reardon et al. 2007). rTMS does appear safe, although it may provoke seizures and mania. Syncope, headaches, and scalp, neck, and facial pain are the most frequently reported side effects (Rossi et al. 2009).

Despite general hope for the procedure, the Achilles heel of rTMS is confirming efficacy. Part of the problem is defining standards for strength of stimulation (stimulating, high frequency ≥10 Hz; inhibitory, low frequency ≤1 Hz), choice of location, and length of treatment. Addressing prefrontal asymmetry theory (Liu et al. 2016; Mayberg 2003), most studies have employed "bilateral" rTMS: high-frequency rTMS and low-frequency rTMS are respectively applied over the left and right dorsolateral prefrontal cortex (DLPFC). More recent alternative approaches include theta bursts continuously inhibiting the right, while intermittently stimulating the left, DLPFC; low-field synchronized TMS; deep TMS; accelerated high-frequency rTMS, in which four or more high-frequency rTMS stimulation sessions are given per day; and priming low-frequency rTMS, which delivers high-frequency rTMS prior to low-frequency rTMS.

An RCT with improved methodology (George et al. 2010) was performed to answer questions about the quality of previous studies and the weak strength of clinical benefit they demonstrated (Brunoni and Fregni 2011). This study used daily left prefrontal treatment with high-intensity stimulation (120% motor threshold), a high number of pulses (3,000 stimuli per session), localization guided by MRI, and active sham comparisons (mimicking the procedure without providing the actual treatment, which helped to maintain a double blind). Earlier studies used lower power and usually only 2 weeks of treatment. Protocol for the George et al. (2010) study also allowed continued open-label treatment for apparent responders. Unfortunately, the study was underpowered for its design, and the remission rate for fully adherent completers was not clinically significant.

Although significance was demonstrated for *all* remitters and responders, the number of both was disappointingly small after 3 weeks of treatment. Another 30% responded with up to an additional 2 weeks of open-label treatment, consistent with the pivotal study for the FDA that saw improvement after 4–6 weeks (O'Reardon et al. 2007). Network meta-analysis (see Chapter 2) has shown mostly comparable safety and outcome for bilateral rTMS, priming TMS, and theta burst stimulation. Deep rTMS, accelerated rTMS, and synchronized TMS were no better than sham treatment in the small number of studies addressing these (Brunoni et al. 2017).

Most responders in these RCTs have also been found to have low antidepressant resistance. Treatment of major depression with TMS is very expensive for patients, often costing $12,000, and is not usually covered by insurance. In view of the weak treatment effect that has so far been demonstrated (number needed to treat 10–12; see Chapter 2), clinicians and patients will need to review the data and decide together if this cost appears justified, given other treatment options.

As with most treatments, TMS is being tried for just about everything, including neuropathic and phantom limb pain, PTSD, dementia, mild cognitive impairment, stroke, substance abuse, and OCD. Evidence thus far, however, has been insufficient to support treatment recommendations for TMS in these areas.

Transcranial Direct Current Stimulation

Another noninvasive treatment is transcranial direct current stimulation (tDCS). Like TMS, it targets the DLPFC and attempts to achieve neuroplasticity in the structural and functional reorganization of neural circuits, but in tDCS, a weak electrical current is applied directly to the scalp (Kuo et al. 2017). tDCS does not induce synchronized action potentials but moderates spontaneous neuronal activity by altering the threshold for spontaneous discharges (Woods et al. 2016). Unfortunately, current evidence only supports possible efficacy in non-treatment-resistant major depression (Lefaucheur et al. 2017). Some studies have shown moderate improvement in bipolar depression but, as with TMS, have also shown a risk of tDCS switching these patients into mania (Dondé et al. 2017).

Deep Brain Stimulation

Psychosurgery has a dubious and sometimes dark history when applied to psychiatric disorders. With few exceptions, such as cingulotomy and capsulotomy for treatment-resistant OCD and major depression, it is generally rejected by practitioners (Lapidus et al. 2013; Staudt et al. 2019).

Because the effects of surgery are static, excitement has increased about potentially reversible surgical procedures that could be studied and attempted with fewer permanent repercussions. Deep brain stimulation (DBS), first applied psychiatrically in 1955 (Heath et al. 1955) and since utilized for movement disorders such as Parkinson's disease, represents a current effort in this regard.

DBS involves implantation of electrodes into target nodes in the brain, followed by microelectrode mapping and intraoperative stimulation. A battery and pulse generator are placed under the patient's clavicle or in the patient's abdomen 1–2 weeks later. Electrical stimulation follows through wireless telemetric programming after another 2–4 weeks (Williams and Okun 2013). A neuromodulating treatment, DBS can have differential effects given the location and electrical frequency chosen: it may inhibit or excite neural elements or lead to a novel equilibrium (Hamani et al. 2017). Work remains to determine the exact interventions that may alleviate symptoms (Graat et al. 2017), and new techniques are being developed, including fractionation of the current along the multipolar lead, selective current steering, and closed-loop adaptive stimulation, which may lead to delivery of stimulation only as needed (Hariz 2014).

DBS has been investigated for the treatment of major depression, addiction, Tourette syndrome, schizophrenia, anorexia nervosa, and OCD but is currently only approved in the United States for OCD under a humanitarian device exemption. Studies are not controlled, sample sizes are limited, and stimulus location has been significantly heterogeneous. Adverse events vary with stimulus location and include nausea, hypomania, psychosis, strabismus, and blurred vision in addition to the risks of neurosurgery. However, adjusting the stimulus should eliminate the nonsurgical risks. The cost of DBS is well over $200,000 and is not reimbursed by insurance. Even following failure of psychotherapeutic and psychopharmacological interventions, DBS is currently considered an experimental treatment limited to clinical studies performed by an interdisciplinary team (Naesström et al. 2016).

Vagus Nerve Stimulation

In spite of multiple treatment options, some patients will show no response to psychotherapy, pharmacotherapy, or somatic therapies. Vagus nerve stimulation (VNS), used for epilepsy since the mid-1990s, has been found useful as a tool for research and for the treatment of major depression in open and naturalistic studies, particularly in cases resistant to multiple treatment attempts (George et al. 2000; Nahas et al. 2005; Rush et al. 2000). Improvement over sham treatment has been noted only with long-term treatment (Rush et al. 2005a, 2005b). Although response and remission can be striking in patients with otherwise treatment-resistant illness, even those with more than eight previous treatment attempts or resistance to ECT, improvement often takes at least 6 months to develop, with response continuing to improve over 5 years in prospective registries (Aaronson et al. 2017; Rush et al. 2005b).

A programmable pulse generator is implanted in the patient's chest wall and connected to electrodes attached to the left vagus (tenth cranial) nerve in the neck. Two weeks later, stimulation is initiated with a stimulus intensity of 0.25 mA, a pulse width of 500 μs, and a frequency of 20 Hz or 30 Hz, with stimulation *on* for 30 seconds every 5 minutes. Stimulus strength can be increased in 0.25-mA increments as tolerated, most commonly to 0.5–1.5 mA. Programming is accomplished in an office setting with a computer or cellphone and a telemetric wand and may be adjusted weekly to every few weeks as clinically indicated. In addition to the risks of surgery, VNS side effects may include switch into mania (3.3% in one report) as well as mild voice alteration or hoarseness (55%), coughing (17%), or dyspnea (15%), especially exertional, all related to stimulus strength and usually reversible (Sackeim et al. 2001; Salloum et al. 2017). Other adverse events may include headache (22%), neck pain (17%), dysphagia (20%), and pain (15%) (Sackeim et al. 2001; Salloum et al. 2017).

Because it is surgically implanted, VNS costs more than $45,000, not including ongoing costs. Although approved by the FDA in 2005, in 2007 it was denied approval for treating major depression by Medicare and thus has been largely unavailable for insurance reimbursement in the United States, significantly limiting its availability. This decision was reversed in 2019 and now large studies have been initiated to further understand its efficacy (Aaronson and Suppes 2020). Noninvasive VNS is also being developed and may offer substantially less expensive VNS treatment (Ben-Menachem et al. 2015; Bremner and Rapaport 2017). If efficacy can be established for this noninvasive form, VNS may become more than a very expensive last option for patients with the most treatment-resistant affective disorders.

Summary

Somatic treatments are available that may compete with or supplement pharmacological treatments. ECT was an early treatment for mood disorders that remains the gold standard. Evidence-based protocols, developed in the past few decades, have helped identify the best practices for sustained response to this safe, now common treatment. rTMS is still early in development, searching for the best methods and confirmation of robust efficacy.

Data are insufficient for its variation, tDCS, beyond non-treatment-resistant major depression. DBS, although helpful in neurology, is an experimental psychiatric treatment limited to clinical studies. VNS is not easily available but may offer hope for patients with treatment-resistant mood disorders, including those who did not respond to ECT. The response, however, takes at least 6 months, with progressive improvement for up to 5 years. Development of noninvasive forms may widen its applicability.

Key Points

- Continuation electroconvulsive therapy is a rapidly effective, safe, and reasonable treatment for mood disorders.
- Repetitive transcranial magnetic stimulation is safe, although its efficacy appears mostly limited to patients who also respond to antidepressants.
- The exceptional costs and risks of some somatic treatments should be openly discussed and compared with the likelihood of benefit.

Self-Assessment

1. Which of these treatments has been found helpful for treatment-resistant OCD? (Choose all that apply)

   A. Anterior capsulotomy
   B. Repetitive transcranial magnetic stimulation
   C. Cingulotomy
   D. Deep brain stimulation
   E. Vagus nerve stimulation

2. Which of these treatments is most likely to show improvement in treatment-resistant major depression?

   A. Electroconvulsive therapy or vagus nerve stimulation
   B. Deep brain stimulation or repetitive transcranial magnetic stimulation
   C. Transcranial direct current stimulation or deep brain stimulation
   D. Repetitive transcranial magnetic stimulation or electro-convulsive therapy

3. Electroconvulsive therapy is effective (choose all that apply)

    A. Acutely for depression, both unipolar and bipolar
    B. Long term with continuation electroconvulsive therapy
    C. Acutely for mania
    D. Acutely for mixed bipolar states

4. Which of the following somatic treatments has demonstrated switch into mania or hypomania for susceptible patients? (Choose all that apply)

    A. Electroconvulsive therapy
    B. Repetitive transcranial magnetic stimulation
    C. Deep brain stimulation
    D. Vagus nerve stimulation

5. Which of the following somatic treatments currently involves surgical implantation? (Choose all that apply)

    A. Deep brain stimulation
    B. Electroconvulsive therapy
    C. Vagus nerve stimulation
    D. Repetitive transcranial magnetic stimulation

Discussion Topics

1. A patient with recurrent major depression and no comorbidities has failed adequate trials of selective serotonin reuptake inhibitors, serotonin-norepinephrine reuptake inhibitors, bupropion, monoamine oxidase inhibitors, and lithium. He responds well to 10 acute electroconvulsive therapy (ECT) treatments and plans to proceed with continuation ECT. Given your knowledge of the literature, what is your recommendation regarding the use of antidepressant medication going forward?

2. A patient with treatment-resistant major depression has failed two trials of medication and wants your opinion on repetitive transcranial magnetic stimulation (rTMS). Her husband plans to take out a loan to finance the treatment, if you recommend it; she abhors the idea of ECT. What is your treatment planning discussion?

Additional Reading

Cleary DR, Ozpinar A, Raslan AM, et al: Deep brain stimulation for psychiatric disorders: where we are now. Neurosurgical Focus 38(6):E2, 2015

Cusin C, Dougherty DD: Somatic therapies for treatment-resistant depression: ECT, TMS, VNS, DBS. Biol Mood Anxiety Disord 2:14, 2012

Rasmussen KG: Principles and Practice of Electroconvulsive Therapy. Washington, DC, American Psychiatric Association Publishing, 2019

References

Aaronson ST, Suppes T: Bipolar disorder: a discussion of emerging understanding. Presented at the American College of Psychiatrists Meeting, Ft. Lauderdale, FL, February 21, 2020

Aaronson ST, Sears P, Ruvuna F, et al: A 5-year observational study of patients with treatment-resistant depression treated with vagus nerve stimulation or treatment as usual: comparison of response, remission, and suicidality. Am J Psychiatry 174(7):640–648, 2017 28359201

Barker AT, Jalinous R, Freeston IL: Non-invasive magnetic stimulation of human motor cortex. Lancet 1(8437):1106–1107, 1985 2860322

Ben-Menachem E, Revesz D, Simon BJ, et al: Surgically implanted and non-invasive vagus nerve stimulation: a review of efficacy, safety and tolerability. Eur J Neurol 22(9):1260–1268, 2015 25614179

Bourgon LN, Kellner CH: Relapse of depression after ECT: a review. J ECT 16(1):19–31, 2000 10735328

Brannon EP, Graham WL: Intensive insulin shock therapy—a five-year survey. Am J Psychiatry 111(9):659–663, 1955 14350085

Bremner JD, Rapaport MH: Vagus nerve stimulation: back to the future. Am J Psychiatry 174(7):609–610, 2017 28669203

Brunoni AR, Fregni F: Clinical trial design in non-invasive brain stimulation psychiatric research. Int J Methods Psychiatr Res 20(2):e19–e30, 2011 21538653

Brunoni AR, Chaimani A, Moffa AH, et al: Repetitive transcranial magnetic stimulation for the acute treatment of major depressive episodes: a systematic review with network meta-analysis. JAMA Psychiatry 74(2):143–152, 2017 28030740

Brus O, Nordanskog P, Båve U, et al: Subjective memory immediately following electroconvulsive therapy. J ECT 33(2):96–103, 2017 27930429

Cooper K, Fink M: The chemical induction of seizures in psychiatric therapy: were flurothyl (indoklon) and pentylenetetrazol (metrazol) abandoned prematurely? J Clin Psychopharmacol 34(5):602–607, 2014 25029329

Dondé C, Amad A, Nieto I, et al: Transcranial direct-current stimulation (tDCS) for bipolar depression: a systematic review and meta-analysis. Prog Neuropsychopharmacol Biol Psychiatry 78:123–131, 2017 28552295

Faedda GL, Becker I, Baroni A, et al: The origins of electroconvulsive therapy: Prof. Bini's first report on ECT. J Affect Disord 120(1–3):12–15, 2010 19268370

Fink M: The seizure, not electricity, is essential in convulsive therapy: the flurothyl experience. J ECT 30(2):91–93, 2014a 24625714

Fink M: What was learned: studies by the consortium for research in ECT (CORE) 1997–2011. Acta Psychiatr Scand 129(6):417–426, 2014b 24571807

Gagné GG Jr, Furman MJ, Carpenter LL, et al: Efficacy of continuation ECT and antidepressant drugs compared to long-term antidepressants alone in depressed patients. Am J Psychiatry 157(12):1960–1965, 2000 11097961

Gálvez V, Hadzi-Pavlovic D, Waite S, et al: Seizure threshold increases can be predicted by EEG quality in right unilateral ultrabrief ECT. Eur Arch Psychiatry Clin Neurosci 267(8):795–801, 2017 28401340

George MS, Sackeim HA, Rush AJ, et al: Vagus nerve stimulation: a new tool for brain research and therapy. Biol Psychiatry 47(4):287–295, 2000 10686263

George MS, Lisanby SH, Avery D, et al: Daily left prefrontal transcranial magnetic stimulation therapy for major depressive disorder: a sham-controlled randomized trial. Arch Gen Psychiatry 67(5):507–516, 2010 20439832

Graat I, Figee M, Denys D: The application of deep brain stimulation in the treatment of psychiatric disorders. Int Rev Psychiatry 29(2):178–190, 2017 28523977

Hamani C, Florence G, Heinsen H, et al: Subthalamic nucleus deep brain stimulation: basic concepts and novel perspectives. eNeuro 4(5), 2017 28966978

Hariz M: Deep brain stimulation: new techniques. Parkinsonism Relat Disord 20(suppl 1):S192–S196, 2014 24262179

Heath RG, Monroe RR, Mickle WA: Stimulation of the amygdaloid nucleus in a schizophrenic patient. Am J Psychiatry 111(11):862–863, 1955 14361778

Jelovac A, Kolshus E, McLoughlin DM: Relapse following successful electroconvulsive therapy for major depression: a meta-analysis. Neuropsychopharmacology 38(12):2467–2474, 2013 23774532

Kellner CH, Knapp RG, Petrides G, et al: Continuation electroconvulsive therapy vs pharmacotherapy for relapse prevention in major depression: a multisite study from the Consortium for Research in Electroconvulsive Therapy (CORE). Arch Gen Psychiatry 63(12):1337–1344, 2006 17146008

Kellner CH, Ahle GM, Geduldig ET: Electroconvulsive therapy for bipolar disorder: evidence supporting what clinicians have long known. J Clin Psychiatry 76(9):e1151–e1152, 2015 26455688

Kellner CH, Husain MM, Knapp RG, et al: A novel strategy for continuation ECT in geriatric depression: phase 2 of the PRIDE study. Am J Psychiatry 173(11):1110–1118, 2016 27418381

Kuo MF, Chen PS, Nitsche MA: The application of tDCS for the treatment of psychiatric diseases. Int Rev Psychiatry 29(2):146–167, 2017 28523976

Lapidus KA, Kopell BH, Ben-Haim S, et al: History of psychosurgery: a psychiatrist's perspective. World Neurosurg 80(3–4 suppl 27):27.e1–27.e16, 2013 23419707

Lefaucheur JP, Antal A, Ayache SS, et al: Evidence-based guidelines on the therapeutic use of transcranial direct current stimulation (tDCS). Clin Neurophysiol 128(1):56–92, 2017 27866120

Leiknes KA, Jarosh-von Schweder L, Høie B: Contemporary use and practice of electroconvulsive therapy worldwide. Brain Behav 2(3):283–344, 2012 22741102

Lisanby SH, Sampson S, Husain MM, et al: Toward individualized post electroconvulsive therapy care: piloting the Symptom-Titrated, Algorithm-Based Longitudinal ECT (STABLE) intervention. J ECT 24(3):179–182, 2008 18708943

Liu W, Mao Y, Wei D, et al: Structural asymmetry of dorsolateral prefrontal cortex correlates with depressive symptoms: evidence from healthy individuals and patients with major depressive disorder. Neurosci Bull 32(3):217–226, 2016 27015663

Mayberg HS: Modulating dysfunctional limbic-cortical circuits in depression: towards development of brain-based algorithms for diagnosis and optimised treatment. Br Med Bull 65:193–207, 2003 12697626

McDonald A, Walter G: Hollywood and ECT. Int Rev Psychiatry 21(3):200–206, 2009 19459094

Naesström M, Blomstedt P, Bodlund O: A systematic review of psychiatric indications for deep brain stimulation, with focus on major depressive and obsessive-compulsive disorder. Nord J Psychiatry 70(7):483–491, 2016 27103550

Naguib M, Koorn R: Interactions between psychotropics, anaesthetics and electroconvulsive therapy: implications for drug choice and patient management. CNS Drugs 16(4):229–247, 2002 11945107

Nahas Z, Marangell LB, Husain MM, et al: Two-year outcome of vagus nerve stimulation (VNS) for treatment of major depressive episodes. J Clin Psychiatry 66(9):1097–1104, 2005 16187765

O'Reardon JP, Solvason HB, Janicak PG, et al: Efficacy and safety of transcranial magnetic stimulation in the acute treatment of major depression: a multisite randomized controlled trial. Biol Psychiatry 62(11):1208–1216, 2007 17573044

Petrides G, Dhossche D, Fink M, et al: Continuation ECT: relapse prevention in affective disorders. Convuls Ther 10(3):189–194, 1994 7834255

Rossi S, Hallett M, Rossini PM, et al: Safety, ethical considerations, and application guidelines for the use of transcranial magnetic stimulation in clinical practice and research. Clin Neurophysiol 120(12):2008–2039, 2009 19833552

Rush AJ, George MS, Sackeim HA, et al: Vagus nerve stimulation (VNS) for treatment-resistant depressions: a multicenter study. Biol Psychiatry 47(4):276–286, 2000 10686262

Rush AJ, Marangell LB, Sackeim HA, et al: Vagus nerve stimulation for treatment-resistant depression: a randomized, controlled acute phase trial. Biol Psychiatry 58(5):347–354, 2005a 16139580

Rush AJ, Sackeim HA, Marangell LB, et al: Effects of 12 months of vagus nerve stimulation in treatment-resistant depression: a naturalistic study. Biol Psychiatry 58(5):355–363, 2005b 16139581

Sackeim HA, Prudic J, Devanand DP, et al: The impact of medication resistance and continuation pharmacotherapy on relapse following response to electroconvulsive therapy in major depression. J Clin Psychopharmacol 10(2):96–104, 1990 2341598

Sackeim HA, Rush AJ, George MS, et al: Vagus nerve stimulation (VNS) for treatment-resistant depression: efficacy, side effects, and predictors of outcome. Neuropsychopharmacology 25(5):713–728, 2001 11682255

Salloum NC, Walker MC, Gangwani S, et al: Emergence of mania in two middle-aged patients with a history of unipolar treatment-refractory depression receiving vagus nerve stimulation. Bipolar Disord 19(1):60–64, 2017 28098427

Sanghani SN, Petrides G, Kellner CH: Electroconvulsive therapy (ECT) in schizophrenia: a review of recent literature. Curr Opin Psychiatry 31(3):213–222, 2018 29528902

Semkovska M, McLoughlin DM: Objective cognitive performance associated with electroconvulsive therapy for depression: a systematic review and meta-analysis. Biol Psychiatry 68(6):568–577, 2010 20673880

Sienaert P: Based on a true story? The portrayal of ECT in international movies and television programs. Brain Stimul 9(6):882–891, 2016 27522170

Squire LR, Zouzounis JA: ECT and memory: brief pulse versus sine wave. Am J Psychiatry 143(5):596–601, 1986 3963246

Staudt MD, Herring EZ, Gao K, et al: Evolution in the treatment of psychiatric disorders: from psychosurgery to psychopharmacology to neuromodulation. Front Neurosci 13:108, 2019 308282889

UK ECT Review Group: Efficacy and safety of electroconvulsive therapy in depressive disorders: a systematic review and meta-analysis. Lancet 361(9360):799–808, 2003 12642045

Van Mensvoort FA, Blok G, Blom JD: Insulin shock treatment in The Hague from 1937 to the end of the 1950s [in Dutch]. Tijdschr Psychiatr 54(10):869–877, 20012, 2012 23074031

Williams NR, Okun MS: Deep brain stimulation (DBS) at the interface of neurology and psychiatry. J Clin Invest 123(11):4546–4556, 2013 24177464

Woods AJ, Antal A, Bikson M, et al: A technical guide to tDCS, and related noninvasive brain stimulation tools. Clin Neurophysiol 127(2):1031–1048, 2016 26652115

Adverse Events

Although the highest hope for treatment with psychoactive medications is resolution or amelioration of targeted syndromes, adverse events still occur at incidences greater than desired. Although the quality of published case reports may sometimes call into question evidence for causation, and therefore accurate estimations of incidence (Talat et al. 2013), adverse events should be anticipated and addressed prior to treatment and not just following their occurrence. The therapeutic alliance between provider and patient is enhanced by early discussions of these possibilities, because patients will understand the depth of their providers' knowledge, have confidence in their guidance, and appreciate the opportunity to make well-informed choices. Informed patients are also more likely to report problems promptly to their prescribing physicians.

General Assessment of Adverse Events

As discussed in Chapters 3 and 12, practitioners should assess, at least, a problem-oriented review of systems at every patient contact. Completing a full review during the initial evaluation helps separate preexisting problems from new, possibly adverse, events. For example, identifying any sexual desire or performance problems that exist *prior to* prescription will help clarify whether reports of sexual problems *during* treatment might be adverse events and how they might be addressed. Once possible adverse events are reported during treatment, rational clinicians take a complete and thorough history of the symptom. Triage based on severity and risk; patients may need to be evaluated in an office or emergency setting prior to their next scheduled visit. Determine their compliance with treatment, searching for missed, inaccurate, or extra doses as well as any changes in brand (e.g., to or from generic or among generic brands; see Chapter 6, "Pharmacokinetics"). Inquire about the use of any new or as-needed medications, because the other agent may be the culprit. As an example, a rash may develop from a long-term medication but is more likely from a new medication added by another practitioner, particularly antibiotics. If the timing is suspicious for the new agent, ask the other clinician to reconsider the prescription, rather than removing it yourself. Providers unfortunately have a bad habit of blaming all problems on medication from other practitioners, but we hope the psychopharmacologist will approach this rationally from both sides.

When you have determined that the patient is safe, and that an adverse event related to the psychiatric treatment plan has occurred, you will need to consider options and discuss these with the patient. If this is an expected event that the patient was forewarned about and he or she consented to the risk, is it still tolerable and acceptable to the patient? Is the degree of benefit from the treatment sufficient to allow the adverse event to continue? What are the risks of stopping the treatment and losing its benefit, such as with a patient treated for psychosis or suicidal ideation? Thoughtful consideration and open discussion of options is essential in ongoing, dynamic treatment planning (see Chapters 4 and 12).

The remainder of this chapter considers special cases.

Serotonin Syndrome

Psychopharmacologists prescribe many different medications that modulate serotonin (see Chapter 7): antidepressants, including monoamine oxidase inhibitors (MAOIs) and trazodone; second-generation antipsychotics; methamphetamine; buspirone; and some weight loss treatments. Many other medications stimulate serotonin in various ways, including cough and cold treatments with codeine, chlorpheniramine, cyclobenzaprine, or dextromethorphan; pain medications such as phenylpiperidines (e.g., tramadol, methadone, fentanyl), hydrocodone, meperidine, and oxycodone; triptans and ergotamine for migraine; dietary supplement and serotonin precursor L-tryptophan; and St. John's wort (see Chapter 8) (Brown 2010; Schenk and Wirz 2015; Vashistha et al. 2017). Serotonin syndrome occurs when high levels of serotonin are achieved in the CNS. Although it is usually thought to result from the combined effects of two or more medications, reports have been published of serotonin syndrome occurring from a single medication, particularly with escalated doses (Gill et al. 1999). Medications with longer effective half-lives, such as fluoxetine, may contribute to serotonin syndrome weeks after they are discontinued when another serotonin agent is given. Serotonin syndrome may also be provoked by concomitant use of medications inhibiting CYP2D6 and CYP3A4, raising the serum level of serotonin drugs (Mitchell 1997).

Serotonin syndrome is not an idiopathic event, although evidence has shown that some genetic polymorphisms may predispose to it (Alusik et al. 2014). It occurs when serotonin levels are high; clinical features range from minimal and overlooked to lethal symptoms, heightening the importance that clinicians actively look for signs of the problem, because deterioration may be rapid. There is no routine presentation, but serotonin syndrome generally involves mental status changes, neuromuscular abnormalities, and autonomic hyperactivity. Associated mental status changes often involve agitation and delirium. Autonomic hyperactivity can present as tachycardia, diaphoresis, mydriasis, nausea, vomiting, diarrhea, and active bowel sounds. Neuromuscular changes often include tremor, which is nonspecific for symptoms, and clonus, which has been suggested as the most specific symptom and may present as spontaneous, inducible, or ocular. Headaches and dizziness are the most common symptoms reported, and gait disturbance is one top reason patients seek help. Hyperreflexia is common, and peripheral hypertonicity may occur, which would suppress clonus; fever is possible, but hyperthermia is less common (Boyer and Shannon 2005; Prakash et al. 2019).

Three tools may assist in making the diagnosis: the Hunter criteria, focusing more on physical symptoms; the Sternbach criteria, including more mental status changes; and its revision, the Radomski criteria, which clarifies severity. The Hunter criteria are the most commonly valued and used, although recent authors have suggested clinicians focus more on awareness of the potential for serotonin syndrome in diagnosis than on individual symptoms or criteria (Dunkley et al. 2003; Radomski et al. 2000; Sternbach 1991; Werneke et al. 2016). As always, full knowledge of the pharmacokinetics and pharmacodynamics of every medication prescribed will mitigate risk (see Chapter 6). Serotonin syndrome may need to be distinguished from neuroleptic malignant syndrome (NMS; discussed later), CNS infection, anticholinergic poisoning, and sepsis (Dosi et al. 2014).

Treatment for all severities of serotonin syndrome begins with discontinuing serotonergic agents. This is essential and will lead to important decisions about alternative treatments once the patient is stable. Even patients with mild cases should be hospitalized for observation and supportive treatment with fluids and vital signs stabilization. Antiemetics that affect serotonin (e.g., ondansetron) must be avoided. In severe cases, respiration and circulation must be supported and hyperthermia addressed with cooling. Treatment with serotonergic antagonists, such as cyproheptadine, may be helpful. These steps are discussed in Wang et al. (2016); practitioners should not delay making appropriate referral for these interventions.

When a serotonergic medication may be prescribed, psychopharmacologists should discuss serotonin syndrome with their patients during treatment planning. Knowledgeable patients will be better able to mitigate the risk from medications they may add as needed, over-the-counter (OTC) medications, or those from another provider, and to alert the clinician about early signs. Again, the best approach is to be aware of the possibility of serotonin syndrome so that even mild, nonspecific clinical features may alert patient and clinician to the risk of worsening—particularly if another serotonergic agent has been added for any reason by anyone.

Tardive Dyskinesia

Tardive dyskinesia (TD) is a late-onset involuntary movement disorder linked to dopamine receptor blockade from antipsychotic medications. An important adverse event, TD is discussed elsewhere in this book (see Chapter 7, "Medications to Treat Psychosis," as well as Chapters 3 and 4). The persistence of TD beyond use of the causative agent, along with its conspicuousness, motivates patients and practitioners to minimize the risk of developing it.

TD typically begins after at least 3 months of dopamine-blocking treatment but may occur earlier. It can develop in any muscle of the body and is most obvious when it affects the upper and lower extremities or facial muscles, a common and distressing presentation. It rarely affects the diaphragm. Withdrawal dyskinesias may also be seen when antipsychotic medication is rapidly discontinued, even when no TD was seen during treatment; these are usually brief and self-limiting, and no other intervention is usually necessary.

TD is distinguished from acute dystonic reaction (ADR) and extrapyramidal syndrome (EPS; also called pseudoparkinsonian side effects or drug-induced parkinsonism) by timing of onset, nature, and response to treatment. ADR is an acute sustained muscle contraction, such as a cramp, or an oculogyric crisis, in which the extraocular muscles fix the eyeballs upward (Solberg and Koht 2017). Although distressing for patients, ADR is rapidly reversed with administration of oral or intramuscular anticholinergic medication, such as diphenhydramine or benztropine. EPS mimics Parkinson's disease, with a resting "pill-rolling" tremor, bradykinesia, flat facies, and cogwheel muscle rigidity (see Chapter 7). It is most commonly treated with minimization of dose (if possible), or benztropine, trihexyphenidyl, or amantadine may be used if necessary. Recall from Chapter 7 that anticholinergic side effects (e.g., cognitive impairment, dry mouth, urinary retention, constipation) may become a problem as well as worsen the symptoms or risk of TD. Amantadine, although it does not exacerbate TD, might worsen psychosis (Ward and Citrome 2018).

Some providers have begun using the ^{123}I-ioflupane dopamine transporter protocol, through in vivo testing with single-photon emission computed tomography, to differentiate Parkinson's disease not only from essential tremor but also from EPS. Dopamine transporter testing requires subjective assessment from the clinician, and many clinicians ordering the test are not experienced enough to interpret it correctly (Brogley 2019; Gajos et al. 2019); this can be quite distressing for a patient who may feel advised to discontinue the antipsychotic based on the clinician's incorrect interpretation, with serious consequences. Also, some neurological consultations regarding movement side effects from neuroleptics result in simple recommendations to solve the problem by discontinuing the offending medication. Mental health practitioners are encouraged to develop working relationships with movement disorder specialists who can appreciate these dilemmas for psychiatric patients and the necessity of treatment, even with side effects, when appropriate.

Old strategies addressing TD involved stopping the medication: after briefly worsening, the symptoms sometimes abated. Alternatively, the dose was raised, temporarily suppressing the TD, which only reemerged later, leading to a cycle in which doses became higher and TD still resulted. Today, TD is minimized by using second-generation antipsychotics and limiting use of anticholinergic medications. Although stopping the medication might work, all antipsychotic medications risk TD, and treatment eventually will need to resume. Only recently have pharmacological treatments for TD shown some success. Both valbenazine, a selective inhibitor of vesicular monoamine transporter 2, and deutetrabenazine, a deuterated version of tetrabenazine, are FDA approved for TD. Randomized controlled trials (RCTs) show improvement in symptoms but not always complete remission (Cummings et al. 2018; Hauser et al. 2017; Lindenmayer et al. 2019; Müller 2017).

Dopamine blocking agents should never be prescribed, even briefly, without fully disclosing the risk of TD and its likely permanence (even with new treatments) and obtaining patient consent. The Abnormal Involuntary Movement Scale (see Chapter 7) or Extrapyramidal Symptom Rating Scale may be used clinically to monitor the appearance and course of TD (Chouinard and Margolese 2005; Gharabawi et al. 2005).

Neuroleptic Malignant Syndrome

NMS is a rare condition (0.02%–0.03%) that carries a mortality of 5.6% (Pileggi and Cook 2016). Originally described as a hyperthermia associated with muscular rigidity that might develop within 72 hours of administration of an antipsychotic, the diagnostic criteria acknowledge a heterogeneous presentation; clinically, NMS is a diagnosis of exclusion. Recent authors have suggested that labeling NMS as being associated only with major tranquilizers is erroneous and risky; all dopamine antagonists, plus the partial agonist aripiprazole (see Chapter 7, "Medications to Treat Psychosis"), have been associated with this syndrome (Belvederi Murri et al. 2015; Menon et al. 2017).

Catatonia may present during psychosis, apart from NMS. This further complicates diagnosis, because altered mental status, including delirium, stupor, or coma, is considered an early sign of NMS. These changes are usually followed by severe systemic "lead-pipe" rigidity in which rhabdomyolysis may occur. Hyperthermia develops, and then autonomic dysfunction (Velamoor et al. 1994). The differential diagnosis includes CNS infections and disease, malignant hyperthermia from anesthetics, abrupt discontinuation of dopamine agonists, heat stroke, serotonin syndrome, central anticholinergic syndrome, and lithium intoxication (Perry and Wilborn 2012; Tse et al. 2015).

Treatment is first and foremost supportive, following immediate discontinuation of the dopamine blocking agent. Respiratory and volume support, with monitoring of electrolytes, is essential. Bromocriptine, dantrolene, and biperiden have been studied as pharmacological treatments, especially bromocriptine, sometimes with dantrolene after. Benzodiazepines have been used in treatment, and amantadine is also an option, although RCTs confirming these choices are not available given the scarcity of the condition. Electroconvulsive therapy is often mentioned, likely more due to the need for treatment of the underlying psychiatric condition (Oruch et al. 2017; Pelonero et al. 1998). As with most adverse reactions, awareness of the possibility provides patients with the most thoughtful care and response should NMS symptoms develop. Emergency hospital-based intensive treatment is always indicated (Ware et al. 2018).

Suicidality

Preventing suicide is a major focus of the mental health profession. Given that psychiatric patients, as a group, carry a higher risk of death from suicide than nonpsychiatric patients and the general population, one goal of psychotropic treatment is to reduce this risk (Bertolote and Fleischmann 2002; Nordentoft et al. 2015). Both psychiatric and nonpsychiatric patients expressing suicidal ideation are at greater risk of dying from suicide than those who have not (Hubers et al. 2018).

Since the early use of antidepressants, clinicians have been aware that profoundly melancholic and psychomotorically retarded patients are less likely to exhibit suicidal behaviors than those who feel just a bit better. For this reason, astute clinicians have always urged caution about an increased risk of suicide in the first few weeks of antidepressant treatment, because patients improve and feel more like getting up and engaging in activities, including suicide (Friedman and Leon 2007). New concerns appeared in the literature during the 1990s that antidepressants might increase the risk of *suicidality* (Teicher et al. 1990), which refers to more than dying from suicide or even making suicide attempts. Patients may also engage in deliberate self-harm that is not intended as suicide, and this behavior showed a ratio to eventual death from suicide of 23 (Singhal et al. 2014) and 36 (Hawton and Harriss 2008; see also Owens et al. 2002). Early literature used the term *suicidality* inconsistently, so the FDA supported research to standardize and refine the data (Posner et al. 2007). Suicidality now includes suicide attempts as well as preparatory behaviors, suicidal ideation, and self-injurious behavior with unknown intent, plus, in RCTs, insufficient information. This has resulted in a reduced estimate of risk (Jurek et al. 2005). In 2011 the Centers for Disease Control and Prevention's National Center for Injury Control and Prevention suggested replacing "suicidality" with the phrase "suicidal thoughts and behavior," yet this parlance remains omnipresent.

Eventually, concerns about increased suicidality extended to soporifics, antianxiety and antipsychotic medications, and anticonvulsants. By 2009, the FDA required black box warnings for 125 prescription medications regarding increased suicidality (Lavigne et al. 2012). As a result of the 2004 FDA warning concerning use of antidepressants in children and adolescents, prescriptions for psychotropic medications dropped, particularly antidepressants, and particularly for children and adolescents. Within 5 years, however, prescriptions for psychotropics had regained their previous levels (Kafali et al. 2018).

Suicidality is often included in exclusion criteria for RCTs, limiting their use for its study (Khan et al. 2018). Nevertheless, RCTs have been analyzed, despite caution urged in interpreting the results, given methodological limitations such as internal and external validity. These analyses have reported evidence that, although rare, an increase in suicidality, along with treatment efficacy, was associated with active antidepressant treatment in children and adolescents. A review of FDA data from RCTs of seven recently approved antidepressants, however, showed no difference in rates of suicide and attempted suicide between active drug, active comparators, and placebo (Khan et al. 2000). Pharmacoepidemiological studies have shown antidepressants to provide protective effects against suicidal events for patients of all ages. Analysis of longitudinal data from the treatment of major depression with fluoxetine and venlafaxine in adults, geriatric patients, and youths showed a significant reduction in suicidality, plus additional clinical benefit; even meta-analyses of RCTs found support for fluoxetine use in children and adolescents. Notably, the longitudinal data also showed that in youths, depressive symptoms sometimes improved without a reduction in pretreatment suicidality (Brent 2016; Gibbons et al. 2012; Hetrick et al. 2012; Julious 2013).

Some authors have argued that because the psychiatric population has a greater incidence of suicidality to begin with, prior to treatment with medication, this confounds the estimates of pharmaceutical risk (residual confounding by indication). Additionally, the general suicide rate in the United States and many other parts of the world has been climbing (Bertolote and Fleischmann 2002; Curtin et al. 2016; Värnik 2012). Many studies fail to adequately exclude patients with mixed or depressed bipolar disorder whose risk of suicidality could be increased with the addition of antidepressants (Rihmer and Gonda 2013; Song et al. 2012). Additionally, calculation of suicidality with nonpsychotropic medications has not been successful, despite considering only death from suicide and suicide attempts (Gorton et al. 2016). Increased risk of suicide with the use of anticonvulsants has not been confirmed due to the heterogeneity of studies and residual confounding (Ferrer et al. 2014; Raju Sagiraju et al. 2018).

Benzodiazepines, as discussed in Chapter 7, may worsen suicidality when used without antidepressants. Comorbid substance abuse significantly increases suicide risk, and other nontreatment factors, including high affective lability, have also correlated with suicidality (Ducasse et al. 2017; Hallgren et al. 2017). Clinicians, particularly nonspecialists, who do not inquire about suicidal thoughts and behavior at every patient contact may see previously undisclosed ideation or planning persist or worsen during treatment. They may misattribute later recognition as an adverse event rather than an inadequate treatment response. Routine inquiry simply removes this possibility, as discussed in Chapters 3 and 12.

While researchers attempt to further clarify the role of medication in suicidality, clinicians hold the ultimate trump card. Every patient must be assessed at every contact for suicidality and given an individualized treatment plan to minimize the risk of self-harm. FDA warnings must be explained to patients and families prior to prescription, but an emphasis on individualized treatment should take precedence. Recovery from psychiatric syndromes with indicated medication largely outstrips any demonstrated risk from utilizing these agents, and proper monitoring, following guidelines from legitimate literature, should offer the best outcome and safest path for most patients (Friedman and Leon 2007).

Summary

Despite our progress in clinical psychopharmacology, adverse events still occur at incidences greater than desired. Clinicians should anticipate and discuss these during initial treatment planning and at every subsequent visit: this offers patients fully informed consent and encourages them to report the smallest concerns during treatment. Once a complete review of systems is documented during initial assessment, a follow-up review during appointments can help clarify the emergence of adverse events. A full history will clarify compliance and the possible interference of new treatments from other providers or of OTC or as-needed medications.

Serotonin syndrome is not idiopathic but is specifically related to high serotonin levels, such as from dose, polypharmacy, or drug–drug interactions. Awareness of the risk, plus a thorough history, are the best tools to aid diagnosis. Begin treatment by discontinuing all serotonin agents and hospitalizing the patient for observation and supportive treatment. TD may develop from the use of all antipsychotic medications and is usually permanent, despite new treatments that reduce symptoms. It is distinguishable from ADR and EPS and worsened by the use of anticholinergic medications. Antipsychotics should never be prescribed for any indication, even briefly, without fully disclosing the risk of TD.

NMS is a rare but potentially lethal complication of dopamine antagonists that is difficult to distinguish from catatonia during psychosis. It may also be confused with serotonin syndrome and is a diagnosis of exclusion. Typified by mental status alterations, hyperthermia, and "lead-pipe" rigidity, NMS emergency treatment begins with discontinuing the dopamine blocking agent and hospitalizing the patient for respiratory and volume support in an intensive care setting.

Suicidality includes suicide attempts, preparatory behaviors, suicidal ideation, self-injurious behavior with unknown intent, and in RCTs, insufficient information. RCTs, due to exclusion criteria, are not particularly suited for the assessment of suicidality, although most of the data we have are obtained from them. Pharmacoepidemiological and other longitudinal studies, which are usually inferior to RCTs for clarifying effective treatments, demonstrate the overall benefit of antidepressant medications and low, or insignificant, enhancement of or failure to treat suicidality. Despite warnings of increased suicidality for many medications, this risk has not always been confirmed. Suicidality should always be discussed with patients and families; clinicians can effectively manage this risk by fully evaluating suicidality at every single patient contact so that individualized treatment plans can be developed and altered as necessary.

Key Points

- Anticipate adverse events.
- Serotonin syndrome may always be provoked when serotonin levels are too high.
- Always discuss the risk of permanent tardive dyskinesia before prescribing any dopamine antagonist or weak agonist.
- Queries about suicidality must be made at every patient contact.

Self-Assessment

1. A patient with schizoaffective disorder presents to the emergency department with altered mental status, headaches, dizziness, tremor, tachycardia, nausea, and moderate fever. Clonus was initially present, but now peripheral hypertonicity is evident. He is taking lithium, aripiprazole, and fluoxetine. Which of the following statements is true? (Choose all that apply)

    A. The differential diagnosis must include, at least, lithium toxicity, serotonin syndrome, and neuroleptic malignant syndrome.
    B. Ondansetron may be given for nausea.
    C. This presentation is most consistent with serotonin syndrome.
    D. His medications should be continued during the hospital stay.

2. Which of the following statements is false? (Choose all that apply)

    A. When considering brief use of a dopamine antagonist, such as for treatment-resistant depression, it is not necessary to mention the risk of tardive dyskinesia.
    B. Euthymic patients with no complaints do not have to be specifically asked about suicidality at every visit.
    C. Generic brands are essentially the same, so changes in them do not need monitoring.
    D. None of the above

3. As standardized by the FDA, *suicidality* refers to all of the following, except:

    A. Suicide attempts
    B. Preparatory suicide behaviors
    C. Suicidal ideation

    D. Self-injurious behavior with unknown intent

    E. Insufficient information in randomized controlled trials

    F. None of the above

4. A patient taking risperidone presents to your office with bradykinesia, "pill-rolling" tremor, and muscle rigidity on examination. If an adverse reaction, this is most consistent with

    A. Acute dystonic reaction

    B. Extrapyramidal syndrome

    C. Tardive dyskinesia

    D. Neuroleptic malignant syndrome

5. Regarding tardive dyskinesia (TD), which of the following statements is true? (Choose all that apply)

    A. Increasing the dose of the dopamine antagonist may suppress TD, but only temporarily.

    B. Stopping a dopamine antagonist may lead to brief withdrawal dyskinesias.

    C. Valbenazine and deutetrabenazine may offer some relief from TD symptoms.

    D. It may occur in any muscle of the body.

Discussion Topics

1. Your long-term patient with a thought disorder, stabilized on risperidone for 3 years, recently consulted a neurologist you are unfamiliar with about her extrapyramidal side effects. You have discussed these at every appointment: the dose cannot be lowered further, and she has not done as well with alternative antipsychotics. Anticholinergic agents have been slightly helpful but not to her satisfaction. She tells you that the neurologist performed a dopamine transporter protocol and determined that she does not have Parkinson's disease. She thinks the neurologist is recommending she stop her antipsychotic, and she is strongly leaning toward doing so. What information do you need to have and what steps can you take to provide the best possible outcome for her?

2. You evaluate a new patient who has brought copies of his medical records from treatment with his previous psychiatrist in another

town. The patient tells you that he is allergic to carbamazepine, lithium, and oxcarbazepine, although only carbamazepine is listed as an allergy in the record. Most of the progress notes are checklists; the absence of suicidal ideation is checked at each visit, but the patient tells you that he began feeling like hurting himself, nonlethally, since starting lamotrigine, his current medication. Would you proceed with a complete initial evaluation? What questions will you ask to understand his history of possible adverse events?

Additional Reading

Sheehan DV, Giddens JM: Suicidality: A Roadmap for Assessment and Treatment. Tampa, FL, Harm Research Press, 2015

Wang RZ, Vashistha V, Kaur S, et al: Serotonin syndrome: preventing, recognizing, and treating it. Cleve Clin J Med 83(11):810–817, 2016

Ware MR, Feller DB, Hall KL: Neuroleptic malignant syndrome: diagnosis and management. Prim Care Companion CNS Disord 20(1):17r02185, 2018

References

Alusik S, Kalatova D, Paluch Z: Serotonin syndrome. Neuroendocrinol Lett 35(4):265–273, 2014 25038602

Belvederi Murri M, Guaglianone A, Bugliani M, et al: Second-generation antipsychotics and neuroleptic malignant syndrome: systematic review and case report analysis. Drugs R D 15(1):45–62, 2015 25578944

Bertolote JM, Fleischmann A: Suicide and psychiatric diagnosis: a worldwide perspective. World Psychiatry 1(3):181–185, 2002 16946849

Boyer EW, Shannon M: The serotonin syndrome. N Engl J Med 352(11):1112–1120, 2005 15784664

Brent DA: Antidepressants and suicidality. Psychiatr Clin North Am 39(3):503–512, 2016 27514302

Brogley JE: DaTQUANT: the future of diagnosing Parkinson disease. J Nucl Med Technol 47(1):21–26, 2019 30683690

Brown CH: Drug-induced serotonin syndrome. U.S. Pharmacist, November 17, 2010. Available at: https://www.uspharmacist.com/article/drug-induced-serotonin-syndrome. Accessed October 4, 2019.

Chouinard G, Margolese HC: Manual for the Extrapyramidal Symptom Rating Scale (ESRS). Schizophr Res 76(2–3):247–265, 2005 15949657

Cummings MA, Proctor GJ, Stahl SM: Deuterium tetrabenazine for tardive dyskinesia. Clin Schizophr Relat Psychoses 11(4):214–220, 2018 29341821

Curtin SC, Warner M, Hedegaard H: Increase in suicide in the United States, 1999–2014. NCHS Data Brief (241):1–8, 2016 27111185

Dosi R, Ambaliya A, Joshi H, et al: Serotonin syndrome versus neuroleptic malignant syndrome: a challenging clinical quandary. BMJ Case Rep 2014 24957740

Ducasse D, Jaussent I, Guillaume S, et al: Affect lability predicts occurrence of suicidal ideation in bipolar patients: a two-year prospective study. Acta Psychiatr Scand 135(5):460–469, 2017 28260234

Dunkley EJ, Isbister GK, Sibbritt D, et al: The Hunter Serotonin Toxicity Criteria: simple and accurate diagnostic decision rules for serotonin toxicity. QJM 96(9):635–642, 2003 12925718

Ferrer P, Ballarín E, Sabaté M, et al: Antiepileptic drugs and suicide: a systematic review of adverse effects. Neuroepidemiology 42(2):107–120, 2014 24401764

Friedman RA, Leon AC: Expanding the black box: depression, antidepressants, and the risk of suicide. N Engl J Med 356(23):2343–2346, 2007 17485726

Gajos A, Dabrowski J, Bienkiewicz M, et al: Should non-movement specialists refer patients for SPECT-DaTSCAN? Neurol Neurochir Pol 53(2):138–143, 2019 30855703

Gharabawi GM, Bossie CA, Lasser RA, et al: Abnormal Involuntary Movement Scale (AIMS) and Extrapyramidal Symptom Rating Scale (ESRS): cross-scale comparison in assessing tardive dyskinesia. Schizophr Res 77(2–3):119–128, 2005 15913963

Gibbons RD, Brown CH, Hur K, et al: Suicidal thoughts and behavior with antidepressant treatment: reanalysis of the randomized placebo-controlled studies of fluoxetine and venlafaxine. Arch Gen Psychiatry 69(6):580–587, 2012 22309973

Gill M, LoVecchio F, Selden B: Serotonin syndrome in a child after a single dose of fluvoxamine. Ann Emerg Med 33(4):457–459, 1999 10092727

Gorton HC, Webb RT, Kapur N, et al: Non-psychotropic medication and risk of suicide or attempted suicide: a systematic review. BMJ Open 6(1), 2016 26769782

Hallgren KA, Ries RK, Atkins DC, et al: Prediction of suicide ideation and attempt among substance-using patients in primary care. J Am Board Fam Med 30(2):150–160, 2017 28379821

Hauser RA, Factor SA, Marder SR, et al: KINECT 3: a phase 3 randomized, double-blind, placebo-controlled trial of valbenazine for tardive dyskinesia. Am J Psychiatry 174(5):476–484, 2017 28320223

Hawton K, Harriss L: How often does deliberate self-harm occur relative to each suicide? A study of variations by gender and age. Suicide Life Threat Behav 38(6):650–660, 2008 19152296

Hetrick SE, McKenzie JE, Cox GR, et al: Newer generation antidepressants for depressive disorders in children and adolescents. Cochrane Database Syst Rev (11):CD004851, 2012 23152227

Hubers AAM, Moaddine S, Peersmann SHM, et al: Suicidal ideation and subsequent completed suicide in both psychiatric and non-psychiatric populations: a meta-analysis. Epidemiol Psychiatr Sci 27(2):186–198, 2018 27989254

Julious SA: Efficacy and suicidal risk for antidepressants in paediatric and adolescent patients. Stat Methods Med Res 22(2):190–218, 2013 22267546

Jurek AM, Greenland S, Maldonado G, et al: Proper interpretation of non-differential misclassification effects: expectations vs observations. Int J Epidemiol 34(3):680–687, 2005 15802377

Kafali N, Progovac A, Hou SS, et al: Long-run trends in antidepressant use among youths after the FDA black box warning. Psychiatr Serv 69(4):389–395, 2018 29241433

Khan A, Warner HA, Brown WA: Symptom reduction and suicide risk in patients treated with placebo in antidepressant clinical trials. Arch Gen Psychiatry 57(4):311–317, 2000 10768687

Khan A, Fahl Mar K, Gokul S, et al: Decreased suicide rates in recent antidepressant clinical trials. Psychopharmacology (Berl) 235(5):1455–1462, 2018 29480436

Lavigne JE, Au A, Jiang R, et al: Utilization of prescription drugs with warnings of suicidal thoughts and behaviours in the USA and the US Department of Veterans Affairs, 2009. J Pharm Health Serv Res 3(3):157–163, 2012

Lindenmayer JP, Marder SR, Singer C, et al: 77 Long-term valbenazine treatment in patients with schizophrenia/schizoaffective disorder or mood disorder and tardive dyskinesia. CNS Spectr 24(1):214–215, 2019 30859992

Menon V, Thamizh JS, Rajkumar RP, et al: Neuroleptic malignant syndrome (or malignant extrapyramidal autonomic syndrome): time to revisit diagnostic criteria and terminology? Aust N Z J Psychiatry 51(1):102, 2017 27565995

Mitchell PB: Drug interactions of clinical significance with selective serotonin reuptake inhibitors. Drug Saf 17(6):390–406, 1997 9429838

Müller T: Valbenazine for the treatment of tardive dyskinesia. Expert Rev Neurother 17(12):1135–1144, 2017 28971695

Nordentoft M, Madsen T, Fedyszyn I: Suicidal behavior and mortality in first-episode psychosis. J Nerv Ment Dis 203(5):387–392, 2015 25919385

Oruch R, Pryme IF, Engelsen BA, et al: Neuroleptic malignant syndrome: an easily overlooked neurologic emergency. Neuropsychiatr Dis Treat 13:161–175, 2017 28144147

Owens D, Horrocks J, House A: Fatal and non-fatal repetition of self-harm. Systematic review. Br J Psychiatry 181:193–199, 2002 12204922

Pelonero AL, Levenson JL, Pandurangi AK: Neuroleptic malignant syndrome: a review. Psychiatr Serv 49(9):1163–1172, 1998 9735957

Perry PJ, Wilborn CA: Serotonin syndrome vs neuroleptic malignant syndrome: a contrast of causes, diagnoses, and management. Ann Clin Psychiatry 24(2):155–162, 2012 22563571

Pileggi DJ, Cook AM: Neuroleptic malignant syndrome. Ann Pharmacother 50(11):973–981, 2016 27423483

Posner K, Oquendo MA, Gould M, et al: Columbia Classification Algorithm of Suicide Assessment (C-CASA): classification of suicidal events in the FDA's pediatric suicidal risk analysis of antidepressants. Am J Psychiatry 164(7):1035–1043, 2007 17606655

Prakash S, Rathore C, Rana KK, et al: Refining the clinical features of serotonin syndrome: a prospective observational study of 45 patients. Ann Indian Acad Neurol 22(1):52–60, 2019 30692760

Radomski JW, Dursun SM, Reveley MA, et al: An exploratory approach to the serotonin syndrome: an update of clinical phenomenology and revised diagnostic criteria. Med Hypotheses 55(3):218–224, 2000 10985912

Raju Sagiraju HK, Wang CP, Amuan ME, et al: Antiepileptic drugs and suicide-related behavior: is it the drug or comorbidity? Neurol Clin Pract 8(4):331–339, 2018 30140585

Rihmer Z, Gonda X: Pharmacological prevention of suicide in patients with major mood disorders. Neurosci Biobehav Rev 37(10 Pt 1):2398–2403, 2013 23022665

Schenk M, Wirz S: Serotonin syndrome and pain medication: what is relevant for practice? [in German]. Schmerz 29(2):229–251, 2015 25860200

Singhal A, Ross J, Seminog O, et al: Risk of self-harm and suicide in people with specific psychiatric and physical disorders: comparisons between disorders using English national record linkage. J R Soc Med 107(5):194–204, 2014 24526464

Solberg M, Koht J: Oculogyric crises. Tremor Other Hyperkinet Mov (NY) 7:491, 2017 28975049

Song JY, Yu HY, Kim SH, et al: Assessment of risk factors related to suicide attempts in patients with bipolar disorder. J Nerv Ment Dis 200(11):978–984, 2012 23124183

Sternbach H: The serotonin syndrome. Am J Psychiatry 148(6):705–713, 1991 2035713

Talat B, Mayers A, Baldwin DS: Quality of case reports of adverse drug reactions with psychotropic drugs: a 25-year review. Hum Psychopharmacol 28(5):413–420, 2013 23754771

Teicher MH, Glod C, Cole JO: Emergence of intense suicidal preoccupation during fluoxetine treatment. Am J Psychiatry 147(2):207–210, 1990 2301661

Tse L, Barr AM, Scarapicchia V, et al: Neuroleptic malignant syndrome: a review from a clinically oriented perspective. Curr Neuropharmacol 13(3):395–406, 2015 26411967

Värnik P: Suicide in the world. Int J Environ Res Public Health 9(3):760–771, 2012 22690161

Vashistha V, Wang RZ, Kaur S, et al: In reply: serotonin syndrome. Cleve Clin J Med 84(5):342–343, 2017 28530903

Velamoor VR, Norman RM, Caroff SN, et al: Progression of symptoms in neuroleptic malignant syndrome. J Nerv Ment Dis 182(3):168–173, 1994 7906709

Wang RZ, Vashistha V, Kaur S, et al: Serotonin syndrome: preventing, recognizing, and treating it. Cleve Clin J Med 83(11):810–817, 2016

Ward KM, Citrome L: Antipsychotic-related movement disorders: drug-induced parkinsonism vs. tardive dyskinesia—key differences in pathophysiology and clinical management. Neurol Ther 7(2):233–248, 2018 30027457

Ware MR, Feller DB, Hall KL: Neuroleptic malignant syndrome: diagnosis and management. Prim Care Companion CNS Disord 20(1):17r02185, 2018

Werneke U, Jamshidi F, Taylor DM, et al: Conundrums in neurology: diagnosing serotonin syndrome—a meta-analysis of cases. BMC Neurol 16:97, 2016 27406219

Rational and Methodical Treatment Monitoring

As we begin the final chapter of this book, we have discussed data: how to determine what is needed and how to obtain it (Chapter 3); how to separate signal from noise (Chapters 2 and 4); a historical review of psychopharmacological treatments and supplements (Chapters 7 and 8); lifestyle changes that are essential to achieve desired psychopharmacological outcomes (Chapter 9); exploring and managing adverse events (Chapter 11); and how to think rationally and turn this information into potentially successful treatment plans (Chapters 1, 4, and 5). These processes must be employed not only during initial evaluation and treatment plan development but also at every subsequent visit. Before reading this final chapter, I strongly suggest that you reread Chapter 3, "Thorough Assessment Techniques," before proceeding. This not only will allow you to review the information that must be obtained, but it will also prepare you to devise a method for monitoring treatment plans developed in therapeutic alliance with your patients. Go ahead, reread Chapter 3. I'll wait.

Done? Wonderful. Lest you feel overwhelmed, practicing this full assessment will quickly make it natural and easy to obtain essential and complete data in a short amount of time. Included in this chapter are checklists you may employ until you are fully familiar with each detail of the assessment. Many clinicians allow 60–90 minutes for the initial outpatient assessment (although in inpatient settings this may be different); slightly more information is gathered in the initial visit, the therapeutic alliance is just forming, and additional time to consider an initial treatment plan is necessary. Unfortunately, follow-up visits, often labeled "med checks," may last only 15 minutes. It is entirely possible to cover all the information necessary, make rational decisions about treatment plan changes, answer questions, and write prescriptions in 15 minutes, but only with foreknowledge of what must be accomplished and with practice. Certainly, if more time is available, use it.

As an aside, psychiatrists in particular often approach med checks in the same way we approach psychodynamic psychotherapy sessions: with fixed start and stop times. Certainly, knowing and respecting the subtexts of transference, countertransference, and acting-in is essential for managing treatment and a therapeutic alliance. Again, however, the techniques of clinical psychopharmacology are not identical to those of psychotherapy. For this reason, a clinic model, in which sessions start when the provider and patient are available and end when tasks are accomplished, is fully consistent with rational practice and not to be discouraged in many circumstances.

To complete all steps required in approximately 15 minutes, two things must occur: 1) the clinician must remain cordially in control of the interview, and 2) *change* must be the key theme of the discussion. As discussed in Chapter 3, some patients may confuse open-ended questions with psychotherapeutic explorations. Begin the session with inquiry into how the patient is doing (also often mistaken as a social pleasantry) and move immediately into specific questions if the answer is not helpful. Never accept "good," "fine," or "okay" as an accurate or sufficient response. Again, asking for specifics is a helpful signal to the patient that you are gathering information, and details are necessary. If we direct the questions toward *change* in symptoms, we will more quickly focus on the key features necessary to evaluate the progress of treatment. Remember, progress notes should reflect *progress*, not just reiterate previously recorded data. While open-endedly seeking changes in the patient's symptoms, lifestyle, medications, compliance, and so on, we reinforce that *change* is our goal and what is to be measured first and foremost.

Symptom Review

First, cover the chief complaint from the initial visit, focusing on *what, when, how long, antecedents, context,* and *change.* Review every neurovegetative symptom: sleep, appetite, weight, memory, concentration, interest in pleasure (hedonia), and physical energy (Table 12–1). Of course, unhelpful changes are every bit as important to discover as helpful ones. Use the criteria delineated in Chapter 3 for your assessment, recording every detail in

TABLE 12–1. Follow-up visit symptom checklist

Appearance	Grooming, clothing, eye contact, motor activity
Orientation	Person, place, time, situation
Speech	Prosody, speed, volume, pitch
Sleep	Degree and quality, daytime drowsiness
Appetite	
Weight	
Memory	Immediate, short, and long term
Concentration	Length
Anxiety	Including avoidance
Interest in pleasure	Including socialization and sex
Motivation for activities of daily living	Such as work, school, cleaning, purchases
Physical energy	Distinguished from sleepiness
Mood	Subjective
Affect	Objective appearance of mood/anxiety with congruence
Irritability	
Thought processing	Associations, speed of thoughts
Thought content	Hallucinations, illusions, delusions
Self-harm	Including suicidal ideation, plan, and intent
Violence	Including homicidal ideation, plan, and intent
Insight	
Judgment	
Reliability	Including cooperation
Compliance	

the progress notes so they can be consulted even years later, should treatment efficacy need to be reassessed. Patients may sometimes recall a treatment as helpful when actually it was not; these data will be useful in preventing retrials of failed treatments. They may also be helpful in determining partial responses if combination treatment becomes necessary.

Second, once the objective symptoms are clarified, move to subjective ones, such as mood, anxiety, motivation, and irritability, recording answers in detail. Again, do not accept a simple answer to "How are you?"

Ask specifically about mood, anxiety, socialization, sexual desire, and distortions of reality.

The third level of symptom review is completing any remaining gaps in the mental status examination with formal questioning. Remember, self-harm, suicidality, and violent ideation should be asked about at every patient contact, no matter how well a patient is doing (recall Chapter 3, "Mental Status Examination" and Chapter 11, "Suicidality"). Has the patient taken any action based on these thoughts? Assess for any steps you must take to guard the safety of the patient or others. The Mini-Mental State Examination (MMSE) may now be repeated, if employed, although formal memory testing need not occur at every follow-up session if memory has been deemed adequate and change is denied and not apparent, nor is asking patients to interpret proverbs and questions about judgment. However, hallucinations and delusions should be queried if not already covered in the chief complaint. Remember that not all hallucinations are auditory and visual; ask about olfactory and tactile hallucinations as well, because these often go unmentioned by patients. Again, make your own assessment of insight, judgment, and reliability, recording these with examples, if available.

Medication Review

Once the chief complaint and mental status examination are complete, review each and every medication and supplement the patient is taking (Table 12–2). Clarify that the patient is actually taking what you thought he or she was, including the dosages you expected. Explore compliance and any reasons for less-than-ideal cooperation. Specifically ask if the patient is using any new medications or supplements, if any have been changed by other practitioners for any reason, and if any have been stopped. Ask specifically about any brand changes, which are likely to affect the bioavailability of the medications you or others are prescribing (see Chapter 6, "Pharmacokinetics"), because these may alter serum levels and tolerability of your medications through drug–drug interactions. If necessary, ask patients to bring prescription bottles with them so that you can detect brand changes; always record the brands in your notes, calling the pharmacy if necessary. Explore the use of any medications used "as needed," again focusing on changes.

Inquire about adverse events and possible side effects, exploring and recording them in detail, again always looking for other medication changes that could also lead to these complaints (e.g., a new antibiotic started at the same time a rash appeared). Ask fertile female patients about menses and birth control (documenting compliance and method, if used) and onset

TABLE 12–2. Follow-up medication, adverse events, and lifestyle checklist

Medications taken	Including nonpsychiatric, over-the-counter, and as-needed
Supplements taken	
New medications	
Stopped medications	Reason
Brand changes	To and from (and to alternative) generics with dates
Dose changes	Timing and reasons
Side effects	Degree, timing
Adverse events	Degree, timing, treatment
Alcohol	Amount
Nicotine	Form, amount
Caffeine	All sources, including chocolate, plus amounts
Psychoactive drugs	Legal and illegal, recreational, and self-treatment
Birth control	Including compliance
Pregnancy	Method of testing, stage, complications
Nursing	Including schedule
Last menstrual period	

of most recent period. Document at every visit whether nursing mothers are still nursing.

Lifestyle Issues

Once medication and supplements are covered, ask specifically about each lifestyle issue: ask about use of alcohol, legal or illegal psychoactive drugs, nicotine, and caffeine, reminding the patient of each source of caffeine; ask about foods containing cannabis, if indicated. Inquiring about these will not only help monitor treatment but reinforce this important part of the treatment plan.

General Medical History

Follow with an update of the patient's general medical history. Determine any changes in active problems and ask about new medical problems. Has the patient sustained any new head injuries, even mild bumps (see Chapter

3, "General Medical History and Review of Symptoms")? Next, complete a review of systems (Table 12–3). This review should cover every area of the body and function and may be done quickly, still allowing time for exploration of any positive responses, and will also help identify any side effects or other adverse events that were not mentioned previously.

Laboratory and Diagnostic Studies

Laboratory and diagnostic study results should then be reviewed and discussed (see Table 12–3). These may include relevant serum levels of therapeutic agents (e.g., lithium and valproate levels); nutritional assessments and supplements, such as vitamin D levels (see Chapter 8); assessments for toxicities (e.g., liver profiles with valproate); and baseline metabolic functions necessary to maintain safe use (e.g., renal function for lithium and gabapentin use and sodium levels for oxcarbazepine). Electroencephalograms, electrocardiograms, and any imaging such as CTs or MRIs should be reviewed and discussed. This is also the time to consider ordering any of these tests.

Assessment of Progress

Once you have this information, ask the patient for his or her assessment of progress. Combine this assessment with yours, and together discuss how successful you feel the treatment plan is thus far. Because most plans take weeks to months to show ultimate improvement, remind the patient of the expected target date for success and ask how you can further support the patient while waiting. Does the patient need social support or assistance from local or governmental agencies? Have referral information readily available. Reevaluate the need for supportive or other psychotherapy.

Using a Bayesian approach (recall Chapter 4), examine your model of the patient's problems and how well your prediction for the treatment plan matches your expectations. If the outcome is not as expected, look first at the model, rather than the treatment. Is the diagnosis correct? By reviewing the chief complaint fully, at every single visit, you have the opportunity to reevaluate your diagnoses every time; do so consciously. Would altering the model (including diagnosis) better fit the data you are obtaining? If so, discuss alterations. A common example is when major depression turns out to be bipolar disorder. An antidepressant given to a patient during a downward mood curve may worsen the mood before it reverses; starting it on the upswing of a cycle, it may merely accompany improvement or lead to excessive mood elevation—the result is dependent on initial conditions, as in chaos theory, another useful concept to keep in mind (see Gleick 1987).

TABLE 12–3. Follow-up visit review of systems and laboratory checklist

Blood pressure	Especially with stimulant and some antidepressant treatment (may include postural)
Weight	
Allergies	Update
New medical problems	Injuries, infections, exacerbations or return of old problems, new diagnoses
Neurological	Including new head injuries (even mild), seizures, syncope, headaches, motor and sensory problems (tremor, weakness, involuntary movements, rigidity, gait, balance, vision [diplopia, blurred vision], olfaction)
Gastrointestinal	Swallowing, nausea, vomiting, diarrhea, constipation, pain, bleeding
Cardiovascular	Abnormal rhythm including tachycardia, chest pain
Respiratory	Dyspnea (a check on allergy), cough, shortness of breath, snoring, sleep apnea
Sexual	Desire, arousal, tumescence, ejaculation, orgasm, infection, changes in menstruation
Orthopedic	Mineralization changes, joint problems (a check on allergy), injury (good check on head injury)
Endocrine	Changes in blood sugar, nocturia, kidney stones, thyroid status
Dermatological	Rash, swelling, pain, pruritis
Relevant serum levels of medications	May include prescription of others; essential when brand or dose is changed or drug interaction is possible
Liver profile	As indicated
Electrolytes and serum creatinine	As indicated
Complete blood count	As indicated
Vitamin D level (as 25[OH]D)	When replacing, otherwise annually
Thyroid-stimulating hormone	Initial screen and as indicated; during replacement every 6–12 months
Thyroid antibodies	Initial screen and as indicated

Beware of errors in extremes: either rigidly adhering to a model that is not fitting your data or impulsively jumping to models with inadequate data (e.g., adding a diagnosis of ADHD based merely on worsening concentration or of OCD based only on worsening of obsessive thoughts). Use the full DSM-5 criteria for any diagnostic changes (American Psychiatric Association 2013).

If your diagnosis still seems valid, what about your modeled expectations of this treatment plan? Have you controlled for as many variables as possible: lifestyle issues discussed in Chapter 9, family and individual history, types and brands of medication, and compliance? Your updated history should alert you to factors compromising success, but you may need to repeat questions or to dig deeper and look more broadly to discover unexpected changes that matter.

One of the most important answers to obtain is why a medication that seemed to be working just fine has suddenly lost its efficacy or does not work with reintroduction. *Never* proceed without determining at least a few reasonable hypotheses about the cause. Although tachyphylaxis with neurons may be demonstrated in vitro (in test tubes), this "tolerance" has been demonstrated in vivo (in patients) mostly in retrospective anecdotes and naturalistic and observational studies in which causes are not defined. Eschew clinical gossip, which is rife about such a "poop-out syndrome," and take it as an essential truth that effective treatments never quit working for no reason—at least one cause should always be discoverable (see Fornaro et al. 2019). The clinician must be an ardent detective, never resting until a plausible hypothesis can be justified. If an interference with one treatment cannot be determined, it also may prevent success with several more. Is the medication being taken? Is this loss of a placebo response? Is the underlying condition worsening or altering? Is the diagnosis incorrect? Has the patient's use of alcohol or cannabis changed? Has fiber been added that is reducing absorption and therefore the maximum peak concentration or other values? Employing patients to detect along with you will teach them to be vigilant for factors that may compromise their treatment (Bosman et al. 2018; Katz 2011; Kinrys et al. 2019; Zimmerman and Thongy 2007).

Once the model is tweaked, if necessary, determine how much change this will lead to in treatment. Should an antidepressant be changed to a mood stabilizer? Should a prescribed stimulant be discontinued? Should caffeine be stopped? Make sure patients are fully aware of any change in model, why, and how accompanying treatment changes must be made. You are not guessing randomly but are applying Bayesian logic, in partnership, maximally utilizing every bit of available data to increase the chances of treatment success. Patients sharing ownership of these plans will be far more compliant and helpful in monitoring than those who feel like passive recipients.

Referrals

Discuss consideration of any necessary referrals. Have new health concerns outside the purview of psychopharmacology been identified that another professional should evaluate or manage? Are health concerns interfering with the chosen treatment plan (e.g., blood pressure so high or low that the current treatment plan cannot be safely continued, such as orthostatic hypotension with antidepressants or antipsychotics or hypertension with stimulants)? If so, the rational psychopharmacologist will shepherd these consultations by making a formal request with specific questions to be answered and following up directly with the professional involved. Document the response and actions of the other professional so they can be reviewed at any time.

Second Opinions

The best psychopharmacologists also know when to ask for second opinions on their own diagnoses and treatment plans. Patient requests for these should always be graciously—in fact, enthusiastically—supported, with suggestions for competent evaluators if the patient is interested. Rational practitioners know that another pair of eyes can help work around unconscious biases, add knowledge or experience they may lack, and even elicit information they were not able to, just as they did for referring primary care providers. As mentioned before, however, a true second opinion is only performed by someone trained and skilled in clinical psychopharmacology. The opinion of anyone else is seldom helpful and may be misguided, confusing the patient. Devote time to explain to the patient why this distinction is essential. Patients are reasonable to want a referring physician, such as their primary care physician, involved in their treatment, and this professional will, we hope, respect your expertise. If not, suggest a second opinion yourself to clarify important issues for the patient and referring provider.

Once a second opinion has been obtained, schedule a visit to discuss the results with the patient. You should have had time not only to review the evaluation prior to this meeting but also to discuss the evaluation with the professional who performed it. Read the report together, and explain it to your patient's satisfaction, noting any questions either of you may have that you can clarify later with the author of the report. Explore your patient's opinion of the report, then give your assessment; discuss how the second opinion fits with the diagnostic model you, together, have crafted. Then discuss how it fits with any treatments that have been attempted or considered. Agree on any adjustment to the treatment plan.

At times, patients may wish to change their care to the clinician who did the other evaluation. Ethically, no provider of a second opinion should accept such a transfer until the patient and the original provider have had the opportunity to explore the issues involved, together, during a session. Certainly, our rational psychopharmacologist would never do so and must encourage the patient not to seek this, for his or her own protection. This can help guard against "provider shopping" and creates the opportunity to discuss any outstanding issues, such as compliance, that may continue to thwart outcome and the therapeutic alliance with each provider. Before beginning a second-opinion visit for the patient of another provider, always clarify that this visit is not initiating a doctor–patient relationship but only providing information for the patient and the referring provider to discuss together.

Reevaluation and Monitoring

Thorough, methodical reevaluation and monitoring are necessary even when things are going well and patients have no complaints. To maintain favorable outcomes, assess their compliance and safety at regular intervals, searching for threats to continued success, such as upcoming work shift changes (see Chapter 9, "Sleep"). Once patients are stable and asymptomatic, most need to be assessed every 90–180 days, sooner when medical changes, self-harm, uncertain compliance, substance abuse, or the prescription of controlled substances is involved. Many patients recovering from substance abuse do well with monthly visits.

Governmental regulation of controlled substances will vary and must also be taken into account when determining proper timing of follow-up. When a patient receiving a stimulant for ADHD requests an early refill or replacement of a lost prescription, these should be denied until the proper time for a refill and then be refilled only for patients maintaining regularly scheduled appointments. Patients receiving benzodiazepines may be given sufficient supplies to reach an upcoming appointment and no more and should be reminded that it is dangerous to stop this medication too quickly, that office visits are essential to continuing the treatment, and that unilateral changes in dosing are not allowed. A clinician whose patient fails to make or attend appointments may prescribe and mail a safe taper schedule to the patient, recording this in the chart and giving it to the pharmacy with the understanding that this is the patient's one chance to safely remove the medication and that further prescriptions will not be forthcoming. Inform patients that emergency department visits may be necessary should they fail to comply. Patients prescribed antidepressants, mood stabilizers, and antipsychotics should not receive repeated refills despite frequently missed appointments; compliance must be addressed. Clarifying such refill policies prior to initial prescription is necessary.

Summary

Having thoroughly evaluated patients and their problems in the initial sessions, clinicians' regularly scheduled follow-up sessions with patients are designed to efficiently recapitulate much of this same information, which will then be applied to successive approximations in refining the model of the problem and the probability of the best solutions. This process increases the chances of good therapeutic outcome and safety. Data should be recorded in detail, making them available for later review. This process is a collaborative effort with the patient in the context of a therapeutic alliance. Opportunities for consultation on primary and secondary issues should be encouraged.

Key Points

- Follow-up assessments must focus on change, desirable and not.
- Fully explain adjustments of treatment models to patients.
- Explanations must be found when medications appear to lose efficacy.
- Second opinions from other psychopharmacologists can be valuable.

Self-Assessment

1. Which of the following statements is false? (Choose all that apply)

   A. Seeming tolerance to the therapeutic benefit of an antidepressant should always be exhaustively investigated.
   B. It is not necessary to repeat a full review of systems in follow-up sessions.
   C. Nonprescription supplements and medications can have a significant influence on treatment efficacy.
   D. Generic medications have the same potency as brand-name medications.

2. Detailed records of symptoms, side effects, treatments, and changes must be maintained to (choose all that apply)

    A. Provide information to future providers
    B. Provide information for second opinions
    C. Allow review by any clinician of past treatments that might be reconsidered
    D. Help alter diagnostic and treatment models in the face of insufficient success

3. Which of the following statements is true?

    A. It is not necessary to always ask about suicidal ideation if the patient is doing well.
    B. A patient saying "I'm feeling well" means he has a good mood.
    C. It is sufficient to ask patients if they have hallucinations.
    D. None of the above

4. Regularly scheduled assessments (choose all that apply)

    A. Allow for rational adjustment of treatment planning
    B. Allow confirmation of working diagnoses
    C. Improve compliance
    D. Help monitor the use of controlled substances

5. Which of the following is important to explore and document during a follow-up assessment? (Choose all that apply)

    A. Blood pressure
    B. Weight
    C. Last menstrual period
    D. Nursing
    E. New head injury
    F. Laboratory and other diagnostic data
    G. Erectile dysfunction

Discussion Topics

1. A patient you diagnosed with major depression and started on an antidepressant comes for follow-up. You discover he is more depressed and spontaneously reports suicidal ideation. Discuss how each of the following may influence this outcome: diagnostic error,

length of treatment, compliance, medication changes (including brand alterations and new medications prescribed by other providers), lifestyle, new injuries, and nonpsychiatric medical changes.

2. A patient is angered by your inquiry about suicidal ideation and lifestyle issues at every visit, thinking you should know her better by now. Would you change this routine? How would you discuss this with your patient?

Additional Reading

Fornaro M, Anastasia A, Novello S, et al: The emergence of loss of efficacy during antidepressant drug treatment for major depressive disorder: an integrative review of evidence, mechanisms, and clinical implications. Pharmacol Res 139:494–502, 2019

Gleick J: Chaos: Making a New Science. New York, Viking Press, 1987

References

American Psychiatric Association: Diagnostic and Statistical Manual of Mental Disorders, 5th Edition. Arlington, VA, American Psychiatric Association, 2013

Bosman RC, Waumans RC, Jacobs GE, et al: Failure to respond after reinstatement of antidepressant medication: a systematic review. Psychother Psychosom 87(5):268–275, 2018 30041180

Fornaro M, Anastasia A, Novello S, et al: The emergence of loss of efficacy during antidepressant drug treatment for major depressive disorder: an integrative review of evidence, mechanisms, and clinical implications. Pharmacol Res 139:494–502, 2019

Gleick J: Chaos: Making a New Science. New York, Viking Press, 1987

Katz G: Tachyphylaxis/tolerance to antidepressive medications: a review. Isr J Psychiatry Relat Sci 48(2):129–135, 2011 22120449

Kinrys G, Gold AK, Pisano VD, et al: Tachyphylaxis in major depressive disorder: a review of the current state of research. J Affect Disord 245:488–497, 2019 30439676

Zimmerman M, Thongy T: How often do SSRIs and other new-generation antidepressants lose their effect during continuation treatment? Evidence suggesting the rate of true tachyphylaxis during continuation treatment is low. J Clin Psychiatry 68(8):1271–1276, 2007 17854252

Answer Key

Chapter 1

1. **Answer: A—A meme.** In the original evolutionary biology usage, *meme* would refer to a cultural belief or system of behavior.

2. **Answer: B and C.** Although the provider and the patient are working together honestly with mutual effort toward only one goal—the health of the patient—only the patient makes the final decision about accepting or rejecting a treatment plan. A provider may refuse to participate and refer for further consultation if he or she thinks the patient's chosen plan is harmful, which reinforces the therapeutic alliance itself.

3. **Answer: D—All of the above.** We are using the term in its simplest nontechnical form (a list of steps or instructions to solve a problem—just what we learn in medicine).

4. **Answer: C—Developing theories from partial information, forming hypotheses, then testing them.** Option A is inductive reasoning; option B is deductive reasoning, valid only if the hypothesis is true; and option D is also Platonic deductive reasoning. Abductive is the form of reason most often used in medical practice.

5. **Answer: D—All of the above.** All are examples of unconscious threats to rational consideration of information.

6. **Answer: A—Generating multiple responses in a free flow of ideas.** Option B is convergent thinking. Divergent thinking may be humans' best contribution in the future.

Chapter 2

1. **Answer: A, B, C, and D.** Last observation carried forward is particularly prone to bias and is discouraged by the FDA. The nature of the missing data in intention to treat can never be known, so bias may al-

ways exist. Bias in meta-analysis may be introduced by heterogeneity and data mining in ill-defined subgroup analysis.

2. **Answer: A and C.** A low number needed to treat (NNT) means the treatment effect is more likely to occur in your practice than with a high NNT. Adverse events are less likely with a higher number needed to harm.

3. **Answer: B—Is never proof of statistical significance.** The *P* value represents a scale along which statistical significance increases or decreases but is never definitive. It is best reported to at least three decimal places.

4. **Answer: A and D.** The null hypothesis must be rejected to show a treatment effect. It can never be proven, however; it can only be disproven (rejected) or *fail to be disproven*. Confidence interval is used to estimate the accuracy and the size of the effect of the odds ratio.

5. **Answer: B and D.** Prospective studies and prospective registries with sufficient scale capture broader data than retrospective studies and retrospective registries, which may suffer from sampling error.

Chapter 3

1. **Answer: A, B, C, and D.** Each may be valid a syndrome symptom if it occurs on a regular basis in the absence of outside interference with sleep.

2. **Answer: B—Immediate memory.** This test might also measure mathematical ability, but its purpose is to measure immediate memory.

3. **Answer: D—A and C.** Rapid thinking may lead to rapid speech or even to speech latency when the patient is unable to keep up with his or her own thoughts enough to speak. Rapid thinking can only be determined through careful questioning and patient report.

4. **Answer: A, B, C, and D.** Attorneys know that hard whacks may produce no damage to the brain, whereas slight taps may cause significant damage—the *eggshell skull rule* of common and some tort law. Clinicians are bound to evaluate each individual for residual brain dysfunction that might be exacerbated by the addition of medication, such as provoking a seizure through the threshold-lowering properties of antidepressants and antipsychotics. Many patients may minimize their injuries because they fear "brain damage."

5. **Answer: A—Consistent with hypothyroidism.** Thyroid-stimulating hormone levels sustained >2.5 mU/L have been consistent with hypothyroidism for the past few decades. Although a patient with these values might be a normal outlier, consultation with an endocrinologist knowledgeable about the thyroid is warranted. Should responses to

antidepressants consistently disappoint, a trial of thyroid supplementation may be considered (in the absence of contraindications). Thyroiditis is detected by measuring antibodies, especially antithyroid peroxidase and antithyroglobulin.

Chapter 4

1. **Answer: A and C.** Medications that are added to target symptoms already being addressed through treatment for the complete syndrome may confound treatment and tolerability; too many variables exist to consider a rigid first, second, and third choice of medication.

2. **Answer: D—All of the above.** Option A is the Keynesian definition of probability theory. For option B, the probabilities of treatment outcomes can help layer the options for planning. Option C involves Bayesian logic, which helps integrate new information rationally and less arbitrarily than only using P tests.

3. **Answer: C—The preponderance of data from randomized controlled trials and postmarketing analysis.** Avoid outlying data such as poorly designed studies, anecdotal case reports, and clinical gossip, remembering that dosages originally suggested for marketing by the FDA may be lowered as well as raised with postmarketing data (as with risperidone, discussed in Chapter 7).

4. **Answer: B—Mechanism of action might be used effectively when changing treatment plans.** Although mechanism of action alone is never sufficient to determine initial treatment choice, it may provide small to significant advantage in view of family history and secondary or tertiary attempts at treatment. A fair number of treatments found effective in randomized controlled trials still lack a clearly understood or agreed-upon mechanism of action.

5. **Answer: A, B, and C.** All available treatments that have data to support reasonable consideration should be discussed and the chances of desired outcome listed in descending order of probability and medical necessity; all risks should be clearly stated, with estimates of probability.

Chapter 5

1. **Answer: D—A and C.** Although lower-level structure informs that of higher scales, the element of chance and other factors prevent explanation by simple reductionist thinking.

2. **Answer: D—All of the above.** These unconscious errors in rational thinking preclude attempts at prediction of clinical response from proposed mechanisms of action.

3. **Answer: C—Binding affinity determines dosage.** There is quite a scatter in the specific receptors targeted by antidepressants, although the clinical response is similar. It is not always perfectly clear that presumed unnecessary or undesirable binding leading to "side effects" is not part of the mechanism of action.

4. **Answer: A—Isoniazid was an early tricyclic antidepressant.** Isoniazid was an early monoamine oxidase inhibitor.

5. **Answer: B and C.** Algorithms are lists of steps for solving a problem and may or may not be designed for pattern recognition.

Chapter 6

1. **Answer: C—30–50 hours.** It takes five half-lives ($t_{1/2}$) to reach steady-state serum level concentration and the same amount of time to leave the body from steady state, assuming no individual interference with normal elimination.

2. **Answer: A—The one with a higher therapeutic index.** The therapeutic index is the ratio of the toxic dose to the effective dose. Therefore, a higher therapeutic index should be better tolerated.

3. **Answer: B and C.** Binding affinity is not a measurement of efficacy, just a determination of how tightly the molecule binds to the receptor and, therefore, how much will need to be present for clinical effect. This is the potency, which informs the dosage. Strong affinity (low K_d) indicates a high potency and lower dose than otherwise.

4. **Answer: A and C.** A drug's effective half-life is the half-life of the parent compound plus the half-lives of all its clinically active metabolites. Therefore, an agent with active metabolites has an effective half-life greater than $t_{1/2}$. The effective half-life for a medication with no active metabolites is equal to $t_{1/2}$.

5. **Answer: A, B, C, and D.** Note, however, that drug–drug interactions are not limited to these factors.

Chapter 7

1. **Answer: A—Sublingual preparations.** These may offer improved absorption over oral, such as with asenapine. The others may help with pill

swallowing problems but otherwise show no benefit for compliance or time to response.

2. **Answer: A, B, C, and D.** Although bupropion has a prominent FDA warning regarding seizure risk, both antipsychotics and antidepressants carry this side effect.

3. **Answer: A and C.** Although only clozapine has mandated FDA monitoring, all antipsychotics and anticonvulsants carry this risk.

4. **Answer: D—All of the above.** All medications, but particularly aromatic anticonvulsants, carry the risk of rash, but lamotrigine has been particularly publicized for its risk of Stevens-Johnson syndrome.

5. **Answer: C—Should not be changed, except for compliance or tolerability.** Acetylcholinesterase inhibitors only delay, not reverse, cognitive impairment. Efficacy in preventing progression from mild cognitive impairment to dementia has not been established, although benefit in mild and moderate dementia is the most robust. The outcome for a single patient can never be measured against not taking the medication, so changes for efficacy are irrational and may allow more rapid cognitive decline.

Chapter 8

1. **Answer: D—All of the above.** Correlation is not causation—please review the references and form your own opinion.

2. **Answer: A and D.** Carbamazepine levels are lowered by these supplements through induction of CYP3A4 (St. John's wort), and phenytoin and valproate are lowered through induction of CYP2C19 (Ginkgo biloba). Phenobarbital and phenytoin are also potent inducers of CYP3A4.

3. **Answer: B—Assist in the treatment of treatment-resistant depression at dosages of 15 mg/day.** Only dosages of 15 mg/day were found effective; Testing for *MTHFR* polymorphism does not reliably predict response in major depression.

4. **Answer: A, B, C, and D.**

5. **Answer: A and B.** Lower serum level ratios of omega-3 to omega-6 are associated with major and perinatal depression. Maternal replacement of omega-3 may not occur by 6 months, and takes much longer with repeated pregnancies. Only replacement of the eicosapentaenoic acid (EPA) form has been shown effective, and only in treating formally diagnosed major depression.

Chapter 9

1. **Answer: None of these statements is true.** Shift work compromises mood stability and increases the risk of cancer and dementia. Missed sleep is never regained, and patients will feel best by getting up and going to sleep within 1 hour of the same time every day of the week (even this 1 hour still has negative effects, such as occurs with the changes around daylight saving time). Cooler rooms help with sleep initiation, and 68°F (20°C) is recommended. Daytime napping, particularly in the afternoon, often interferes with adequate nighttime sleep.

2. **Answer: D—All of the above.** Exercising close to bedtime may interfere with healthy sleep. Some patients with anxiety disorders may find their symptoms are provoked by exercise if they exercise without adequate and progressive training; this effect may be the result of lactate buildup from both aerobic and anaerobic exercise. Depletion of brain-derived neurotrophic factor may be associated with major depression and corrected by routine, moderate aerobic exercise.

3. **Answer: A and C.** The body mass index (BMI) is invalid in patients with eating disorders. It may overestimate fat in cases of excessive muscle mass and underestimate it in muscle wasting. BMIs for children and adolescents must be corrected for sex and age.

4. **Answer: A, B, and C.** The alcohol in beer or wine does not have a milder effect on the brain than that in distilled spirits. Cannabis, natural or synthetic, should not be considered a current treatment option for psychiatric, developmental, and neurodegenerative disorders. Due to lipophilic storage, it may take 12 months for cannabis to completely leave the body after cessation of use; weight loss may lead to spikes in serum concentration. The half-life of MDMA is 8 hours.

5. **Answer: A and C.** Mediated by strong inhibition of CYP1A2, fluvoxamine and verapamil significantly elevate serum levels of caffeine, with clinical consequences. Duloxetine, imipramine, amitriptyline, clomipramine, clozapine, and olanzapine are also metabolized by CYP1A2. "Herbal" is a marketing term for many teas and does not necessarily indicate the absence or partial removal of caffeine. Green tea is not low in caffeine; in fact, it has the same caffeine as most teas and more than some soft drinks. Avoidance of caffeine is often essential in the treatment of anxiety and bipolar disorder. Chlorogenic acid, quinic acid, caffeic acid, quercetin, and phenylindane in coffee have been implicated in the inhibition of amyloid-β or tau aggregation associated with dementia, but caffeine has been specifically eliminated as a factor.

6. **Answer: A, B, C, and D.** Sudden death from smoking while wearing the nicotine patch was reported early on, but subsequent evaluation has found the use of transdermal nicotine patches safe in the absence of smoking. The patches may also be combined with varenicline or bupropion, each of which, when used alone, has shown efficacy and safety when used appropriately (although varenicline may lead to insomnia and abnormal dreams). Recall that bupropion is an antidepressant and usually should not be used in bipolar disorder or without concomitant anticonvulsant medication when seizures are a risk and used carefully in combination with other antidepressants.

Chapter 10

1. **Answer: A and C.** Some evidence also exists for vagus nerve stimulation.

2. **Answer: A—Electroconvulsive therapy or vagus nerve stimulation.** Electroconvulsive therapy remains the gold standard for the treatment of major depression, and vagus nerve stimulation shows significant response and remission in patients with treatment-resistant depression, progressively, after 6 months. Deep brain stimulation is a yet-unproven experimental treatment for major depression; transcranial direct current stimulation has shown improvement only in non-treatment-resistant major depression, and the response to repetitive transcranial magnetic stimulation is weak and mostly evident in patients whose illness is less resistant to medication.

3. **Answer: A, B, C, and D.**

4. **Answer: B, C, and D.** Electroconvulsive therapy is a treatment for mania. Repetitive transcranial magnetic stimulation, deep brain stimulation, and vagus nerve stimulation all have published reports of switching in bipolar patients.

5. **Answer: A and C.** Noninvasive vagus nerve stimulation is under development.

Chapter 11

1. **Answer: A and C.** Given the patient's exposure to lithium, altered mental status, and nausea, toxicity must be considered. His symptoms include those of neuroleptic malignant syndrome as well as serotonin syndrome; he has exposure to both a serotonin agent and a dopamine antagonist, so each should also be suspected. Ondansetron is a sero-

tonin agent and must be avoided. Serotonin syndrome is the most likely explanation, because headache and dizziness are the most common symptoms, and clonus, prior to suppression by peripheral hypertonicity, is also a common feature. The fever in neuroleptic malignant syndrome is usually very high. The first step in treating any of the diagnoses in your differential is stopping the offending medication, so all should be stopped while supportive, intensive hospital treatment is given.

2. **Answer: A, B, and C.** Permanent tardive dyskinesia can develop from even brief use of dopamine antagonists or weak agonists. It would be unethical to not warn patients of this risk. Suicidality must be explored at every single patient contact to maintain safety and accurately monitor the progress of treatment, including long-term, stable success. As discussed in Chapter 6, the bioavailability of generic medication varies and may be responsible for drug–drug interactions and toxicities as well as the loss of benefit.

3. **Answer: F—None of the above.** All are defined as suicidality by the FDA, based on the Columbia Classification Algorithm of Suicide Assessment. *Suicidality* actually refers to the presumed risk of suicide, not just completed events. To say a medication increases the *risk* of suicidality is not synonymous with saying it increases the *rate* of suicide. This may be an important distinction to clarify for patients.

4. **Answer: B—Extrapyramidal syndrome.** Also referred to as pseudoparkinsonian side effects or drug-induced parkinsonism, extrapyramidal syndrome may be addressed by minimizing dosage, if possible, or adding anticholinergic medication if the risks of side effects, including a greater risk of TD, are accepted.

5. **Answer: A, B, C, and D.** Routinely increasing the dose to suppress TD is an archaic practice that only leads to higher doses with the same symptoms. Withdrawal dyskinesias often do not lead to TD. Valbenazine and deutetrabenazine have demonstrated relief from symptoms in randomized controlled trials, although not necessarily complete remission. TD is most obvious in the face, hands, and extremities but can occur in any muscle.

Chapter 12

1. **Answer: B and D.** So-called poop-out has been reported mostly in anecdotal case reports and naturalistic and observational studies. A thorough search for an explanation of loss of previous benefit is essential. A full review of systems at every visit is important for uncovering new

medical factors that influence treatment and safety, as well as providing a check on unreported adverse events. Supplements and nonprescription medications can influence absorption, bioavailability, and tolerability and therefore compliance and outcome. As discussed in Chapter 6, each brand of a medication carries a different bioavailability that may affect serum levels, pharmacodynamics, and ultimately, efficacy.

2. **Answer: A, B, C, and D.** This information can be a gold mine to be utilized rationally in any context, reducing uncertainty.

3. **Answer: D—None of the above.** Ideas about self-harm and violence *must* be asked about at each and every patient contact, for safety and to monitor progress. Initial statements are often considered pleasantries by patients; mood, like any other symptom, must be asked about at every visit. A patient may not accurately understand what a hallucination is; ask if the patient has seen, heard, or smelled things that others thought were not really there or has felt something touching him or her when it is not.

4. **Answer: A, B, C, and D.** The absence of data is the absence of data—without detailed regular assessments, providers will be unaware of errors in diagnosis and treatment. Regular contact may improve the therapeutic alliance; reinforce important details of a treatment plan; allow for monitoring patients' use of controlled substances and the timing of refills; and support accountability within the therapeutic alliance.

5. **Answer: A, B, C, D, E, F, and G.** Last menstrual period and nursing practices are relevant to female patients; inquire about erectile dysfunction at each visit with male patients. Check blood pressure for all patients receiving stimulants and (especially with, but not limited to) geriatric patients receiving antidepressants and antipsychotics. Assess head injuries for all patients, laboratory and other data when indicated and available, and weight unless an eating disorder contraindicates.

Index

Page numbers printed in **boldface** type refer to tables and figures.